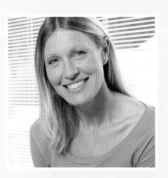

YOUR
menopause
BIBLE

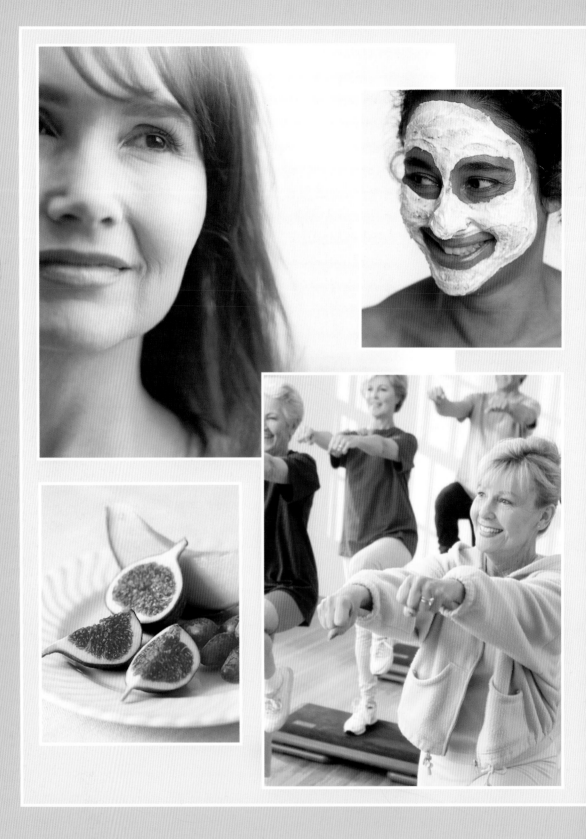

YOUR
menopause
BIBLE

Consulting editor
Dr. ROBIN N. PHILLIPS

CARROLL & BROWN PUBLISHERS LIMITED

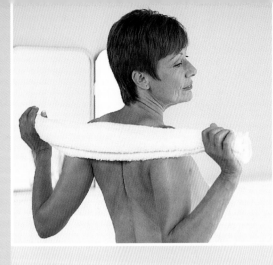

First published in 2005 in the United Kingdom by

Carroll & Brown Publishers Limited
20 Lonsdale Road
London NW6 6RD

Managing Art Editor Emily Cook

Copyright © Carroll and Brown Ltd 2005

A CIP catalogue record for this book is available
from the British Library.

ISBN 1-904760-12-0

10 9 8 7 6 5 4 3 2 1

All rights reserved. No part of this publication may be
reproduced in any material form (including photocopying
or storing it in any medium by electronic means and
whether or not transiently or incidentally to some other
use of this publication) without the written permission of
the copyright owner, except in accordance with the
provisions of the Copyright, Designs and Patents Act of
1988 or under the terms of a licence issued by the
Copyright Licensing Agency, 90 Tottenham Court Road,
London W1P 9HE. Applications for the copyright owner's
written permission to reproduce any part of this
publication should be addressed to the publisher.

Reproduced by Colourscan, Singapore
Printed in China by C&C Offset Printing Co., Ltd.

Publisher's note: the information contained in this book
should be used as a general reference guide and does not
constitute, and is not intended to substitute for, an expert's
medical advice or legal advice. Consult your doctor or
healthcare professional prior to following any treatment or
exercises contained in this book.

CONTENTS

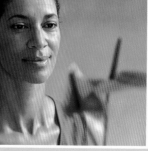

CONSULTANTS AND CONTRIBUTORS

Robin N. Phillips, M.D.
Assistant Clinical Professor of Obstetrics,
Gynecology and Reproductive Medicine, and
Assistant Clinical Professor of Geriatrics and
Adult Development at the Mount Sinai School
of Medicine, New York

Dr. Penny Preston
Medical author and journalist on women's
health issues

Carlos A. Widgerowitz, M.D.
Senior Clinical Lecturer, Director of Research,
Consultant Orthopaedic Surgeon at the
University of Dundee

Dr. Amanda Roberts
Specialist in genito-urinary medicine, sex
therapist and author

Fiona Hunter
Nutritionist, author and journalist

Anne Hooper
Accredited sexual and marital therapist, author
and journalist

Anji Jackson-Main
Accredited herbalist

Alison Mackonochie
Health writer, author and editor

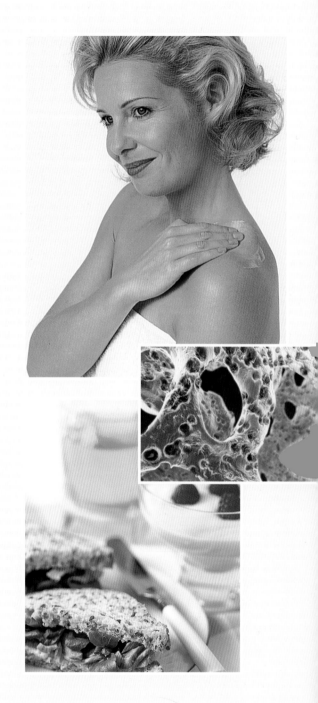

INTRODUCTION

Menopause is a fact of female life. All women will go through it (if they live long enough!), but some will feel the effects profoundly, others will feel some of the effects, and still others may feel nothing whatsoever and glide through the whole experience, oblivious to the whole 'change of life' apart from the obvious cessation of menstrual periods. As an inescapable fact of life, it's essential that women know what to expect and when to expect it, and understand the issues that may arise and the options that are open to them.

What May Happen

With the approach of menopause, production of the female sex hormones oestrogen and proges-terone declines, causing menstruation to cease. This, in turn, can cause a number of symptoms. Some of these may be short-term, such as hot flushes, fatigue, night sweats, loss of libido and headaches. Others are usually longer term, such as vaginal and urinary problems, and may become permanent but are not life-threatening, and can be remedied or at least alleviated by several therapies.

However, there are other consequences of the decrease in sex hormones at menopause that are dangerous and may be unnoticed, until they pose a serious problem. One of the main risks at menopause is the development of osteoporosis, a loss of bone mass that can be seriously debilitating and even life threatening. Other conditions that more readily arise after the decline in oestrogen production are coronary heart disease leading to heart attacks, cerebrovascular disease leading to strokes, and certain cancers.

On the positive side, there are many treatment options available depending on your symptoms, from hormone therapy (HT) to nutritional supplements and from dietary changes to beneficial exercises. HT has proved invaluable to millions of women around the world, but the debate surrounding it is controversial and ongoing, and the guidelines on its use have changed in light of recent research. We have used the term 'HT' rather than 'HRT' throughout this book because the amount of hormone actually used in HT drugs is only a fraction of that produced previously by the ovaries, making the word 'replacement' a misnomer.

Reviewing the Options

Creams, patches, tablets, suppositories, implants, even nasal sprays are widely available, and they have given relief from menopausal symptoms and long-term protection from certain conditions.

However, getting to grips with the advice being offered by different experts is at times mind-boggling, so it is essential that every woman considering HT is fully informed of her options, and discusses these with her healthcare provider to ascertain what each treatment can offer, and to balance any potential benefits against any possible risks.

In addition, as we approach midlife, other life changes begin to take place – at home, at work and at play. For women with families, this is often a time when children leave home and when partners may also be going through a time of transition in their own lives, both of which can cause anxieties. New light is often thrown on the work-life balance, and women begin to look forward to lessening (or, sometimes, strength-ening) their commitments at work. Also, whereas younger adults are driven by personal ambition, adults entering midlife tend to find intellectual pursuits and interests far more inspirational. With all this turmoil and activity, it's no wonder this time of life is referred to as 'the change'!

Your Life Your Way

Along with providing you with information on various therapies and techniques, this book can help you overcome the negative aspects of menopause and has been written to inform you of the positive changes that can happen at this time. For far too long menopause has been seen in a bad light – the end of something rather than the beginning of something new. A century ago, female life expectancy in the UK was just 50 years, and many women were not expected to live to experience the symptoms of menopause. Now, females are expected to live well into their eighties – which means that for many of us, almost half our lives will be spent as postmenopausal women – one very good reason to explore all the possible avenues to make your experience of menopause a good one.

In addition to an increased lifespan, women are now more vocal and more curious about things they can do for themselves. Menopause was never a subject for discussion or comparison in our grandmothers' or even our mothers' generations. Information was limited and 'grin and bear it' was the maxim to live by – what other options were there? However, breakthroughs in science and medicine, along with new thinking about alternative therapies have changed all that. Moreover, women are eager to know more and to put that knowledge to use. Unwilling to simply place their trust in doctors who 'know what's best', women are much more determined to take control of their health issues and find workable alternatives to complement or replace traditional medicine.

The Aim of This Book

These are the most important reasons why *Your Menopause Bible* has been created. It has been designed to bring you the most up-to-date information from experts in the various fields of female health. Most health books written for the layperson provide a single point of view and therefore present the author's own biases and perspectives. In most cases this is fine – you want your information to come from a respected specialist source. However, because of the complex nature of the physical, emotional, psychological and intellectual changes that occur at menopause, it's not always possible to ensure that one author has expertise in all related fields. In *Your Menopause Bible*, a team of respected authorities from a variety of fields have written on their specialist subjects. The team ranges from physicians and psychologists to sex therapists, herbalists and nutritionists, and their common goal is to inform you about the preventive medicines, therapies and self-help techniques that will help you at this time. They provide in-depth information on what you can expect, when you can expect it, and what to do when symptoms or situations occur.

Overall, their goal is to provide reassuring information that will help you navigate this important period in your life and to empower you to come through it healthy and revitalized and ready to deal with whatever life holds from then on.

Robin N. Phillips, M.D.

MENOPAUSE QUESTIONNAIRE

Answer these questions to assess your experience of menopause and to find your way quickly to the information in this book that can help you.

Part 1 Symptoms   YES   NO

1 Are you experiencing hot flushes or night sweats?   [✓]   [ ]
2 Are you feeling less energetic?   [ ]   [ ]
3 Are you having difficulty sleeping, or once getting to sleep staying asleep?   [ ]   [ ]
4 Are you feeling low or depressed?   [✓]   [ ]
5 Are you more forgetful?   [✓]   [ ]
6 Are you experiencing headaches more frequently?   [✓]   [ ]
7 Are you experiencing more vaginal dryness or itching?   [ ]   [ ]
8 Are you experiencing trouble controlling your urine?   [ ]   [ ]

These are all well-known menopausal symptoms and there are many things you can do to alleviate one or all of them. Go to chapter 2 for medical treatment options as well as natural therapies and self-help techniques that can provide immediate relief. Chapter 5 outlines simple but highly effective nutritional changes you can adopt; chapter 8 gives information on the different types of hormone therapy that can help; while chapter 9 outlines alternative therapies.

Part 2 Sex   YES   NO

1 Do you feel that your libido is flagging?   [ ]   [ ]
2 Are you experiencing less sexual desire or having fewer sexual fantasies?   [ ]   [ ]
3 Are you experiencing more discomfort when engaged in intercourse?   [ ]   [ ]
4 Have you noticed changes in your genital area?   [ ]   [ ]
5 Do you think your partner finds you less attractive?   [ ]   [ ]
6 Have you noticed any changes in your sexual responsiveness?   [ ]   [ ]
7 Is the sex you are having less fun than it used to be?   [ ]   [ ]
8 If you are still menstruating, are you up-to-date on contraceptive methods available?   [✓]   [ ]

Always a sensitive subject, often if your feelings of sensuality are diminished for any reason your self-esteem also takes a knock, and suddenly your sex life shudders to a halt. It doesn't have to be this way. See chapter 4 for the physical, psychological and emotional reasons why this can happen and how to counteract them. Also, see chapter 7 for ways to combat negative thought processes and chapter 10 for simple strategies to make you feel fantastic.

Part 3 Emotions

1 Are you feeling less motivated and less confident?   [✓] [ ]
2 Do you cry more easily?   [ ] [ ]
3 Are you more anxious or irritable?   [✓] [ ]
4 Do you feel more aggressive or hostile?   [ ] [ ]
5 Are you experiencing more mood swings?   [ ] [ ]
6 Are you feeling afraid or apprehensive for no apparent reason?   [✓] [ ]
7 Are you having trouble remembering things?   [✓] [ ]
8 Do you feel more fatigued in general?   [✓] [ ]

Some of these questions relate directly to recognized menopausal symptoms as seen in chapter 2, while others relate to psychological or emotional issues, such as stress and lifestyle choices, that can be reviewed and adapted (see chapter 7). Whatever your experiences, there are decisions you can make that will give immediate results (such as reviewing your stress levels) and others that may be more long-term (such as giving up smoking), but recognizing the problems in the first place is a step in the right direction.

Part 4 Physical I

1 Do you notice more lines and wrinkles around your mouth and eyes?   [ ] [ ]
2 Is your skin more prone to spots and pimples?   [✓] [ ]
3 Does the skin on your hands, arms and legs feel less toned?   [✓] [ ]
4 Does your hair feel more brittle and lack lustre? Is it falling out?   [ ] [ ]
5 Are your nails more likely to split and crack?   [ ] [ ]
6 Are your teeth more sensitive?   [ ] [ ]
7 Are you developing more facial hair?   [ ] [ ]
8 Do your eyes feel more gritty and dry?   [ ] [ ]

The loss of hormones and the natural aging process can lead to some unwelcome changes in appearance. But don't despair, read chapter 2 for self-help ideas to combat many common menopausal problems and chapter 10 for positive and effective ideas that will encourage you to devote time to yourself and look after your body.

Part 5 Exercise

		YES	NO
1	Are you overweight?	☐	☐
2	Do you have a regular exercise routine that you practise for at least 20 minutes at least 3 times a week?	☐	☐
3	Do you feel as if your muscles have lost their tone?	☐	☐
4	Are you experiencing more joint pain when exercising?	☑	☐
5	Do you feel exhausted and out-of-breath when undertaking light exercise such as walking?	☐	☐
6	Are you prone to falls?	☐	☐
7	Do you feel less flexible when you exercise?	☐	☐
8	Do you complete a warm-up and cool-down routine after you exercise?	☐	☐

Exercise is something that will benefit both body and mind at menopause, so it's well worth reviewing your exercise routines. Take heart from the fact that any exercise is better than none at all, so by beginning with small changes in your routine and building up you can be doing yourself a great deal of good. Chapter 6 contains all the information you need to get on the move, while the information on bone and joint health in chapter 3 will give you the impetus to do so. The nutritional information in chapter 5 will help you shed that extra weight.

Part 6 Physical II

		YES	NO
1	Are you experiencing more aches and pains?	☑	☐
2	Do you feel generally weaker?	☐	☐
3	Are your allergies getting worse?	☐	☐
4	Are you feeling less energetic?	☐	☐
5	Have you been told, or do you think, you are anaemic?	☐	☐
6	Are you experiencing more muscle cramps or spasms?	☐	☐
7	Are you more susceptible to inflammations and swellings?	☐	☐
8	Are you experiencing spotting or breakthrough bleeding?	☐	☐

The information throughout this book will help you to understand what's happening to you and why, and give you the tools and encouragement to ask your healthcare professional all the right questions and decide on the right course of action for you. Some of the complaints listed here can be alleviated by the advice given in chapter 2; others will benefit from the nutritional advice found in chapter 5; others may require exercise solutions (chapter 6), hormone therapy (chapter 8), medication or other medical interventions (chapter 11). The important thing is not to panic – the symptoms of menopause vary hugely from woman to woman, and only you know what's normal for you and what's not.

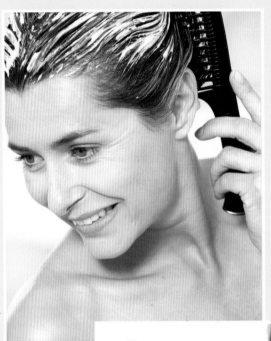

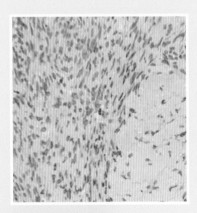

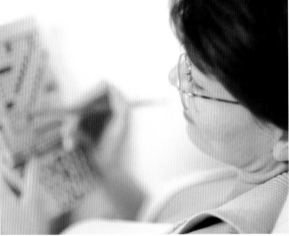

1

WHAT HAPPENS DURING MENOPAUSE?

Menopause is medically defined as one straight year without periods. But the time leading up to this year – which varies from woman to woman, and may be of up to 15 years' duration – as well as the year itself are considered part of the experience. This chapter outlines the physical changes you might expect at this time and the other changes, including mood swings, memory loss and emotional upheaval that can occur as a direct result of the body's decreased production of oestrogen.

CHANGES TO THE MENSTRUAL CYCLE

It has become usual to refer to all the changes that take place at the end of a woman's fertile time as 'menopause'. In fact the word menopause simply means 'the last menstrual period', and no one can say when this is until a year has passed since that last period. Once a year *has* passed after the last menstrual bleed, a woman can say her menopause was on that date. Any subsequent bleeding is not considered normal, and a thorough investigation is advisable (see pages 26–27).

The proper name for the period of about five years around the time of the last menstrual bleed is 'the climacteric'. This term covers the time when women's hormone levels fluctuate and many can experience problems as their bodies adapt.

OVARIES AND PERIODS

During the reproductive years, most women's ovaries release one or two eggs per month, and this regular ovulation takes place under the control of the menstrual cycle.

As menopause approaches, your menstrual cycle will usually change. A very few women just stop having periods without the cycle length changing in some way – but for most women periods become heavier or sparser, or stop and start over a few months. Not all women's periods are the same, but all are considered normal as long as they happen fairly regularly and the bleeding lasts from two to eight days (usually about four to six days). The average cycle length is 28 days, but anything from 21 to 36 days is still considered normal. Your

WISE WOMAN
Follicle production

•

By the time a baby girl is 6 months old her ovaries are full of primordial follicles (about 4–500,000); each of which has the potential to develop into an ovum or egg. No more new ones will be made, and only a small percentage of these primordial follicles will develop into mature ovarian follicles and ova.

menstrual cycle may change throughout the course of your life, with many outside factors affecting it, including illness, contraception methods, weight gain or loss, stress or pregnancy.

To fully understand what changes your body goes through in the time leading up to menopause, it is important to grasp just how your monthly cycle has been controlled and what exactly your ovaries have been doing.

What Has Been Going On?

Every month at the beginning of your menstrual bleed, the area of the brain called the hypothalamus detects low oestrogen levels and sends a signal, via gonadotropin-releasing hormone, to another area of the brain, the pituitary. The pituitary in turn signals to the ovaries by releasing follicle-stimulating hormone (FSH) and luteinizing hormone (LH). FSH stimulates around 10–20 ovarian follicles to begin maturing. Usually only one

The Frequency of Periods

Women today have more menstrual periods than ever before. Most women will have between 400 and 500 periods in their lifetime. This is partly because we live longer, thanks to better health-care and nutrition; partly because girls start their periods earlier than in the past; and mainly because women have fewer pregnancies.

or two will become mature ova ready for fertilization. The others degenerate and are reabsorbed. The developing follicles release the hormone oestrogen, which in turn acts on the lining of the uterus, causing it to grow and thicken. This first phase of the menstrual cycle is called the follicular phase.

When one of the follicles is ripe enough, oestrogen levels in the blood reach a peak, signalling to the pituitary to release LH. This acts on the ripe follicle to cause ovulation and the release of the mature egg, as well as production of the hormone progesterone. The egg is released from the follicle in the ovary and is drawn into the funnel-shaped end of one of the fallopian tubes, where it starts its journey to the uterus.

Most women do not notice when they ovulate, but a few notice a slight abdominal twinge or cramp known as Mittelschmerz or 'middle pain'. Some women notice that they feel most in the mood for sex around the time of ovulation. The subsequent phase is called the luteal phase, when the ovary makes both progesterone and oestrogen, and is usually a constant 14 days in length. In the time leading up to menopause it is this phase in the cycle that becomes erratic, as egg quality and quantity

WISE WOMAN
Cycle length

The follicular phase of the menstrual cycle varies in length. If you have a 28-day cycle you will be ovulating on day 14 and the follicular phase will be 14 days long. If you have a 36-day cycle you will be ovulating on day 22. The follicular phase will be 22 days long, but the luteal phase will stay constant at 14 days.

▶ PREMENSTRUAL SYNDROME (PMS)

Some perimenopausal symptoms resemble the symptoms of PMS. During the first phase of perimenopause, progesterone levels are declining and the oestrogen levels are unopposed. This corresponds to the luteal phase of your menstrual cycle – the time during which some women suffer from PMS. Symptoms such as mood swings, bloating, cramps and tender breasts, as well as feeling irritable, depressed, nervous, anxious and tearful – or the rare condition of premenstrual dysphoric disorder (PMDD) in which symptoms are so severe that they badly disrupt a woman's working and social life – may come and go during perimenopause. Unlike with PMS, however, they do not resolve when your period arrives. Unfortunately, women who suffer from PMS tend to have more severe symptoms around menopause than those who don't.

Taking calcium has been shown to help premenstrual symptoms – so grandma's remedy of a warm milky drink at night to relieve period pains and cramps seems to have a scientific explanation after all.

Many women recognize that they crave chocolate in the week before their period is due. It was once thought this was for the iron that dark chocolate contains, but chocolate also contains magnesium. This mineral helps to relieve anxiety and works with calcium to help reduce symptoms of PMS.

Evening primrose oil, which is rich in omega-6 fatty acids, and Vitamin B_6, which helps with the formation of the body's 'happy' chemical, serotonin, are also recommended for PMS.

If the mood symptoms are severe enough to disrupt normal functioning, a selective serotonin reuptake inhibitor (SSRI) like fluoxetine (Prozac) should definitely be considered.

3 stages of menopause

There is quite a lot of confusion about some of the terms used to describe the time around menopause. The word 'menopause' is popularly used to describe the whole time span in which women experience symptoms from changing hormone levels. In fact, the word simply describes the last menstrual period, just as 'menarche' describes the first.

Premenopause is used by some to refer to the time when menstruation is regular and before hormone levels start to decline. Some people use the word to define the time within the perimenopause before the last period.

Perimenopause includes the whole time before and after the last actual menstrual bleed – after hormone levels have started to fluctuate and before they settle, and there are no more symptoms due to this fluctuation. This is the same time span as the 'climacteric'. It is more and more usual for women to refer to this time as their menopause.

Postmenopause actually starts the day after the last menstrual bleed and describes any time after that. It includes some of the perimenopause, and a woman after her last period is described as postmenopausal, although the term will not be used until a year after the last period because no one will be sure which was the last one until a year has passed. Ninety percent of women in the perimenopause who have not had a period for six months do not have another one.

decline and ovulation may not be taking place at all. During the luteal phase, the follicle that released the egg forms a corpus luteum, or 'yellow body', and produces progesterone. This hormone prevents other follicles from developing and keeps the lining of the uterus prepared in case the egg is fertilized and pregnancy occurs. It takes a few days for the egg to travel down the fallopian tube to the uterus, and it is during this time that the egg may become fertilized if there are sperm present.

If fertilization, or conception, does not take place, the corpus luteum degenerates and disappears, and the progesterone and oestrogen levels fall. The uterine lining starts to disintegrate and finally is shed as a menstrual bleed. The low hormone levels feed back information to the hypothalamus in the brain, and the whole cycle starts again.

AS WE GET OLDER

As early as age 35 the egg follicles may stop ripening in a predictable way, and even if regular menstruation occurs, not all cycles will involve ovulation, and therefore not all cycles will have the usual rise in progesterone to follow the rise in oestrogen. The oestrogen levels become lower as fewer egg follicles grow and ripen, and if none mature enough to be released no corpus luteum is formed to produce progesterone. This means that the uterus builds up a thick lining in response to oestrogen but no progesterone is released. The endometrial lining of the uterus gets thicker and thicker and when menstruation occurs there can be heavy bleeding.

The cycle will probably be longer or shorter than usual. The first sign of the perimenopause is nearly always a change in the menstrual pattern. The very first sign of ovarian decline is a shortening of the cycle. Most women have a shorter cycle in their early 40s than they did in their 20s. Subsequently, around the perimenopause they experience longer cycles and less bleeding. Some have longer cycles and then very heavy bleeds, and others continue with the shorter cycles but with very short, scanty periods – and the unlucky ones get short cycles and very heavy bleeds. These are all normal changes, but

Hormone levels

Until menopause, oestrogen and progesterone are produced and released over an approximately 28-day cycle. As the supply and quality of eggs declines in midlife, hormone production from the ovaries becomes erratic. With progression towards menopause, levels of progesterone and oestrogen diminish.

Premenopausal Oestrogen levels peak in the first half of the cycle, then fall off after ovulation, as progesterone levels start to rise. Both levels decline if the egg is not fertilized, and this starts the menstrual bleed.

Perimenopausal Oestrogen is still being produced by the ovaries, but ovulation is sporadic, so progesterone is not produced every cycle and there may not be a monthly bleed.

Postmenopausal The small amount of oestrogen now present is mainly produced by fat cells breaking down and converting the male hormone androstenedione.

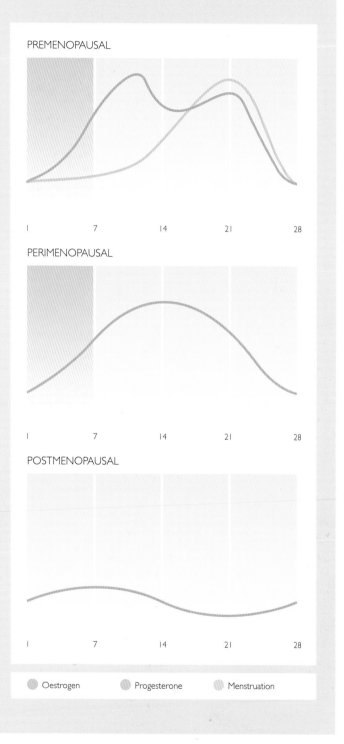

PREMENOPAUSAL

1   7   14   21   28

PERIMENOPAUSAL

1   7   14   21   28

POSTMENOPAUSAL

1   7   14   21   28

Oestrogen   Progesterone   Menstruation

Changing ovaries

These two light micrographs show the premenopausal ovary (top) and a postmenopausal ovary (bottom). In the post-menopausal example, there are no egg cells (primary follicles) present. All that remains is the scar tissue where the egg cells used to be. In time, the scar tissue will shrink, causing the ovaries to become smaller. In the normal ovary many egg cells are visible and they are more regular in shape.

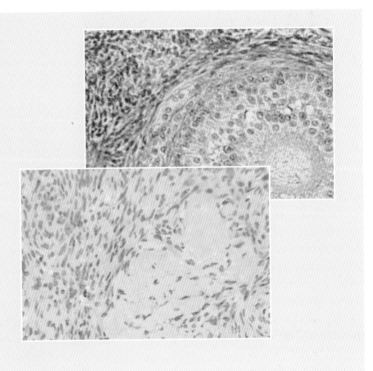

should never be assumed to be perimenopause until other problems have been excluded (see pages 26–27).

Eventually, hardly any egg follicles ripen and virtually no oestrogen or progesterone is released from the ovaries. This in turn causes high levels of FSH and LH to be released from the hypothalamus and pituitary gland, in an effort to stimulate the unresponsive ovaries. It is these two hormones that are measured in the blood to determine if a woman is in perimenopause. The FSH and LH levels fluctuate as the occasional follicle will respond, making it impossible to diagnose from a single test where in the perimenopause a woman is.

Upsetting the Balance

The low level of oestrogen in the blood starts to affect organs all over the body and may produce symptoms. High levels of FSH and LH may also produce symptoms, in particular affecting the metabolism of fats and carbohydrates and the chemistry of the brain. The ovaries do not stop

working and continue to produce some oestrogen after menopause, as well as androgenic hormones. The type of oestrogen produced is known as estrone and is less active than the estradiol produced by developing follicles. Estrone is also produced in fat cells throughout the body. With less oestrogen to balance the androgenic (or 'male-type') hormones produced, the balance tips towards a more masculine-type hormone profile, leading to symptoms such as male pattern hair loss and growth, a thicker waist and an increased risk of heart disease.

CHANGES TO ORGANS AND SYSTEMS

Perimenopause refers to the years before and after the last menstrual bleed, when symptoms come and go, and you notice physical and emotional changes. This can last anywhere from two to 15 years.

SKIN

The decline in oestrogen levels has a dramatic effect on the skin, causing it to lose elasticity all over the body. Skin starts to sag and wrinkle, losing its natural moisture and texture. This is a direct result of a reduction in oestrogen, as the capillaries, connective tissue, glands and hair follicles in the skin are all affected by this hormone. The skin starts to become thinner and the layer of fat cells just under the skin diminishes.

Collagen in the skin is destroyed by ultraviolet light and the skin becomes more sensitive to the sun as it ages. Melanocytes in the skin are lost and so the ability to make pigment and produce a tan diminishes. This makes the skin more likely to burn and increases the risk of permanent damage and skin cancer.

Because the natural moisture in the skin is reduced, women who suffer from psoriasis or eczema may find that their condition becomes worse. A few women in perimenopause experience problems with pimples or acne as their oestrogen levels drop and testosterone causes the sebaceous glands to produce more oily secretions (see page 52).

HAIR

Around menopause, hair may fall out and it may also grow in unusual places. As with glands in the skin, falling oestrogen levels mean less oil is produced in the scalp and hair can become dry and brittle. The hair breaks more easily and seems to be falling out. Eventually some hair follicles cease to function and naturally lost hair is not replaced. This is due to the action of the hormone testosterone circulating without oestrogen (see pages 57–58).

Some women notice the hair thinning all over the scalp; this may be due to a hereditary condition

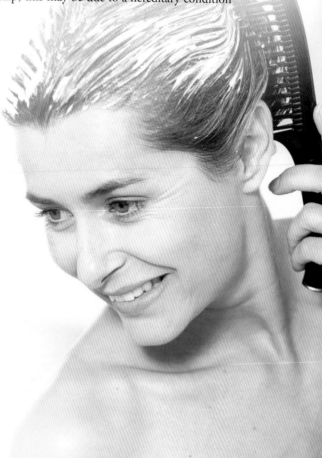

Keeping Hair Healthy

When choosing hair care products look for cleansing agents other than the harsh chemical cleanser sodium lauryl sulphate, and choose those made from nut oils, honey, healing plants and marine extracts (see pages 57–58 and 212).

known as androgenic alopecia. In a few women, testosterone also causes more hair to grow, but not usually where they want it. This phenomenon is known as hirsutism, and hair can start to grow on the face, chest and abdomen (see pages 57–58 and 213).

MIDDLE-AGE SPREAD

One thing almost all women notice around this time is the change in their shape. Until menopause, the oestrogen and progesterone that girls start producing at puberty have helped maintain a feminine shape. Fat is distributed on the hips and buttocks, giving an hourglass silhouette, or pear shape, with a narrow waist and rounded hips. During perimenopause, the fat distribution changes; the hips become less defined and the waist becomes thicker, with more fat being deposited on the abdomen. This is the characteristic 'middle-age spread'. It is considered more masculine and described as the apple shape.

Oestrogen influences enzymes that both break down and deposit fat in different areas of the body, and as oestrogen levels decline the shape change becomes more noticeable. The more the waist measurement increases in relation to hip size, the greater the risk of heart disease. There is a direct relationship between the waist to hip ratio and a healthy heart. The ratio should be less than one – and the lower the better. To work out your waist to hip ratio, measure the waist and then hips at the largest part, then divide your waist measurement by your hip measurement. Recent research has shown that waist size alone can indicate risks to health. As a general rule, a waist circumference above 89 cm (35 inches) is unhealthy for women.

In perimenopause, many women notice that their weight increases despite them not changing the way

WISE WOMAN
Skin and bone
•
Because skin and bone share the same type of oestrogen-sensitive collagen, there is a parallel change in skin thickness and bone density. This knowledge may help in the development of a new, easier test for osteoporosis.

they eat or exercise. This is due to a change in metabolic rate, and from middle age onwards the metabolic rate continues to slow. As menopause approaches, changes in the levels of progesterone affect carbohydrate metabolism. Around perimenopause there is an increased risk of developing Type 2 diabetes. The changes that take place in the body – and in particular any increase in weight – contribute to the development of insulin resistance, and sugars and starches are no longer metabolized efficiently (see pages 122–125).

HEART AND BLOOD VESSELS

There has been a lot of discussion recently about the pros and cons of hormone therapy (HT) and in particular its effect on cardiovascular disease in post-menopausal women.

Before menopause, most women have a much lower risk of heart disease than men of the same age. If they do have a heart attack under the age of 50, however, they are twice as likely to die from it as a man is. The reason for this is still not clear. We do know that a woman whose ovaries are still producing oestrogen has a much lower risk of coronary artery disease, and hence a lower risk of heart attack, than a woman of the same age whose ovaries have been removed or no longer function. Oestrogen seems to protect against heart disease, and nearly all deaths from heart attack in women are in those who have passed menopause.

Oestrogen is said to have a direct effect on the muscles of the heart, improving heart function by increasing its ability to pump efficiently. Oestrogen also has a direct effect on blood vessels, and oestrogen receptors are found in the muscular tissue in the walls of blood vessels. Oestrogen will cause this muscular tissue to relax and thus keep the blood vessels flexible and dilated, and the blood pressure low. When oestrogen levels in the blood fall, the blood vessels constrict, raising blood pressure and reducing the flow of blood. As blood pressure rises, more and more damage occurs to the inner surface of the blood vessels – in particular the arteries, which carry fresh oxygenated blood to the heart, brain and other essential organs. The damaged surfaces then attract fatty deposits, which can further narrow the artery, encouraging clots to form and block the artery, eventually causing heart attack or stroke (see pages 247–248).

The mechanism by which female hormones affect the vascular system is still poorly understood and is an area of active medical research.

The Cholesterol Factor

We know that there are two different types of cholesterol circulating in our blood and that the low-density lipoprotein (LDL) cholesterol is the harmful one. After menopause, the amount of LDL cholesterol in the blood increases and the amount of the beneficial high density lipoprotein (HDL) cholesterol decreases. LDL cholesterol is associated with atherosclerosis and hardening of the artery walls. HDL cholesterol seems to protect against heart disease by helping to remove LDL cholesterol from the blood. Oestrogen helps to keep the overall level of cholesterol down and maintain the correct ratio of LDL to HDL cholesterol.

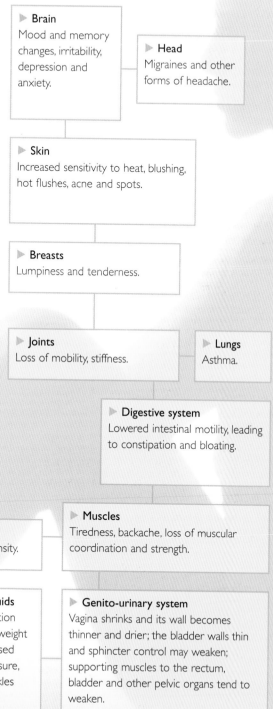

▶ **Brain**
Mood and memory changes, irritability, depression and anxiety.

▶ **Head**
Migraines and other forms of headache.

▶ **Skin**
Increased sensitivity to heat, blushing, hot flushes, acne and spots.

▶ **Breasts**
Lumpiness and tenderness.

▶ **Joints**
Loss of mobility, stiffness.

▶ **Lungs**
Asthma.

▶ **Digestive system**
Lowered intestinal motility, leading to constipation and bloating.

▶ **Muscles**
Tiredness, backache, loss of muscular coordination and strength.

The Changing Female Body
Some of these changes may happen to us all – many affecting men and women. Most occur as a result of the aging process rather than menopause *per se*. The key is to be aware of potential problems and informed about methods to avoid them wherever possible.

▶ **Bones**
Loss of density.

▶ **Body fluids**
Fluid retention leading to weight gain, increased blood pressure, swollen ankles and face.

▶ **Genito-urinary system**
Vagina shrinks and its wall becomes thinner and drier; the bladder walls thin and sphincter control may weaken; supporting muscles to the rectum, bladder and other pelvic organs tend to weaken.

After menopause, blood cholesterol levels tend to go up and so do insulin levels. Insulin not only affects sugar levels in the blood, but it also helps control lipid metabolism. One of oestrogen's direct effects is to lower blood insulin levels; as oestrogen levels fall, insulin levels go up and so does the risk of developing diabetes – a further risk factor for heart disease. Women treated with oestrogen after menopause have shown a lower risk of developing Type 2 diabetes.

BONES

Bone is being formed and resorbed (removed and reabsorbed) all throughout our lives. It is said that the skeleton replaces itself every 10 years, with some bones taking much more wear and tear than others.

Brittle Bones and Osteoporosis

About half of all women in the Western world have a serious degree of osteoporosis by the age of 70, and around age 60 – only 10 years after the average age of menopause – nearly a quarter of women will already have brittle bones. The lower level of oestrogen circulating in the bloodstream is directly responsible for this.

The metabolism of calcium, the mineral mainly involved in bone building, is in part dependent on oestrogen and there are oestrogen receptors in the osteoclasts and osteoblasts. The levels of available calcium circulating in the bloodstream are partly controlled by the hormones calcitonin and parathyroid hormone. Most of our calcium is stored in our bones, and if blood calcium levels fall the parathyroid hormone will act to break down bone and release calcium into the blood. Low oestrogen levels make bone more sensitive to parathyroid hormone, causing it to be broken down more rapidly after menopause (see pages 68–72).

When we are still children the rate of growth exceeds the rate of resorption; bones will get bigger, longer and firmer, and any knock or damage to bones will cause new bone to be formed and then be resorbed as it is modelled to the right shape. The cells that form new bone are called osteoblasts, and those that resorb old or badly formed bone are called osteoclasts. The decline of oestrogen around menopause causes bones to become less dense and therefore more brittle and likely to break. This thinning of the structure of the bones is called osteoporosis, one of the main problems women may experience after menopause (see pages 68–72).

Men generally have much stronger bones than women. From a young age men are relatively heavier than women, and their bones become much stronger and denser to support this weight. Men do suffer from osteoporosis as they get older, but far fewer men than women have fractures or serious problems, as their bones, having started stronger, take that much longer to become weak. Heavier women tend to have less serious osteoporosis than slimmer ones. This is in part thanks to their carrying extra weight, but also to the extra oestrogen produced by the fat cells.

MUSCLES AND JOINTS

Collagen is present all over the body, and all body systems containing this important structural protein change as oestrogen levels fall. Collagen is made by oestrogen receptors in the cells. Muscle mass is reduced as less supporting collagen is made, and this can put a strain on joints. Weaker muscles mean less support for the skeleton, and as we feel weaker we move less. The less we move the weaker our muscles and bones become.

During perimenopause, some women complain of muscle cramps at night; one cause of this can be low levels of calcium circulating in the blood. Since oestrogen helps the absorption of calcium from food, falling oestrogen levels can also lead to less calcium being available for normal muscle function.

BRAIN, EMOTIONS, MEMORY AND MOOD

One of the most common difficulties women experience in perimenopause is failing short-term memory, loss of concentration and loss of recall. Women report not being able to remember names and walking into a room and forgetting why they went into that room, or going out and then not being able to remember if they turned the oven off. To some degree, this deterioration happens to everyone as they get older; it is known as 'benign senile forgetfulness'. When there seems to be a sudden increase in the frequency of these incidents, many women become alarmed and think that they are going mad, and this in turn can have an adverse effect on mood and emotion. There are many things we can do to improve and maintain brain function throughout our lives. The more our brains are stimulated and challenged the more regeneration and repair is stimulated.

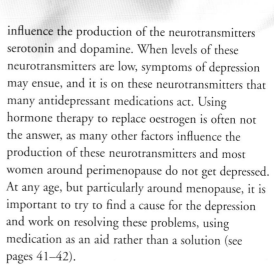

Along with the effects of natural aging, increased forgetfulness can be exacerbated by a decrease in oestrogen production. There are oestrogen receptors all over the brain, and one of the highest concentrations of receptors is found in the hippocampus, the area of the brain concerned with memory. Oestrogen can influence the activity of the brain in many ways: it improves blood flow to the brain by acting on the blood vessels, and this in turn maintains the high oxygen supply needed by brain cells to function efficiently (see page 39).

The Brain's Chemical Messengers

Oestrogen also has a direct effect on the production of the brain's neurotransmitters, the chemical messengers that enable one brain cell to communicate with others. This function is particularly vital for memory. One of the most important of these neurotransmitters is acetylcholine, the levels of which are directly affected by oestrogen. Acetylcholine also affects the regeneration, growth and replacement of neurons.

The area of the brain most concerned with mood is the hypothalamus. This is where oestrogen acts to influence the production of the neurotransmitters serotonin and dopamine. When levels of these neurotransmitters are low, symptoms of depression may ensue, and it is on these neurotransmitters that many antidepressant medications act. Using hormone therapy to replace oestrogen is often not the answer, as many other factors influence the production of these neurotransmitters and most women around perimenopause do not get depressed. At any age, but particularly around menopause, it is important to try to find a cause for the depression and work on resolving these problems, using medication as an aid rather than a solution (see pages 41–42).

Many of the symptoms relating to brain function result from the fluctuation in levels of oestrogen and not just the decline. Once the levels of oestrogen in the blood stop changing and stabilize – even though they are at a lower level than before – mood swings and emotional instability improve. This may partly be because the woman knows by then what has happened and knows that she has been through perimenopause: the changes she was experiencing have been explained, and things do not feel so out of control.

PREMATURE OR EARLY MENOPAUSE

An early menopause can occur naturally or it can be induced by medication, radiotherapy or surgery. Around 10 percent of women have their menopause before the age of 45. Of these, less than two percent will have a true premature menopause, which means their periods will have stopped by the age of 40. Most experiences of true early menopause will have been induced and are the result of surgical or medical intervention. Induced menopause can take place at any age, but the younger the woman, the more traumatic and difficult it will be for her to come to terms with it.

SURGICAL MENOPAUSE

A surgical menopause occurs when both ovaries are removed completely, and its effects start to be felt the day the ovaries are removed. The sudden drop in hormone levels, both oestrogen and androgens, means a rapid adjustment is necessary by the whole body, and severe and distressing symptoms can occur. Most premature menopause is the result of this type of surgery, and it may be performed for a number of reasons. For example, tumours and cysts can destroy the ovaries, and whether these are cancerous or non-cancerous, they may need to be removed. Likewise, in cases of severe or chronic pelvic inflammatory disease, the ovaries may have been destroyed by infection and will have to be removed. In very severe cases of endometriosis, removal of the ovaries is sometimes an option, but symptoms may recur when hormone treatment is given afterwards.

Hysterectomy

Not long ago many gynaecological surgeons used to recommend removing the ovaries when performing a hysterectomy. They justified this by saying that the ovaries were unnecessary if there was no longer a uterus to support a pregnancy, and that the ovaries should be removed to reduce the risk of future ovarian disease, ovarian cancer in particular. The majority of surgeons now feel that there is no point removing a healthy organ – which does have a very important function in continuing to produce essential hormones until a natural menopause occurs. If you are having a hysterectomy, make sure you know whether the surgeon is planning to remove the ovaries and, if so, that the reasons for this decision are clearly explained. After a hysterectomy, women tend to experience menopause around five years earlier than they otherwise would. This is thought to be the result of surgery reducing the blood supply to the ovaries, but the reason is not yet fully understood.

Problems from Induced or Natural Early Menopause

The symptoms surrounding menopause, such as hot flushes (see pages 30–33) and reduced libido (see pages 84–85), are usually felt more intensely when menopause is induced.

Loss of fertility, particularly in women who have not yet had children, can be traumatic and may leave them prone to depression and concerned over their sexuality.

The earlier menopause is experienced the greater a woman's risk of osteoporosis or thinning of the bones. When the protective effect of oestrogen on the cardiovascular system is lost early, cardiovascular problems, including heart disease and stroke, become more likely.

OTHER CAUSES OF PREMATURE MENOPAUSE

The other main medical reason for induced menopause is the effect of chemotherapy or radiation treatment for cancer in the pelvic area. Both of these treatments can damage the ovaries – sometimes temporarily, but often permanently – and menopause may occur immediately or a few months after treatment. Younger women may be offered the chance to have some ovarian tissue removed before treatment, and have it kept frozen for future in vitro fertilization. Women undergoing menopause at a younger age will require greater help in coming to terms with their 'change' and more intensive treatment to control their symptoms.

When premature menopause occurs without being induced, its cause is often unknown. One of the recognized but very rare causes is related to the effects of autoimmune disease. Your own immune system can start making antibodies to tissues in the body, as in rheumatoid arthritis and lupus (systemic lupus erythematosus, or SLE). Auto-antibodies have been known to start to attack the ovaries and eventually cause ovarian failure and menopause.

Oestrogen and progesterone therapy, delivered by various methods, has proved successful in replacing hormones. This preserves the uterus and makes it possible to try implanting a donated ovum or some of the woman's own previously saved eggs if the woman wishes to try to become pregnant.

REVERSIBLE MENOPAUSE

Some drug treatments can cause a temporary reversible menopause. This 'false' menopause may be a side effect of medications or an intended part of the treatment, as in the drug treatment for endometriosis or to shrink fibroids. Early drug treatments

WISE WOMAN
Maintaining fertility
•
Only complete removal or destruction of both ovaries results in menopause. Even a part of one ovary will be enough to continue the production of hormones in the cyclical pattern necessary to maintain the menstrual cycle and potential fertility.

for breast cancer, which used to cause premature menopause, have now been improved to enable a reversible menopause and allow the preservation of ovarian function. During the drug treatment women may still suffer menopausal symptoms.

SMOKING, DRINKING AND DIETING

These are all factors that can influence the timing of menopause. In general, the more you smoke, the more alcohol you drink and the less fat you have on your body, the earlier your menopause will be. None of these factors are likely to cause real premature menopause, but they may mean that your periods end a year or two earlier than they would otherwise have done (see pages 165–169).

▶ THE MUMPS VIRUS

The virus that causes mumps can damage and destroy the ovaries at any age. The virus can cause inflammation of the ovaries and irreversible damage to egg follicles. A girl who has never had a period may suffer from mumps and lose some or all of the function of her ovaries before the onset of menstruation. It is, however, already an extremely rare disease, and it will become rarer still now that there is a vaccine to protect against the mumps virus.

ABNORMAL BLEEDING

For most women, the changes in the pattern of menstruation around this time will be entirely explained by fluctuating hormone levels. It is normal to have irregular periods for anything from four to eight years before the actual last period. It is also normal for periods to be lighter or heavier, a bit longer or a bit shorter. When your cycle starts to change, it is important to see your doctor to make sure the change in pattern is explained by peri-menopause and not anything else. It is not normal for bleeding to occur more than one year after the last period. If bleeding occurs even six months later it should arouse suspicion and you should see your doctor quickly to find out the cause.

INVESTIGATION OF ABNORMAL BLEEDING

When you visit your doctor complaining of any of the above and you are approaching 50, he or she will want to give you a complete examination and do tests to exclude any serious causes.

Testing Methods

Your GP will perform a vaginal examination and cervical smear, and arrange blood tests for anaemia and thyroid function.

You may be referred for an ultrasound examination of the pelvic organs (a transvaginal scan or TVS). This can be done in the ultrasound department of the hospital, but more commonly you would see a gynaecologist who specializes in ultrasound investigation. If the scan shows the lining of the uterus is thickened or irregular, you may have an endometrial biopsy, when a small sample of the lining is taken using using a thin plastic tube. This can be carried out at the same time as the scan and takes two minutes.

Alternatively, you may need a hysteroscopy and/or a D&C (dilatation and curettage, see page 230) under anaesthetic. Hysteroscopy involves examining the uterine cavity with a thin fibreoptic hysteroscope. A D&C involves dilating the cervix, scraping out the lining of the uterus and sending it for further tests. This method is often used as a treatment for heavy bleeding, and sometimes solves the problem.

Either method will help diagnose any abnormality of the endometrium, including polyps, infection, endometrial hyperplasia and cancer.

A cervical smear will help to diagnose the cause of any spotting or bleeding after sex. The test involves scraping some cells from the cervix and examining them for any signs of pre-cancer or cancer. Regular cervical smears after the age of 20 will help to ensure that any abnormality will be found early and can be dealt with before it becomes serious. If the smear is abnormal, further

See your doctor if you experience

Very heavy bleeding, or 'flooding', with clots being passed, or when tampons or sanitary pads need to be changed every half hour or so.

Very long periods with bleeding lasting more than five days on more than one occasion, or when the interval between periods becomes shorter (generally less than 21 days). Fibroids, polyps, endometrial hyperplasia and, rarely, endometrial cancer may be the cause.

Continual spotting, spotting between periods, and spotting or bleeding after intercourse. This is especially important if you have an IUD for contraception or are using HT, or if there is any chance you may be pregnant. Infection in the uterus or fallopian tubes, an ectopic pregnancy, or pre-cancer or cancer of the cervix can all cause this type of bleeding.

examination of the cervix, using a colposcope to magnify the area, will be necessary. Biopsies are done of any visualized abnormalities and sent to the pathologist.

Blood tests will help to show whether the abnormal bleeding is due to hormone imbalance. There is some concern that if you are bleeding heavily due to unopposed oestrogen, your risk of certain hormone-sensitive cancers is increased.

When bleeding patterns change it is important to have blood tests to check the thyroid gland. Thyroid disease can give many of the same symptoms as perimenopause, and if left untreated can cause serious illness.

TREATMENT OF ABNORMAL BLEEDING

The type of treatment depends on the cause of the abnormal bleeding and whether it is coming from the uterus or cervix.

Uterine Bleeding

Most of the time the cause of uterine bleeding (prolonged and irregular) is hormonal. In otherwise healthy perimenopausal women the treatment of choice is a slow-release progesterone coil called the IUS (intra-uterine system) or Mirena. This can be fitted by your GP or after a D&C while under anaesthetic. This lasts for at least three years, and has the added advantage of also acting as a contraceptive. A low-dose progesterone is delivered directly to the endometrium and prevents it from thickening. Periods become much lighter and may stop altogether. In the past, progesterone tablets have been tried to reduce and regulate the cycle, but these are less effective and more likely to cause unwanted side effects.

Other drugs used to help the blood to clot more quickly, such as tranexamic acid, can be effective.

Polyps and Fibroids

If the cause of bleeding turns out to be a problem with the lining of the uterus or polyps within the uterus, they can be destroyed or removed by curettage, by freezing or with cautery.

Fibroids tend to shrink and cause fewer problems after menopause, but if they are very troublesome in perimenopause surgery may be the only solution. The operation to remove fibroids is called a myomectomy and is usually done through an abdominal incision along the bikini line. If the fibroids are not too big they can be removed using only a laparoscope, or occasionally a hysteroscope (see page 230).

Cervical Bleeding

Bleeding from the cervix is treated after evaluation by colposcopy (see page 228) and biopsy using laser electrocautery, freezing or excising the abnormal tissue.

When the cause of abnormal bleeding has been diagnosed and serious disease excluded, there are many complementary treatments and self-help alternatives to help deal with different bleeding patterns (see page 59).

Bleeding with severe pain, even if it is only spotting, needs rapid investigation. The cause could be an infection, an ectopic pregnancy or a fibroid problem.

Bleeding associated with fever is most likely to be caused by an infection, and the uterus and fallopian tubes need to be excluded as the site of infection.

If your periods stop suddenly, unless you have been using adequate contraception, there is a chance you are pregnant, even if you are over 50.

Any bleeding that occurs even six months after periods appear to have stopped should be taken seriously and reported to a doctor.

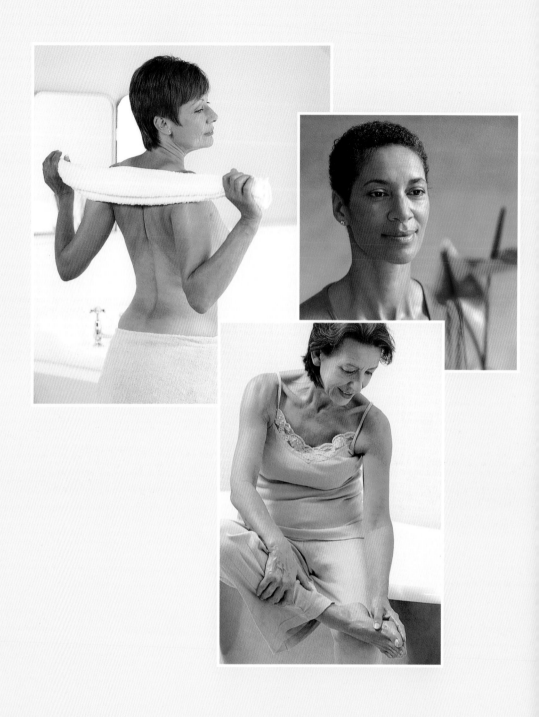

2

SELF-HELP FOR SYMPTOMS OF MENOPAUSE

Every woman's experience of menopause is different. Many women have one or more symptoms – hot flushes, changes to skin and hair, loss of concentration and memory, and emotional upheaval – that they find troublesome; some notice a few slight changes, but nothing that impacts on their everyday lives, and a few sail through the whole experience feeling no different. However, if you know what you might experience, you can take action to recognize these symptoms – and perhaps even prevent some from occurring.

HOT FLUSHES

A widespread discomfort of perimenopause, hot flushes affect about 75 percent of menopausal women. These women report various experiences of the phenomenon, ranging from a glowing sensation to a burning heat, usually with some sweating, which may be particularly bad at night (night sweats). The frequency of the experience also differs greatly: some women have a few mild flushes a week for a short period, while others may experience up to 50 a day for many years. In very severe cases, they may occur six or seven times in an hour. Many women experience hot flushes well before their last menstrual period. Initially, these are infrequent and are on the face, neck and chest only. Over time, these flushes can become more frequent, last longer, and they may continue to occur, with occasional flush-free periods, for up to five years.

HOW YOUR SKIN RESPONDS TO A HOT FLUSH

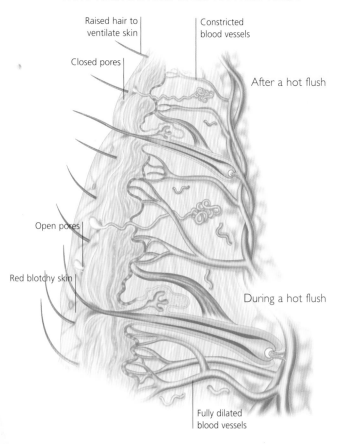

Raised hair to ventilate skin

Constricted blood vessels

Closed pores

After a hot flush

Open pores

Red blotchy skin

During a hot flush

Fully dilated blood vessels

What Causes a Hot Flush?

The underlying physiology is complex, but the onset of a flush may correspond with an increase in the level of the pituitary hormone, follicle stimulating hormone (FSH). Significant changes in levels of FSH secretion are common as menopause approaches, and they appear to be a response to the shrinking of the ovaries and decreased oestrogen secretion. The loss of oestrogen itself makes the blood vessel muscles more unstable, hence the term 'vasomotor instability', which is sometimes used to describe a hot flush. Other internal secretions also surge during a hot flush. For example, there is a significant rise in the blood level of some of the adrenal hormones.

More simply stated, a hot flush occurs because the brain decides your body is overheated. During menopause, your temperature-regulating system changes. Your sweat glands may work less effectively than before because lack of oestrogen changes the way they are programmed. Not only do your sweat glands not cool as efficiently as before, but there also appears to be a change in brain chemistry that affects the temperature control centre in the hypothalamus. The temperature set point becomes lower than normal, and this triggers a dilation of blood vessels in the skin and sweating as your body attempts to reset its thermostat. The adjustments aren't always smooth and your body often overcompensates, hence hot flushes.

To reduce the unpleasantness and potential severity of the experience, there are a number of self-help measures to try, including dietary and lifestyle changes, regular exercise, meditation and complementary therapies.

DIET

Certain foods are suspected of triggering hot flushes: sugary, salty and spicy dishes; acidic foods such as pickles and tomatoes; hydrogenated or saturated fats; chocolate; very hot drinks of all kinds, as well as alcohol and caffeinated beverages such as cola drinks. Other foods can improve your body's ability to withstand the changes. Citrus fruits, such as oranges and grapefruit, contain bioflavonoids, which have a mild oestrogenic effect on the body. Soya-based foods such as tofu contain helpful isoflavones (45-60 mg daily); Linseed is also beneficial.

Vitamin E may help the proper functioning of blood and aid the production of sex hormones. Vegetable oils, leafy green vegetables, whole grains and beans are good sources. If you try a supplement, don't exceed 1,000 units a day. If you suffer from hypertension, heart disease or diabetes, consult your health professional.

Hot flushes deplete the B vitamins, vitamin C, magnesium and potassium, so make sure you eat plenty of foods containing these nutrients or take supplements. General guidelines for a healthy menopause diet can be found on pages 106–121.

Eat smaller meals; large meals dilate blood vessels and cause the body to become warmer. Be sure to drink plenty of water – particularly if you suffer night sweats; if your urine becomes a dark yellow, rather than a light straw colour, it's a sign you're probably dehydrated.

Finally, if you are very thin you might think about putting on some weight. Thinner women have fewer fat cells producing oestrogen, so they generally tend to experience more hot flushes.

EXERCISE

Regular physical exercise is instrumental in preventing hot flushes because it vastly improves circulation, and it can make the body more tolerant of temperature extremes and better able to cool down quickly. Exercise also helps to increase the amount of endorphins circulating in your blood. Try to exercise at least three times a week for 20-minute sessions. One study has shown that aerobic exercise reduces the severity of hot flushes in 55 percent of menopausal and postmenopausal women. Weight-lifting and other strength-training exercises are also effective. Their other benefit is to increase bone density (see pages 130–151 for recommended

ways to cool down quickly

▶ Take a shower.
▶ Run cool water over your wrists.
▶ Have a cooling drink.
▶ Spray water over your face or use wet wipes.
▶ Use a small battery-operated fan.
▶ Apply a cooled gel pack around your neck.
▶ Open your freezer and put your head inside.

Do not use cold or iced water. Both can cause you to overheat after you have applied them. Tepid water will evaporate on your skin, removing the heat, which will make you feel cooler and bring the feeling of fever to a more rapid end.

exercise regimes). However, very intense exercise can trigger a hot flush.

LIFESTYLE

Smoking tobacco or marijuana intensifies hot flushes because it affects your circulation. If you smoke, now is an excellent time to stop.

Stress is thought to contribute to the occurrence of hot flushes. Try to ease the stresses in your life and find time to relax, as relaxation may help to prevent hot flushes from occurring and can decrease their intensity when they do. During a hot flush move to a cool, peaceful place where you can sit or lie quietly. Breathe deeply and slowly, and practice visualization and calming thoughts (see overleaf). If you can, when you inhale, think about cool air filling your body, and when you breathe out, visualize heat rushing out through your hands and feet.

Choose your clothes carefully. Synthetic fabrics, such as polyester and nylon, trap perspiration and those with high collars and long sleeves intensify feelings of suffocation. It's preferable to wear natural fibres such as cotton or linen, and garments that are loose-fitting. Many women choose short sleeves, round or v-necks, or clothes that can be unbuttoned at the neck. Avoid roundnecks or any garment or jewellery that is tight-fitting around the neck.

Maintaining a regular and active sex life can also help. A Stanford University research study in the United States has shown that women who have intercourse regularly, at least once a week, have fewer or less intense hot flushes.

Stay away from hot tubs and saunas. Be on the alert in hot weather, as heat can trigger flushes. Some women keep a fan in their handbag.

HERBAL AIDS

The long-term treatment for hot flushes, as for other menopausal side effects, is achieved by balancing and toning the hormonal system. For this, herbs such as *vitex agnus-castus* (chasteberry) and dong quai (Chinese angelica), which balance the pituitary gland, and black cohosh and red clover blossoms, which contain plant hormones that can act as herbal hormone therapy are very useful. These may be combined in a formula – equal parts of each, to which your herbalist may add other herbs according to your individual condition. (Red clover should not be used if you are being treated for breast cancer.) See pages 188–198 for more information on natural HT.

For hot flushes, sage tincture should make up part of the formula. If your flushes are severe, you may take sage tincture on its own – 15–20 drops three times daily or as needed.

Herbalists believe that an aging liver can contribute to menopausal problems. The naturo-

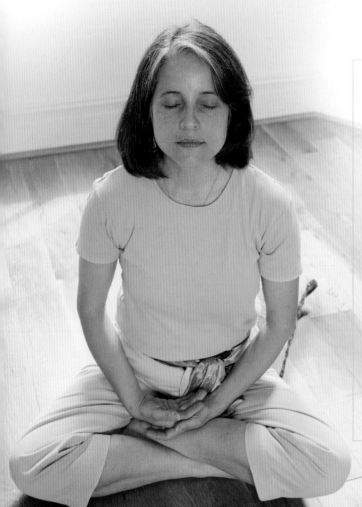

Paced Respiration

Two studies have found that slow, deep breathing reduced the frequency of hot flushes. To develop this skill, find a quiet, private place where you can sit and practise without distraction – at least 15 minutes morning and evening. You need to master diaphragmatic breathing, which involves keeping the ribcage still and inhaling and exhaling by using your stomach muscles, to enable the diaphragm to move up and down.

Without moving your ribcage but distending and retracting your abdominal muscles, inhale for 5 seconds and then exhale for 5 seconds.

Once you are accustomed to the technique you can put it to use. As soon as you feel a flush developing, start the paced breathing and continue until you feel the experience has passed.

pathic liver flush may help hot flushes. First thing in the morning, before eating anything, blend the juice of a whole lemon, half a pint of apple juice, a minced clove of garlic, a small piece of fresh ginger, grated, and a tablespoon of olive oil. Drink this, then prepare enough hot herbal tea (dandelion, nettle or peppermint) to make up two mugs. Sip the hot tea during the following two hours, and do not eat until this time has elapsed.

You can also add a liver herb, such as dandelion or milk thistle, to your tea. Perform the flush for five days, rest two days and then repeat for five days. Traditional Chinese Medicine (TCM) characterizes menopause as a deficiency or stagnation in the blood, liver or kidney, and a practitioner will prescribe specific herbs depending on your symptoms. Proponents of TCM claim that it is very effective in treating hot flushes, using herbs that are gentle yet potent.

HOMEOPATHY
Naturopathic physicians find homeopathic remedies very beneficial in treating menopausal symptoms. They can recommend a wide variety of remedies depending on your pattern of sweating, where sweating manifests itself and any accompanying symptoms. Lachesis, pulsatilla, sepia and belladonna are some of the most commonly prescribed treatments. Lachesis is used for hot flushes that affect the head and face; pulsatilla for hot flushes together with sweating on the face; sepia for hot flushes accompanied by anxiety attacks; and belladona for a sweaty face.

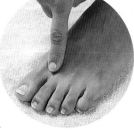

ACUPRESSURE AND ACUPUNCTURE
Both these therapies apply pressure to specific body points – acupressure with the

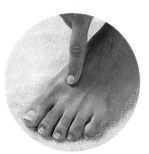

fingers, acupuncture with needles. Acupressure points are situated on meridian lines and are named after them, i.e., Liver. As a hot flush begins, try massaging Liv 2. This is the point at the juncture of the big toe and the second toe (below left, top). This pressure may cool you down by drawing heat away from the top of your body.

To prevent hot flushes, try massaging Liv 3, which is two finger-widths up from the juncture between the big and second toe (below left, bottom).

Acupuncture may also be useful for relieving hot flushes and the insomnia that often accompanies night sweats (see page 34). In this case, it works by rebalancing the hormonal system.

CHEMICAL TREATMENTS
The most effective way to treat hot flushes is with hormone therapy, using the lowest dose of oestrogen that will be effective for your flushes. As time goes by, you may be able to slowly tail off the treatment, but this may take several years.

Some studies have shown that in addition to hormonal remedies, antidepressants can significantly reduce the severity and duration of severe hot flushes. SSRIs (selective serotonin reuptake inhibitors) such as fluoxetine and venlafaxine, in low doses, can help, although this is not a use approved by the Committee on Safety of Medicines. These drugs are believed to work because of the role that serotonin plays in regulating body temperature.

Other drugs tried include clonidine, a drug sometimes used to treat high blood pressure, but studies have not proven its efficacy.

NIGHT SWEATS

Do make sure the temperature of your bedroom is only 65°F (18°C), which is sufficient for a comfortable sleep. If you have a fan or air conditioner, you may want to use it from time to time. Use a few lightweight blankets for flexibility.

Do drink more water. You'll need at least 12 glasses per day at room temperature to cool down your core temperature without shocking your system. Drink one glass before going to bed. Herbalists recommend adding 30 drops of sage tincture to a glass of water placed by your bedside. Simply take a sip or two as needed.

Do wear sleepwear made of natural fibres only and make sure your bedding is also made of cotton or linen. Be prepared to abandon sleepwear, top sheets and blankets.

Do shower or sponge with cool water just before going to bed.

Do avoid all hot baths and showers.

Don't do any heavy physical activity before going to bed.

Don't eat before going to bed. Have your dinner several hours before going to bed.

Don't drink coffee or alcohol, or smoke late in the evening.

A hot flush at night is called a night sweat, and along with soaked bedding and sleepwear, it may be accompanied by feelings of anxiety or terror. Not everyone experiences night sweats along with hot flushes, but many women do experience both. In addition to feeling chilled after a night sweat, it is also quite common to experience insomnia. In fact, most women initially experience disturbed sleep before the sweating begins, which points to the involvement of the nervous system. For more information on sleeping problems, see pages 37–38.

As night sweats can be symptomatic of other, more serious conditions, make certain yours are correctly diagnosed. If you are in any doubt about your symptoms, contact your doctor.

To Lessen the Severity of Night Sweats

If you wake up feeling feverish, try tepid sponging to help cool your face and chest. Simply soak a sponge or washcloth in cool water and then pat your body with it. Do not use cold water since it would cause the small blood vessels beneath your skin to constrict and preserve body heat.

Some naturopaths recommend a hydrotherapy treatment in which you direct alternating hot and cold jets of water up and down your spine. This stimulates your circulation, cooling the blood nearest the surface of the skin, and leaves you with a pleasant, invigorating, tingling sensation.

Along with the natural and chemical remedies suggested for hot flushes on the previous pages, there are a few additional measures that can help to prevent night sweats or lessen their severity (see box, left).

FATIGUE

This is one of the most frequently reported symptoms of menopause, and perhaps unsurprisingly, its most common cause is sleep deprivation (see insomnia, pages 37–38), which is largely due to fluctuating hormone levels. Around this time, androgen, the 'male' hormone we produce – associated with energy levels and a sense of well-being – begins to decrease. A drop in oestrogen levels can also produce sleeping problems. Another common culprit is diet. A high-carbohydrate, low-fat diet can play havoc with your metabolism. It encourages high levels of insulin, which lead to low blood sugar levels. If you drink fizzy drinks, tea or coffee, the caffeine content leads to a release of adrenaline, which further upsets the insulin–sugar balance.

Fortunately, there are a number of things you can do to bring your energy levels up.

SKIN BRUSHING

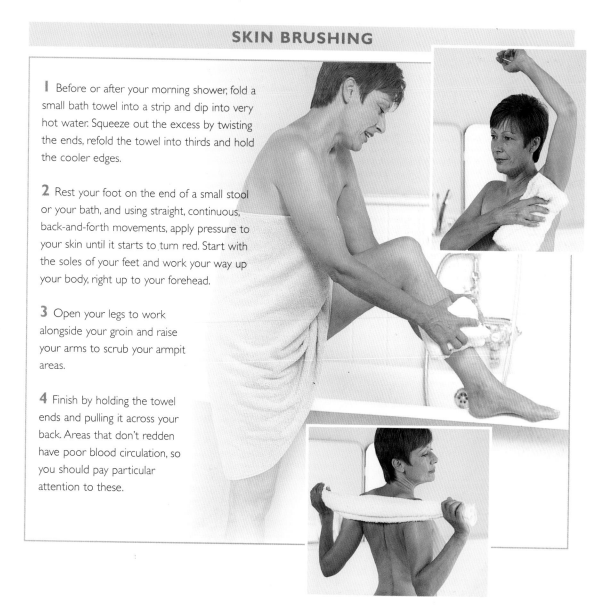

1 Before or after your morning shower, fold a small bath towel into a strip and dip into very hot water. Squeeze out the excess by twisting the ends, refold the towel into thirds and hold the cooler edges.

2 Rest your foot on the end of a small stool or your bath, and using straight, continuous, back-and-forth movements, apply pressure to your skin until it starts to turn red. Start with the soles of your feet and work your way up your body, right up to your forehead.

3 Open your legs to work alongside your groin and raise your arms to scrub your armpit areas.

4 Finish by holding the towel ends and pulling it across your back. Areas that don't redden have poor blood circulation, so you should pay particular attention to these.

DIET

To raise blood glucose levels it is important to eat carbohydrates with a low or medium glycaemic index (see pages 124–125). These provide a gradual and sustained release of energy. Be sure, too, to include plenty of foods containing B vitamins, particularly if you eat a high carbohydrate diet. Sufficient fat and protein are also needed to maintain healthy cellular function; choose healthful fats like linseed, avocado or olive oil, and protein in the form of lean meats, poultry or soya products.

Seaweeds of all kinds can nourish your nervous, immune and hormonal systems. Try eating a portion as a vegetable at least once a week and get into the habit of adding some to soups and salads.

Eating several small meals or snacking through-out the day can reduce the energy-sapping drops in blood glucose levels that occur between meals – as can cutting down on caffeine drinks and alcohol.

HERBAL REMEDIES

Siberian ginseng is commonly taken to increase stamina and boost the immune system. Traditional Chinese Medicine (TCM) treats exhaustion with energy tonics that contain ginseng.

EXERCISE

Lack of exercise leads to inactivity, while keeping active and fit gives you more energy and stamina. Even a brisk 10-minute walk will shift your mood and raise your energy levels.

Many eastern-based practices, such as meditation, yoga, t'ai chi, qi gong and shiatsu, are based on moving energy around your body to revitalize you. Another effective practice is skin brushing (see page 35). Several minutes of scrubbing in the morning will boost your circulation and raise your energy levels. If you have an existing skin problem you can still scrub, just avoid the affected area. Adding the juice of a tablespoon of grated ginger will boost the beneficial effects.

STRESS REDUCTION

Overdoing anything, even something as good as exercise, can also lead to fatigue, so make sure you pace yourself. Take more breaks and, if necessary, cut back on some of your activities. Include plenty of enjoyable activities, even socializing, which can relieve the stress of a hectic schedule. Many thera-pists suggest that clearing your life of clutter – whether it's clearing up your desk or learning to let go of situations beyond your control – will stop your energy from being sapped. Nicotine is also an energy sapper, so if you smoke you should stop.

CHEMICAL TREATMENTS

Testosterone supplements in patch or cream form have been tried, but this use of the drug is not licensed in the UK, nor have studies shown it to be effective.

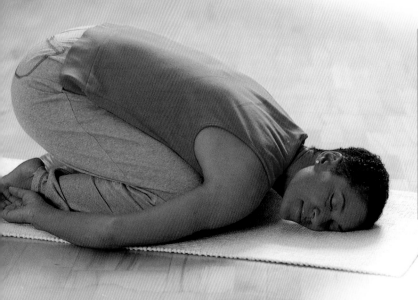

The Child's Pose
To help relieve the symptoms of exhaustion, kneel down on a soft surface and let your head sink to the floor. Rest your arms loosely by your sides with your palms facing upwards. Breathe in and out deeply.

INSOMNIA

With increasing age, sleep problems become more and more common. Menopause is a time when many women begin losing sleep or, if they've been losing sleep before, to lose even more. Insomnia, which is defined as difficulty getting to sleep or getting back to sleep after awakening, is a frequent side effect of menopause.

Another common and annoying disorder is restless leg syndrome (RLS), in which unpleasant tingling or painful sensations in your legs make you jerk or twitch them to relieve discomfort. This may be curtailed by making sure you have plenty of magnesium, B-group vitamins, vitamin E and iron in your diet.

The drop in oestrogen that causes night sweats (see page 34) is also responsible for frequent awakenings, but an inability to fall or stay asleep is often aggravated by unhealthy eating and drinking habits, medications, chronic anxiety, stress and depression.

DIET
The traditional late-night snack of a glass of warm milk before bed has a lot to recommend it. Milk contains the sleep-inducing chemical tryptophan. Other good sources of tryptophan are bananas and peanut butter. On the other hand, cured meats, mature cheeses, chocolate, pickles and tomatoes contain tyrosine, a chemical from which your brain makes the neuro-transmitter noradrenaline,

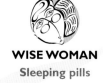

WISE WOMAN
Sleeping pills

Sleeping pills are drugs of dependence, which means that you need to increase the dose to maintain the same effect as time goes by, and you may suffer withdrawal symptoms when you stop taking them.

which is responsible for alertness. These foods should be avoided late in the evening.

Caffeine is a stimulant that affects individual organs as well as your overall metabolism, and it is a major cause of sleep disturbances. If you suffer from sleeping problems, you should cut your intake right down. You should not drink excessive amounts of liquids at bedtime, as these will fill your bladder and disturb your sleep.

Try not to eat a heavy meal before bedtime; it's best if you can eat no later than 7 p.m. – but don't go to bed on an empty stomach either.

HERBAL REMEDIES
Passionflower can help to calm restlessness and anxiety. Take it as an infusion (2 to 5 grams of dried herb three times a day), as a fluid extract (10 to 30 drops three times a day), or as a tincture (1:5 in 45 percent alcohol). Alternatively, try valerian in capsule form; 150–300 mg may be taken an hour before bedtime.

Food or drink	Caffeine (milligrams)
I cup brewed coffee	100–150
I cup instant coffee	85–100
I cup tea	60–75
I 8-oz glass cola	40–60
I cup cocoa	40–55
I chocolate bar	25
I cup decaffeinated coffee	2–4

6 ways to get a better night's sleep

▶ Make sure your bedroom is quiet and cool.
▶ Use your bed only for sleeping or sex. Don't read, watch TV or listen to music in it.
▶ Go to bed and wake up at regular times; try not to vary them.
▶ Avoid exercising within 5–6 hours of bedtime, caffeine after noon and alcohol in the evening.
▶ Before bed, eat a light snack of tryptophan-rich yogurt, cottage cheese, milk or bananas.
▶ Close to bedtime, do something relaxing like folding laundry or reading something easy.
▶ Once you're in bed, don't look at your clock after you lie down or if you get up at night.

CHEMICAL TREATMENTS

Short-acting sleeping pills may be effective in the short term, but there is always the risk of habituation (addiction) with these drugs, and you may find you begin to need an increasingly larger dose to reach the same effect, leading eventually to being unable to sleep without them.

Melatonin supplements – which mimic the action of the brain hormone of the same name, producing drowsiness – are used in the United States for treating sleep disturbance. However, they are not available in the UK except over the internet and for restricted psychological problems.

If you are looking for medication to treat persistent insomnia it is best to consult your healthcare professional.

SCALP AND SOLE MASSAGE

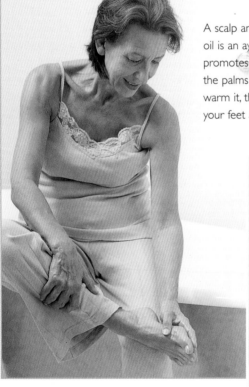

A scalp and sole massage with coconut oil is an ayurvedic remedy that promotes sleep. Rub the oil between the palms and fingers of your hands to warm it, then stroke along the soles of your feet and through your hair.

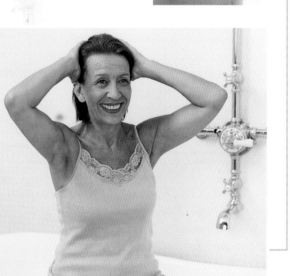

CONCENTRATION AND MEMORY PROBLEMS

While 'senior moments' tend to characterize the perimenopause and menopause, science has not been able to state definitively that changes in hormone balance are to blame: some studies indicate that oestrogen aids memory and problem-solving skills; others have failed to corroborate this. Most doctors believe that the 'fuzzy thinking' many women report has more to do with a temporary overload situation due to stress and the normal decline in cellular processes that accompanies aging. Around the time of perimenopause and menopause, women often experience both physical stresses (for example, night sweats that interfere with sleeping, see page 34) and psychological ones, such as relationship difficulties, problems with children and elderly parents, and self-image.

From around the age of 20, memory starts to decline in everyone. Strategies to deal with loss of concentration and memory lie in keeping your brain 'in shape' and reducing stress.

EXERCISE

Not only does physical activity improve your circulation – thus helping your blood to deliver energy and oxygen to your brain to make you more alert and able to concentrate – but it also releases endorphins, the 'feel-good' chemicals in your brain. You should try to do aerobic exercise (a brisk two-mile walk, for example) three times a week. Keep your brain active by learning something new, doing crossword puzzles or reading interesting books. Yoga and t'ai chi, which calm both the body and mind, are also beneficial.

DIET

As well as a balanced diet with adequate amounts of vitamins (see A New Look at Nutrition, pages 106–127), it's important to include oily fish in your meals. Omega-3 fish oils, the fatty acids in oily fish, have been shown to contribute to memory. Foods rich in choline – eggs and soya products – can boost the neurotransmitter acetylcholine, which is key in maintaining memory. Antioxidants, found especially in fruits and vegetables, can protect your brain from free radical damage. On the other hand, alcohol hinders concentration and interferes with your brain's ability to store and retrieve information, so should be avoided. Caffeine, too, is a known stressor; it will increase symptoms of anxiety and make it difficult to sleep.

RELAXATION AND POSITIVE THINKING

Now, more than ever, it's important to be aware of your own needs as well as those of others. Stressful situations can become much more manageable if you approach them with greater tranquillity by using relaxation and positive thinking techniques. Non-competitive recreation, such as gardening or a craft, can be restful, as will the following practices.

Meditation (see page 42) helps to slow the mind; your actual brainwaves change from the quick beta ones (14–30 Hz) to slower, calmer alpha waves (8–13 Hz). These waves induce feelings of calm and relaxation. Deep abdominal breathing (see page 40) is another calming technique.

Aromatherapy offers a number of treatments that induce relaxation. Lavender essential oil produces feelings of calm. Add a few drops of it to your bath, massage oil or to your pillow before sleep.

Neurolinguistic programming (NLP) involves techniques that help you observe your mind's processes and then allows you to adjust them to create a more positive outlook (see also pages 201–202).

Breathing exercises are useful for achieving a sense of calm. Just taking long, deep breaths can ease a stressful situation, like being caught in a traffic jam. However, if you practise deep abdominal breathing for at least 10 minutes a day, you'll experience much greater benefits.

Lie down in a warm place, where you won't be disturbed, with your head and neck supported. Close your eyes and place one hand on your chest and the other on your abdomen. Inhale deeply into your abdomen, then breathe out slowly. As you near the end of your exhalation, start to pull in your abdominal muscles. The hand on your abdomen should move, not the hand on your chest, if you are breathing in and out correctly.

When you are breathing sufficiently deeply, place your hands by your sides, palms facing upwards. Try not to fall asleep.

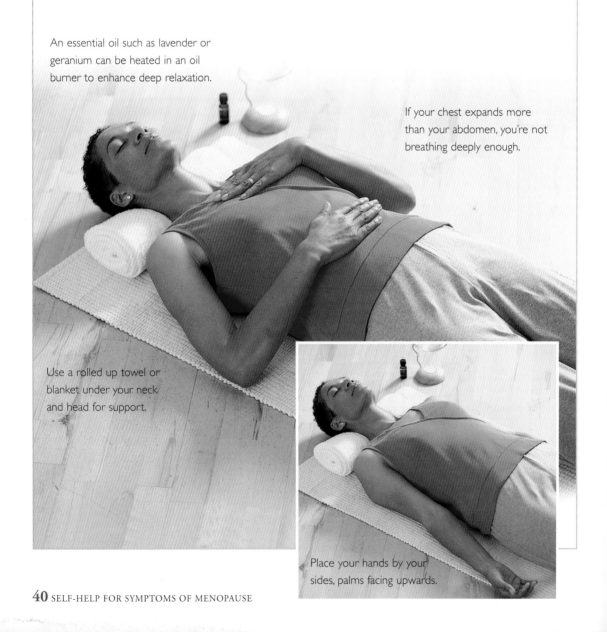

An essential oil such as lavender or geranium can be heated in an oil burner to enhance deep relaxation.

If your chest expands more than your abdomen, you're not breathing deeply enough.

Use a rolled up towel or blanket under your neck and head for support.

Place your hands by your sides, palms facing upwards.

MOOD SWINGS

Although there is no proven link between menopause and clinical depression, many middle-aged women do experience periods of sadness, discouragement, anxiety and irritability, which may be the result of hormonal changes and situational developments. Mood swings appear most often during perimenopause, when changes in hormonal balance are at their greatest, and become less frequent in the menopausal and postmenopausal periods. The good news is that many women who have gone through menopause feel much more positive and have a great zest for life.

Your brain produces a neurotransmitter, serotonin, that is very important in regulating mood. Oestrogen seems to increase the concentration of serotonin, so its lower levels during menopause may be responsible for mood shifts. Serotonin nerve cells (neurons) in the brain have progesterone receptors, and progesterone levels dramatically decrease in menopause due to the lack of ovulation. This progesterone/serotonin connection may explain why depression is so common with PMS sufferers and why

SSRIs like fluoxetine (Prozac) can help PMS. Sleeping problems resulting from hormonal changes (see pages 37–38) and the unpredictability of hot flushes can also result in chronic fatigue and low mood.

Midlife is also a time when there can be stressful life events. Problems with relationships, such as divorce or widowhood; issues with children, whether they're leaving home or returning as adults, or are still young and needing to be looked after; concerns about elderly relatives, whether they need care and will accept it; feelings about your own future – is now the time to retire or try something new? … and all this coming at a time when your self-esteem and body image may also be in question.

If your healthcare professional believes your mood swings are a result of hormonal imbalances, he or she may recommend short-term hormone therapy, which can provide a constant level of hormones and help to stabilize mood. Self-help measures include making sure your diet contains sufficient helpful nutrients, herbal remedies and various techniques to dispel negative feelings.

Natural Light

Light has a strong effect on mood: being outside in the sun is generally cheering. Natural light affects melatonin, the body's neurotransmitter that controls our sleep–wake cycle. People often become miserable as the shorter days of winter approach. Some are so affected by light changes that they are said to suffer from SAD (seasonal affective disorder). Since natural light can lift mood, an easy thing to do is to replace your ordinary light bulbs with natural light ones, particularly in the room where you spend the most time. If this proves effective, particularly if your symptoms are severe, you might want to invest in a light box.

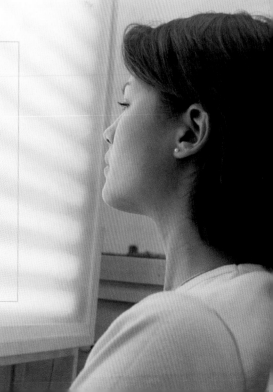

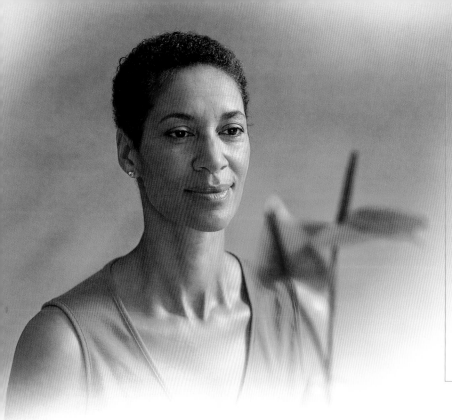

DIET

Certain types of low mood are associated with nutritional deficiencies. Many women have low levels of vitamin B_6, which helps the brain take up serotonin. Vitamin B_{12} and folic acid also have profound mood-stabilizing effects.

The amino acid phenylalanine, abundant in milk, cheese, meat and fish, plays an integral role in maintaining a healthy balance of brain chemicals.

Selenium (found in Brazil nuts and mushrooms), zinc (present in seafood and eggs) and chromium (as a supplement, chromium picolinate) also have a positive effect on mood. Whole grains can supply many of the vital nutrients that will relieve tension and moodiness.

HERBAL REMEDIES

St. John's wort is an effective treatment for mild to moderate depression. It contains hyperforin, which has similar properties to the most prescribed and well-known antidepressants.

Ginkgo biloba also has mood-enhancing effects. It increases microcirculation to the brain and improves the brain's ability to metabolize glucose.

EXERCISE

Aerobic exercise has been found to improve mood. It is a natural and effective way to raise levels of endorphins – brain chemicals that counteract feelings of anxiety and depression. A brisk two-mile walk can be sufficient, or 30 minutes of your chosen exercise at least three times a week.

Some women find the meditative and energy-balancing qualities of yoga and t'ai chi have a positive effect on mood.

PSYCHOTHERAPY

Professional counselling can help women learn better coping strategies. 'Talk' therapy can be very effective, not only in helping you to deal with particular problems, but also in making you feel better about yourself.

CHEMICAL TREATMENTS

SAMe (S-adenosyl methionine) is a supplement that, in large doses (600 mg+ per day), is a promising antidepressant without the side effects of tricyclics and SSRIs. When symptoms are severe, however, a course of other antidepressants may be prescribed.

HEADACHES

For many women going through menopause, headaches are not all in the mind; once women pass puberty and produce higher levels of female hormones, they suffer more from headaches of all types than men. Whereas in the past headaches and migraines were considered separate disorders with separate causes (headaches brought on by muscle contractions; migraines resulting from constriction and dilation of blood vessels in the head), they are now believed to belong to the same continuum, with headaches leading to migraines.

There are many reasons that headaches occur, such as disease, strong emotions, medications, eating and sleeping patterns, environmental factors, physical exertion and hormones. Fluctuating hormone levels are a characteristic of the peri-menopause and they can increase the intensity and/or prevalence of headaches. Women who had headaches before or during their menstrual periods, or who are extra-sensitive to hormone fluctuations, are much more likely to suffer from them after menopause. And if menopause has been surgically induced, migraines, in particular, are much more likely to increase in intensity and severity. Self-help measures to combat headache pain have a lot to do with what, when and how you eat.

DIET

Migraines, in particular, may be triggered by many different factors but among the most common are certain foods. The foods that can trigger a migraine vary from person to person, but there are a number of common ones (see right). Missing meals is another common migraine and headache trigger.

Keeping a diary in which you write down what you eat and drink each day, and the circumstances in which you do so (like on the run), as well as environmental changes (noise, bright lights, changes in weather), may help you to link your headaches to possible causes.

6 **ways** to soothe a headache

- Rub a drop of lavender or chamomile oil briskly between your hands. When your palms are warm and tingly, place them on the part of your head that aches.
- A blinking red light can relieve migraines; for the maximum effect, wear goggles that restrict side vision.
- Make a tea or infusion of fresh sage leaves.
- Stay cool; being hot is a common headache trigger. Avoid hot tubs, saunas and going out in hot weather.
- Soak your feet in cool water to which you add a few drops of rosemary oil and inhale deeply.
- Migraines are most common in the morning. Take any headache remedies before bed and on awakening for maximum benefit.

Migraine triggers

Dairy products	Corn and corn
Chocolate	products
Eggs	Apples
Citrus fruits	Bananas
Meat and fish	Red wine
Wheat and wheat	MSG
products	Pickled or cured
Nuts and peanuts	foods
Tomatoes	Artificial sweeteners
Onions	Alcohol

Whole grains contain high levels of vitamin B and E, which help to regulate hormonal levels, so include plenty of them in your diet. Substances that boost the circulation may be effective in staving off or relieving a migraine (as long as these are not trigger factors). Calcium- and magnesium-rich foods such as nuts, beans and brewer's yeast help to reduce widening of the carotid arteries, while lecithin granules also are beneficial to circulation. Serotonin, a neurotransmitter in the brain, has a big part to play in preventing headaches. People who have headaches are often found to have low serotonin levels, but eating foods rich in tryptophan, such as turkey, fish and bananas, can lead to an increase in brain serotonin. On the other hand, salt leads to water retention, which is a known cause of headache, so it's important to restrict salt in your diet along with caffeine and alcohol. Make sure, also, that your water intake is adequate.

EXERCISE

A brisk walk gets your circulation going, and fresh air can ease headache pain. Although exertion may trigger headaches, regular aerobic exercise can reduce the severity of future attacks. Exercise also stimulates the pain-regulating substances in the brain. Muscular tension can cause or exacerbate a headache. You could try t'ai chi, yoga or the Alexander technique – therapies that promote relaxation and reduced physical stress.

HERBS

Ginkgo extract (*Ginkgo biloba*) can improve circulation and help to prevent headaches, and feverfew (*chrysanthemum parthenium*) is a long-standing headache remedy. Eating a sprig of the fresh plant daily makes it an effective preventative, while brewing 2–4 fresh leaves as a cup of strong tea can help with acute headache.

COMPLEMENTARY THERAPIES

Shoulder tightness and neck problems often lead to headaches, so it's worth consulting a chiropractor to rule out a physical cause for your problems. If your

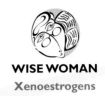

WISE WOMAN
Xenoestrogens

Foreign oestrogens are present in substances outside the human body and, if ingested or absorbed through the skin, can interfere with the normal hormonal balance and produce migraines. Common culprits are pesticides; plastic bottles and wraps; spermicides; detergents; metal cans; commercially raised beef, chicken and pork; preservatives in skin lotions and gels; and shampoos. To protect yourself do not use plastic wrap when heating foods and liquids, use an enzyme-free detergent, and eschew fabric softener. Make sure your lotions, soaps, shampoos and make-up are parabens-free, and buy organic.

vertebrae or cranial bones have become misaligned, you might consider consulting a cranial osteopath, who can make minute adjustments to the bones of your skull. Acupuncture and reflexology can also be helpful.

CHEMICAL TREATMENT

The seesaw pattern of oestrogen production during perimenopause may be helped with hormone therapy. Natural progesterone, in particular, is said to combat hormonal headaches. However, headaches can be a side effect of certain forms of HT, so if you are currently taking HT, ask your doctor whether your dose might be lowered, or whether you should switch to another form that can help you avoid hormone fluctuations.

Your doctor may consider prescribing anti-migraine drugs like sumatriptan and naratriptan.

VAGINAL DRYNESS AND ITCHING

Around the time of menopause almost half of all women have some sort of problem involving vaginal dryness and itching. Even before the levels of oestrogen start to fall significantly, some women notice that less lubrication is produced during intercourse, and sexual arousal is more difficult. They may put it down to 'tiredness' and loss of interest in their partner, but the mucous membranes around the genitals are actually changing.

There are a number of remedies, apart from hormones, for vaginal dryness, but itching normally signals an infection that will require a doctor's attention. (For ideas on improving libido, see pages 86–91.)

What Causes Vaginal Dryness?

When oestrogen levels start to fall, the walls of the vagina become thinner, drier and less elastic; most of this is a direct result of reduced blood flow. Oestrogen is a vasodilator, which means that it increases the size and flexibility of the blood vessels, so with less of this hormone around, the blood supply is diminished, and the cells in the vaginal walls get thinner, drier and more prone to itchiness and irritation. The epithelial tissue in the vagina is dependent on oestrogen and, in the absence of this hormone, the superficial protective layer thins or disappears altogether, making it more prone to damage if extra lubrication is not used during sex. The lubrication of the vagina is also affected by circulation, as a lot of the moisture is produced by fluid seeping out of blood vessels and into the vagina rather than direct secretion

from glands. When there is not enough lubrication, sex can lead to irritation, even pain, and post-coital bleeding. If you experience discomfort or bleeding during intercourse, it is important to do something about it.

Non-Menopausal Causes

Bear in mind that any medicines warning of a dry mouth as a side effect are going to dry up all mucous membranes, including your vagina. Anti-histamines are the biggest culprits, and they include medications for hay fever and travel sickness. Many antidepressants can decrease libido and thus affect lubrication, in particular fluoxetine, the tricyclics and monoamine oxidase inhibitors (MAOIs). If vaginal dryness coincides with or starts soon after you commence any medication, check with your doctor in case the medication is the problem.

If you notice dry eyes, nose and mouth as well as a dry vagina, it is important to check that you don't have an autoimmune disorder known as Sjogrens syndrome. Your doctor will need to do a blood test to diagnose this, and the symptoms can be treated with lubricants and artificial tears and saliva.

Liquid douche preparations can disrupt the normal chemical balance and may lead to a feeling of dryness in your vagina.

DIET

Phytoestrogens (see pages 112–114), particularly iso-flavones found in soya products, produce a mild oestrogen-like effect and may be helpful in increasing moisture in the vagina. Make sure you also drink plenty of water. If your urine is dark

TAKE CARE

Once your periods have stopped, it is very important that any bleeding after sex or for no apparent reason is investigated. It may be due to lack of lubrication, but it is not all right to assume this without excluding infection and having a cervical smear.

yellow and has a strong smell, or if you pass urine fewer than four times a day, you may need to increase your fluid intake.

HERBAL REMEDIES

Black cohosh (*cimicifuga racemosa*) is widely prescribed by herbalists to reduce vaginal dryness and other symptoms of menopause.

A topical cream made from licorice root (*Glycyrrhiza glabra*) has proved extremely effective in counteracting vaginal dryness.

HOMEOPATHIC TREATMENTS

Bryonia 6c and Lycopodium 30c are the two remedies most frequently used.

VAGINAL LUBRICANTS

There are now many lubricants commercially available that can help. Sometimes a special vaginal moisturizer – like Replens – is adequate, but if more lubrication is required, KY jelly or aloe vera gel are recommended. The brands are slightly different, so

WISE WOMAN
More sex please...

At this time in life women can be feeling less attractive and less interested in sex, but studies have shown that sexual activity, if continued through and past menopause, actually helps to prevent degeneration of the vaginal and vulval tissues without any other treatment required. The less often women have sex, the less these tissues respond to stimulation. Even having sex just three times a month involves significantly less degeneration than having sex only once a month, and frequent masturbation helps in lieu of actual intercourse. A healthy vaginal membrane is definitely related to frequent lovemaking.

try a few before deciding on the one that's best suited to your needs.

Don't forget: if you are using condoms it is very important to choose a lubricant that is water-soluble, as any oil-based lubricants can damage the condom and cause it to split.

HORMONAL TREATMENTS

Vaginal oestrogen preparations are very effective in treating symptoms of vaginal dryness and lack of lubrication, and are often more successful than oral treatments.

Preparations are available in the form of creams, suppositories and rings. With most preparations, the dose of hormone entering the bloodstream and reaching other areas of the body is very low, and while this form of hormone therapy does not have the same side effects or carry the same risks as systemic replacements, nor does it have all the same benefits. For example, there is only one vaginal ring that delivers enough oestrogen to affect hot flushes.

Creams result in significant levels of oestrogen in the blood because oestrogen is easily absorbed through the thin vaginal mucosa. They are used with an applicator and are applied daily at first then less frequently. Creams can be messy and are sometimes avoided for long-term use. A vaginal ring may be preferable. The ring can stay in the vagina, delivering a constant dose of oestrogen, for up to three months. Some women prefer to remove it before sex and reinsert it themselves afterwards, although less than 10 percent of male partners report being able to feel the ring during sex. If treatment is started early the vaginal tissues are quickly restored to normal. If treatment is delayed, improvement will take longer, but it will happen and atrophied tissue can return to a healthy state.

Another excellent alternative is a small vaginal oestrogen tablet called Vagifem. They are supplied in a pre-filled applicator and are easily inserted into the vagina. Like the ring, the oestrogen they provide is only minimally absorbed into the blood.

Oral hormone therapy restores vaginal tissue and lubrication but is not as effective as local preparations.

What Causes Vaginal Itching and Irritation?

Due to falling oestrogen levels, perimenopausal women are especially susceptible to vaginal infections. When oestrogen is at premenopausal levels, the cells in the superficial layer of the vaginal epithelium are plump and thick and produce glycogen. When these cells are shed into the vaginal cavity during normal bodily functions, they are consumed by lactobacilli, innocuous organisms that live in the healthy vagina and produce lactic acid. This acid is very important to ensure that the pH balance in the vagina is between 3.5 and 4.5 – a level of acidity at which many other organisms are unable to grow. As oestrogen levels drop, less lactic acid is produced, and the pH level can rise. When the pH rises to between 6 and 8 other organisms can cause problems. One of the most common conditions caused by this change in the bacteria is called bacterial vaginosis (BV). Several organisms may be involved. BV does occur in women who are not sexually active, but it is found far more

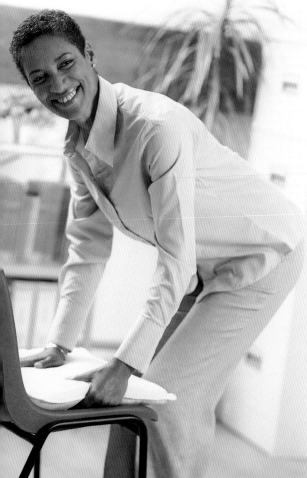

6 **ways** to avoid vaginal infections

▶ Never douche as this disrupts the normal balance of vaginal organisms and should be avoided; it also encourages any infection to ascend into the uterus and fallopian tubes.

▶ Always take care to wash and wipe your genital area from 'front to back' to avoid spreading bacteria from your bottom into your vagina and urethra.

▶ Avoid using soap or shower gel to wash between your legs and don't put perfumed or bubble products into your bath. The number of women complaining of a yeast infection reaches a peak just after Christmas, when all those nice smelling presents get used.

▶ It helps to use mild detergents recommended for babies when washing your underwear and to avoid those with biological or enzyme action.

▶ Whenever possible, wear loose fitting clothes made from natural fibres and, if you have to sit on a plastic or synthetic covered chair all day at work, take a cotton cushion.

▶ If necessary, start local oestrogen therapy early rather than late.

frequently in women who have multiple sexual partners or who have recently changed partner. The infection is easy to treat, usually with the antibiotic metronidazole or clindamycin gel, available on prescription. Another common infection is a yeast infection called Candida albicans, often known as yeast infection, yeast vaginitis or 'thrush'. This yeast can grow in almost any warm, moist area of the body if the normal balance of bacteria is upset. Treatment is available over the counter, usually as suppositories and cream but sometimes as oral therapy. Neither of these infections is considered to be a sexually transmitted disease and both are easily treated.

Rarely, an infection with a bacterium known as haemolytic streptococcus can cause a very sore and painful vulval area. This needs to be diagnosed by your doctor and treated with antibiotics.

Keep in mind that these types of infection, if experienced around the time of menopause, are mainly a result of falling or low oestrogen levels. Local oestrogen treatment will help to restore the natural balance and prevent infection.

Other Causes of Irritation

Lichen sclerosus is an uncommon disease of the skin that in women can cause vulval itching, soreness and discomfort. It is accompanied by a gradual thinning and loss of colour or whitening of the skin, which is more marked than the natural lightening of the area that occurs due to a reduced blood flow around menopause. The condition can affect women of any age but it is not clear why certain people develop it and not others. In men it affects the penis. It may be an inherited risk and is certainly not something that can be passed from one person to another, and it does not present any risk to fertility. It can be the cause of pain during sexual intercourse, as the opening to the vagina may become tight. Usually the condition causes very little problem and is treated with simple steroid creams, moisturizers and occasionally creams containing testosterone.

There is a very small risk that cancer can develop in the abnormal skin, so a check by your doctor once or twice a year is recommended. Any split or ulcer in the skin of the vulva that does not heal properly should be investigated.

Because of the increasing divorce and separation rate, many women are entering new relationships at this time and may find themselves at risk from sexually transmitted diseases (STDs) such as chlamydia, gonorrhoea, syphilis, genital warts, HIV etc. (see page 92).

	Bacterial vaginosis	Yeast vaginitis (thrush)
Odour	Vaginal discharge has an unpleasant fishy or musty smell	Vaginal discharge has no odour
Discharge	Watery, milky white or grey	Thick and white (similar to cottage cheese)
Itching/irritation	Not always present	Vaginal itching or burning is usually present
Cause	Bacteria	Yeast
Treatment	Requires specific antibacterial treatment available only on prescription from your doctor	Once diagnosed by a doctor, recurrent infections can be treated with over-the-counter products from a pharmacy

BLADDER PROBLEMS

Frequent urination, nocturia (needing to get out of bed to urinate several times during the night), incontinence (the involuntary leakage of urine) and painful urination, resulting from urinary tract infections, become increasingly common as we age. These can be brought on by changes that occur during menopause – the thinning of the lining of the urethra, the outlet of the bladder, due to lack of oestrogen – and by the gradual weakening of the pelvic musculature over time. Happily, there are some remedies.

Lifestyle Factors

Drinking a lot of fluids or drinking late at night; irritating your bladder by smoking or drinking alcoholic or caffeinated beverages; eating high-acid foods (such as tomatoes and oranges); and being overweight are all contributing factors within your control. However, don't cut back too much on your fluid intake. It's essential to remain hydrated otherwise incontinence may worsen and constipation result.

If your exercise programme involves heavy weights or high impact exercises, you should modify it.

KEGEL EXERCISES

The pelvic musculature supporting the bladder can be strengthened using a series of exercises shown on page 50. Done regularly, they are very effective in combatting stress incontinence.

BIOFEEDBACK

Measuring devices can help you become aware of your body's functioning. By using electronic devices or diaries to track when your bladder and urethral muscles contract, you can gain control over these muscles. Biofeedback can be used with Kegel exercises and electrical stimulation.

WISE WOMAN
Urinary incontinence

Stress incontinence, the leakage of urine upon coughing, laughing, sneezing, or lifting is most common during the perimenopause but usually does not worsen over time. However, experiences of urge incontinence, where you have an urgent need to urinate but there is insufficient "warning" so you can't get to a toilet on time, appears to increase after menopause.

ELECTRICAL STIMULATION

Brief doses of electrical stimulation can be used to strengthen muscles in the lower pelvis in a way similar to exercising the muscles. Electrodes are temporarily placed in the vagina or rectum to stimulate the contraction of urethral muscles. Electrical stimulation can be used to reduce both stress incontinence and urge incontinence.

TIMED VOIDING OR BLADDER TRAINING

These are techniques that make use of biofeedback. In timed voiding, you fill in a chart noting down when you urinate and when leakages occur. From the patterns that appear in your chart, you can plan to empty your bladder before you would otherwise leak. Biofeedback and muscle conditioning or bladder training can alter the bladder's schedule for storing and emptying urine.

MEDICAL AND SURGICAL TREATMENTS

Incontinence should never be viewed as an inevitable result of aging. Even if a cure is not possible, comfort and frequency can be improved. There are many strategies to treat the problem. Medications can reduce many types of leakage. Some drugs inhibit contractions of an overactive bladder. Others relax muscles, leading to more complete bladder emptying during urination. Some drugs tighten muscles at the bladder neck and urethra, preventing leakage. And some, especially

Kegel exercises are two exercises that should be performed five times a day. This seems a lot but they can be done almost anywhere – sitting down at work, in a lift, while waiting at a bus stop. If you find it necessary, your doctor can prescribe small cone-shaped devices that you place and hold in your vagina to help you isolate the appropriate muscles. Once you've strengthened these muscles, try to consciously use them when you cough, sneeze or laugh.

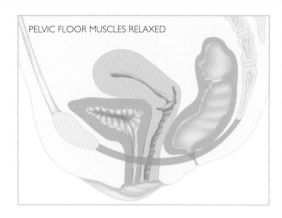

PELVIC FLOOR MUSCLES RELAXED

Exercise 1

You want to contract the pubococcygeal muscle. To identify this muscle, try stopping the flow of urine in mid-stream. Contract the muscle for 5–10 seconds,

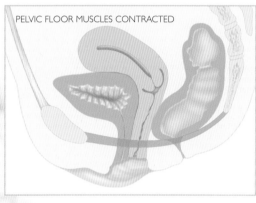

PELVIC FLOOR MUSCLES CONTRACTED

making sure not to contract your stomach muscles at the same time, then release. Focus on both the contracting and relaxing. Repeat 10 times. You can put your fingers on your lower abdomen, right above your pubic bone, to make sure you're not 'cheating' and contracting your abdomen instead of your pelvic floor.

Exercise 2

Do 10 contractions, holding them as long as possible before releasing.

hormones such as oestrogen, are believed to cause muscles involved in urination to function normally.

A pessary can be inserted by a doctor or nurse into the vagina. This is a stiff ring that presses against the wall of the vagina and the nearby urethra. The pressure helps reposition the urethra, leading to a reduction in stress leakage. If you use a pessary, watch for possible vaginal and urinary tract infections, and see your doctor regularly.

Implants Injected into tissues around the urethra, a collagen implant adds bulk and helps to close the urethra to reduce stress incontinence. Implants can be injected by a doctor in about half an hour using local anaesthesia.

Surgery If other treatments prove unsuccessful it is possible to pull the bladder up to a more normal position through surgery. For severe cases of stress incontinence, the surgeon may secure the bladder with a wide sling. This not only holds up the bladder but also compresses the bladder's bottom and the urethra's top, further preventing leakage.

In rare cases, a surgeon implants an artificial sphincter, a doughnut-shaped sac that circles the urethra. As fluid fills and expands the sac, it squeezes the urethra closed. Pressing a valve implanted under the skin causes the artificial sphincter to deflate. This removes pressure from the urethra, allowing urine from the bladder to pass.

BLADDER INFECTIONS

Cystitis and other urinary tract infections occur more commonly during and after menopause because the urethra and bladder, which are located next to the vagina, contain similar oestrogen-sensitive tissues, and these become thin as well. When organ walls are thinned they more easily become irritated and susceptible to infection. You should suspect a urinary infection if you begin to need frequent trips to the toilet, or you feel pressure in your bladder to urinate even when you don't have to or are not able to. Once urination is painful, the infection has established itself and you will need antibiotics. Not all doctors

ways to prevent bladder infections

▶ Make sure you urinate after sexual intercourse and, when you feel the urge, to void as soon as possible, and certainly within an hour.

▶ Wear underwear with a cotton crotch to minimize moisture retention.

▶ Avoid tight jeans and other tight trousers and tights; these can hold in heat and moisture.

▶ Stop using douches, hot tubs, whirlpool baths and highly chlorinated pools.

▶ Don't use coloured toilet paper or bath products that are perfumed.

▶ Drink unsweetened cranberry juice; it can maintain the pH balance of your urine.

▶ Don't use tampons or a diaphragm and particularly a diaphragm with a spermicide.

▶ Eat yogurt frequently.

agree that HT can prevent infections but some feel that a natural form of oestrogen, such as estriol or estradiol, used vaginally, is worth a try.

Natural strategies

Arctostaphylos uva-ursi (called bearberry, kinnikinnick and uva ursi) is an evergreen shrub that has long been popular for fighting urinary tract infections. It can be taken in teas, tinctures, capsules and extracts. The recommended dose is 500 mg, or ½ tsp liquid extract, four times a day for one week. To effectively fight a urinary tract infection with uva ursi, your urine must be alkaline. You may be able to help maintain an alkaline pH by consuming plenty of dairy products and non-citrus fruits. By the same token, don't take uva-ursi with substances that acidify the urine, such as citrus fruits, tomatoes and vitamin C supplements.

Unless you are taking uva-ursi, a high dose of vitamin C can help you fight the infection. Taking ¼ tsp of the powdered form every hour while symptoms are acute can help.

SKIN CHANGES

The hormonal changes that characterize peri-menopause and menopause will also affect your skin. Diminished levels of oestrogen contribute to a decline in elastin (a protein within the fibres of connective tissue that accounts for the elasticity of the skin and other organs) and skin collagen (which gives skin its rigidity). They also cause an increase in wrinkles. The decline in collagen is greatest in the years just after menopause: about 30 percent of skin collagen is lost during the first five years after menopause and about two percent every year thereafter.

Plummeting oestrogen levels also result in your skin's sebaceous glands producing less oil, so there is a tendency for your skin to dry out more quickly, and for its texture to coarsen. Some women complain of irritating skin sensations, including severe itching and formication (the feeling that ants are crawling on the skin).

The fat layer below your skin will thin out, as will the protective layer on top of your skin; it therefore becomes more prone to developing thread veins, which are broken capillaries, more liable to becoming irritated and infected, and less able to heal quickly. Similar changes will be reflected in the state of your vaginal tissues (see page 84).

The swing of the hormone balance between androgen and oestrogen in favour of androgen may cause acne, particularly in women who had acne in their teen years. Typically, this appears on the lower face along the chin and neck.

As well as following the skin care routines on pages 206–209, the following self-help measures can be of benefit to your skin.

WISE WOMAN

Free radicals

These are unstable molecules formed naturally in the body that target and destroy healthy cells. They also result from the exposure to environmental toxins such as tobacco and exhaust smoke, ozone, fluorescent lights, video- and TV-watching, and chemicals in food and home furnishings.

DIET

Because aging skin is less capable of holding moisture, it's important to be continually hydrated. Drink at least eight glasses of water per day.

A number of nutrients are vital to keeping the skin in good shape. Zinc and copper are essential for keeping the skin supple, and vitamin A can be used internally and externally to protect skin from damage and to promote repair. Vitamins C and E, selenium, coenzyme Q_{10} and alpha-lipoic acid are important antioxidants and protect the skin from free radicals. Fruits and vegetables are good sources of vitamins and minerals, while co-enzyme Q_{10} and alpha-lipoic acid can be taken as supplements.

Make sure your diet contains sufficient fibre; constipation can affect the appearance of your skin. Adding 50 g ground golden linseed to your diet will supply the fibre you need and other supporting nutrients. Increase your consumption of fish rich in omega-3 fatty acids and soya products.

SKIN CREAMS AND EMOLLIENTS

Cocoa butter, apricot kernel oil, and almond and olive oils are natural substances that can be used to add moisture to the skin.

Liposomes are microscopic hollow vessels able to transport dermatological agents. Found in certain skin-care products, they target and transport moisture to the skin.

Alpha-hydroxy acids (AHAs) present in many skin products help to remove dead skin cells, increase the hydration of the skin and promote the repair of elastin and collagen.

This self-massage helps clear energy blockages to leave you with clear, glowing skin.

1 With your hands either side of your trachea, make upward strokes with your fingers towards your chin; finishing with your hands behind your ears.

2 With thumbs and index fingers touching, place them in the centre of your chin, index fingers on top, thumbs underneath. Sweep up and around your jawline. When your fingers reach your ears, press just below your lobes. Repeat 3 times.

3 Place your ring fingers on both cheekbones where they meet your nose. Draw them along your cheekbones and up to your temples; press in and repeat 3 times.

4 Press the area between your forehead and eyebrows with your right thumb. Pinch your eyebrows with your thumbs and index fingers, drawing them outwards. Press again at your temples with your index fingers. Repeat 3 times.

5 Place your fingertips in the centre of your forehead and draw them out to your hairline, pressing at your temples. Repeat 3 times.

6 Rest the fleshy part of your palms over your eye sockets for 30 seconds. Do not press on your eyeballs. Relax and release.

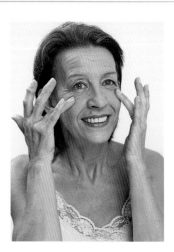

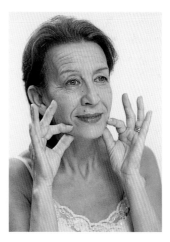

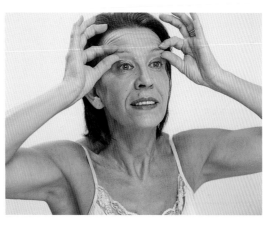

SUN PROTECTION

Ultraviolet radiation from the sun is one of the most significant causes of premature skin aging as well as skin cancers. Sun damage causes the skin to lose its resiliency and elasticity. You must use a sunscreen with an SPF of 15 or higher every day – even in winter – on your face as well as your neck and hands. If you use sun protection, it can block vitamin D from the sun from reaching your skin, so think about taking vitamin D supplement (see page 111).

AYURVEDA

This holistic life science from India proposes that we are a combination of three doshas: *vata, pitta* and *kapha*. Each of us is a specific combination, but good health, and great-looking skin, is a result of keeping your doshas in balance. Ayurvedic practitioners use herbs, massage techniques (see previous page) and meditation (see page 42) to encourage balance and the movement of helpful energy around the body.

CHEMICAL TREATMENTS

Retinoic acid derivatives (retinoids) are derived from a form of vitamin A, and they can help prevent or reduce fine lines and wrinkles, reverse sun damage and heal acne. They are available on prescription from a dermatologist, but may not suit everyone as there are side effects such as dryness, itching and increased sun sensitivity. Some over-the-counter products contain retinoic acid, or Retin-A, in a weaker form.

ROSACEA, SKIN TAGS AND AGE SPOTS

During middle age a number of specific skin conditions may also appear.

Rosacea is a common skin condition that causes facial redness and swelling. Both men and women can suffer from it, but it most commonly affects women and generally develops around age 40–50. At first it may seem like a tendency to blush easily, but it can lead to pus-filled spots and a plethora of blood vessels on the skin's surface. Dermatologists can propose a variety of treatments to stop its progress, and sometimes reverse it, but it is important that it is diagnosed as early as possible. Certain over-the-counter medications can make it worse.

There are also a number of self-help measures you can follow, such as avoiding hot drinks, spicy foods, caffeinated and alcoholic beverages; exercising in a cool environment; avoiding rubbing the skin; and using cosmetics and facial products for sensitive skin.

Skin tags, common and harmless skin growths, become much more prevalent with age, particularly in women. They frequently develop on the eyelids, neck, chest, armpits and groin. They can be frozen, tied or cut off by a dermatologist.

Age spots usually start to appear in our early 30s. They put us at a higher risk of developing skin cancer, so it is important to have them checked out if they change in appearance. Both over-the-counter and prescription medications are available that will gradually lighten them.

WISE WOMAN
Smoking

Nicotine prevents nutrients reaching the skin and interferes with the skin being able to rid itself of the toxins caused by cell metabolism. The result is slower skin growth and rejuvenation so that women who smoke have dark circles around the eyes, a paler skin tone, and more lines and wrinkles, particularly around the lips, than non-smokers.

BREAST TENDERNESS

A great many women suffer from breast pain, the majority cyclically around the first two weeks before menstruation. Though breast pain generally disappears during menopause, it can still be problematical during peri-menopause, particularly when oestrogen levels are dominant. While the cause has not been determined exactly, cyclical breast pain has a strong hormonal association; most breast discomfort occurs in the second part of the menstrual cycle, and medications that are effective against it commonly interrupt the hormonal events during the premenstrual time period. Also, the fact that it disappears with menopause points towards a hormonal connection.

Women who have large breasts are more likely to suffer pain, not only in their breasts but also in their necks, shoulders and backs.

Taking up a new sport or leisure pastime can sometimes result in breast pain.

DIET

Because hormone levels have a lot to do with breast tenderness, a diet that helps to balance hormones may help to reduce discomfort. Such a diet is one in which fat makes up less than 20 percent of the total calorie intake. It also needs to contain an adequate amount of the B vitamins, foods containing omega-3 fatty acids and soya products. Linseed acts as an anti-oestrogen on breast tissue, so including it in the diet will also be helpful. Additionally, supplemental vitamin E (400–800 units per day), has been shown to be effective in reducing breast pain.

Stopping, or at least cutting back, on caffeine in coffee, tea and chocolate during the premenstrual period can be very effective in lessening pain. Breast

WISE WOMAN

Cyclic breast pain

Cyclic breast pain usually involves both breasts. The entire breast may be affected as well as the underarm area. Noncyclic breast pain tends to occur more often in one breast and may be more centrally located in the breast.

pain may be related to fatty acid imbalance within the cells, which can make breast tissue more sensitive to circulating hormones. Taking evening primrose oil, which contains gamma-linolenic acid, a type of fatty acid, may help to normalize fatty acid content in the tissues of women who are particularly likely to suffer from cyclic breast pain.

Blackcurrant seed oil is rich in essential fatty acids. These are converted to prostaglandins to fight infection and help to reduce breast tenderness.

HORMONES

Oral contraceptives can be helpful, though breast tenderness usually increases during the first few cycles, as is the case with HT. In fact, as many as 30 percent of women taking hormone therapy experience breast tenderness when they first start their medication.

4 ways of easing breast discomfort

- ▶ Wear a supportive bra and make sure it has been properly fitted by a professional.
- ▶ During exercise, wear a sports bra, and when your breasts are particularly painful, wear it while sleeping.
- ▶ Simple pain relievers such as paracetamol and nonsteroidal anti-inflammatory agents such as ibuprofen may be effective.
- ▶ Apply hot or cold compresses.

BLOATING AND GAS

A very common symptom of menopause – over two-thirds of menopausal women experience it – is bloating in the intestinal tract due to the production of gas. While gas and bloating are very common during menopause, it's not certain whether this is due to hormonal action or simply the normal processes of aging. Some researchers see a relationship to decreasing hormone production, while others think it has to do with dietary changes around the time of menopause. The recommended menopause diet (see pages 106–127) is high in grains, vegetables, dairy products, legumes and soya proteins – all of which are gas-producing substances!

Lactose intolerance, an inability to digest significant amounts of lactose, the predominant sugar in milk, is another very common problem that increases with age. This is also associated with gas

Gas-producing foods

Vegetables	Legumes	Grains/cereals /seeds/nuts
Beetroot	Black-eyed	Barley
Broccoli	peas	Oat bran
Brussels	Broad beans	Oat flour
sprouts	Chickpeas	Pistachios
Cabbage	Lentils	Rice bran
Carrots	Lima beans	Rye
Cauliflower	Mung beans	Sesame flour
Sweetcorn	Peanuts	Sorghum grain
Cucumbers	Peas	Sunflower
Leeks	Pinto beans	flour
Lettuce	Red kidney	Wheat bran
Onions	beans	Whole wheat
Parsley	Soya beans	flour
Sweet		
peppers		

8 ways to prevent gas

▶ When eating gassy foods (see chart), try taking a digestive aid to eliminate gas. These contain enzymes that break down problem complex sugars that cause gas.

▶ Gas-reducing agents that contain simethicone may also be helpful. They do not eliminate gas production but break up already existing gas bubbles in the stomach.

▶ Give up carbonated beverages like fizzy drinks and beer. If you choose to drink them, let them go flat first.

▶ Include more ginger in your diet. This herb relieves pain and can ease digestive upset.

▶ Try to stay relaxed; stress can worsen any bloating.

▶ Eat three to five small meals per day. Eating large quantities of food at a single meal can elevate your insulin level and make bloating worse.

▶ Drink plenty of water to clear the body of toxins.

▶ Don't go to bed on a full stomach; leave at least three hours between your last meal and bedtime.

and bloating and can be alleviated by drinking lactose-free milk or avoiding dairy products altogether. Severely lactose-intolerant women need to ensure that they get sufficient calcium from other sources.

While it is true that proteins and fats cause little gas, and soya products, fibre- and carbohydrate-rich foods do, it is still possible to maintain a healthy diet by following the suggestions above.

HAIR, NAIL AND TOOTH PROBLEMS

Hair and nails both depend on the protein keratin for their health so, if you have hair problems, you may also find your nails need attention, too. Both not enough hair (alopecia) and too much hair (hirsutism) can characterize the menopausal period, and both are a result of hormonal imbalance. Hormone fluctuations can also greatly affect your teeth and change the way your mouth looks or feels.

Alopecia and Hirsutism

While hair loss and thinning has a lot to do with genetics, it also may occur as a result of the shift in balance between the hormones oestrogen and androgen. When the androgen-to-oestrogen ratio is tipped in favour of androgen, you might not only experience hair loss and thinning but also excessive hair in areas such as the chin, upper lip and cheeks, which are more androgen sensitive. A surgically caused menopause can make matters worse.

Excess hair can be removed by waxing, plucking, shaving and even by electrolysis and laser treatment, but the right diet and avoiding stress will also help.

Hair loss in women generally involves widespread thinning rather than the development of bald patches as with men, so sometimes a new hairstyle or hair preparations that temporarily thicken hair with a coating may be sufficient.

SELF-HELP

A healthy diet (see pages 106–127) can help, along with a multivitamin and mineral supplement. If you are overweight, this might give an incentive to slim down; fat is the ideal environment for androgens to form.

Traditional Chinese Medicine (TCM) claims success with hair growth using certain herbs, like Shou Wu Pian. Consult a practitioner, who can determine the right herbal combination for you.

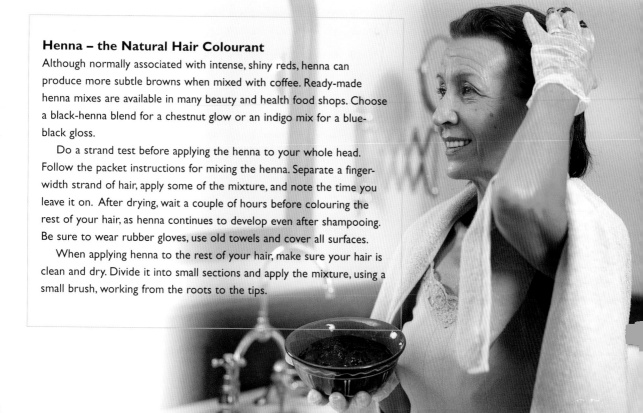

Henna – the Natural Hair Colourant

Although normally associated with intense, shiny reds, henna can produce more subtle browns when mixed with coffee. Ready-made henna mixes are available in many beauty and health food shops. Choose a black-henna blend for a chestnut glow or an indigo mix for a blue-black gloss.

Do a strand test before applying the henna to your whole head. Follow the packet instructions for mixing the henna. Separate a finger-width strand of hair, apply some of the mixture, and note the time you leave it on. After drying, wait a couple of hours before colouring the rest of your hair, as henna continues to develop even after shampooing. Be sure to wear rubber gloves, use old towels and cover all surfaces.

When applying henna to the rest of your hair, make sure your hair is clean and dry. Divide it into small sections and apply the mixture, using a small brush, working from the roots to the tips.

It is possible to increase circulation to the scalp, which will increase the flow of blood to the head and help nutrients reach the hair follicles. Make up a massage oil using 10 drops of essential oils to 1½ tbsp of carrier oil. Camomile or lavender essential oils can be added to avocado carrier oil, or sandalwood can be added to sweet almond and coconut carrier oils.

Avoid harsh chemical treatments such as perms and dyes, and wear a bathing cap when swimming in a chlorinated pool.

CHEMICAL TREATMENTS
If you are perimenopausal, your doctor may prescribe HT in order to balance your hormones. Minoxidil (Regaine) is an anti-hypertensive medication that can increase hair growth when applied topically. A dermatologist should be consulted for this and other treatments.

NAIL PROBLEMS
As we get older, our nails grow more slowly, and may become dryer, thicker and harder, or develop ridges. Sometimes, such problems are related to a remediable vitamin or mineral deficiency in your diet (see chart below).

Some nail problems, however, may signal another condition that might need medical attention: greenish nails may indicate an infection in your nail bed, while bluish nail beds can be a sign of breathing problems or malnutrition.

SELF-HELP
Take care to keep your nails moisturized. Use a specialist nail oil and avoid over-using nail polish removers that contain acetone. Wear gloves when washing dishes.

If a vitamin or mineral deficiency is indicated, you should take an appropriate supplement, but at the same time, make sure your diet contains lots of green leafy vegetables and protein.

MOUTH AND TOOTH PROBLEMS
During menopause you may experience discomfort in your mouth, including pain and burning sensations in your gums; increased sensitivity to hot and cold; altered taste, especially salty, peppery or sour; and sometimes a dry mouth. More seriously, you may experience bleeding gums and even tooth loss.

While lowered levels of oestrogen may be to blame, calcium and vitamin deficiencies may also contribute (as well as the side effects of prescription medications and certain medical conditions). If you experience any of the following – swollen, tender or bleeding gums, or gums that pull away from your teeth; persistent bad breath; loose teeth, changes in your bite or denture fit – it's important not only to seek dental advice, but also to advise your health care professional. Oral health changes can be indicators of serious health problems elsewhere in the body. For example, gum disease can increase your risk of heart disease, stroke and pneumonia.

Good dental hygiene is covered on pages 213–214.

Menopausal Gingivostomatitis
This condition is marked by dry and shiny gums that bleed easily and range in colour from a very pale pink to a deep red. If you experience these symptoms, consult your dentist for treatment as soon as possible.

Problem	Deficiency
White lines or spots	Zinc or iron
Thin, flat nails	Vitamin B_{12}
Ridged nails	Iron
Brittle, dry nails	Calcium
Frequent hangnails	Vitamin C
Yellowish or discoloured nails	Vitamin B_{12}

HEAVY OR IRREGULAR BLEEDING

Until periods cease altogether, you may experience heavier and/or irregular menstrual periods. By the time you are in your 40s at least half your cycles will not produce an egg, but the cells that surround them still respond to FSH (follicle stimulating hormone) and produce normal to even higher levels of estradiol. However, due to the lack of ovulation, progesterone levels will be low, and the oestrogen-driven build-up of your uterine lining will continue unopposed. When the lining breaks down and you menstruate, it may be accompanied by heavy and prolonged bleeding at unpredictable times.

As you go through perimenopause, your periods will become more variable in flow, duration and spacing. However, if you experience really heavy, prolonged vaginal bleeding with clots; periods that last more than seven days or are two to three days longer than usual; periods that arrive more frequently (21 days from one to another); spotting or bleeding between menstrual periods; and bleeding from the vagina after intercourse, you must see your doctor immediately to have your symptoms diagnosed and controlled.

SELF-HELP
Eating the right diet (see pages 106–127) can help. Make sure you eat plenty of vitamin B-rich foods, which can help to strengthen your blood vessel walls. Vitamins E, C and A will also help.

If you feel tired as well, you may be suffering from an iron deficiency. Get your blood levels checked, and if they are low in iron start taking a supplement. You'll need at least 15 mg per day.

WISE WOMAN
Heavy bleeding

Because heavy bleeding can be symptomatic of a wide number of conditions, it's important to have a physical examination and a cervical smear to determine the cause before undergoing any treatment.

HORMONAL HELP
A new option recently introduced is an IUD that contains progesterone. It substantially reduces the bleeding in perimenopausal women and, in some cases, even stops the bleeding completely.

SURGICAL TREATMENT
Although hysterectomy, the removal of the uterus, is now the last resort for intractable bleeding, dilatation and curettage (D&C, see page 230) may be recommended. This involves scraping the uterine lining and removing excess tissue.

Endometrial ablation is another treatment, in which a laser or cauterizing instrument is used to obliterate the uterine lining. It can prevent future pregnancies, so any woman contemplating having more children should not opt for this procedure.

FIBROIDS
A large number of women develop benign growths in the uterus known as fibroids. These growths are stimulated by oestrogen, so that after menopause they usually shrink dramatically. Normally, they don't cause symptoms, but occasionally they can cause heavy bleeding depending on their position in the pelvis.

Laparoscopic or hysteroscopic surgery can remove some small fibroids; more extensive surgery may be required to remove larger ones.

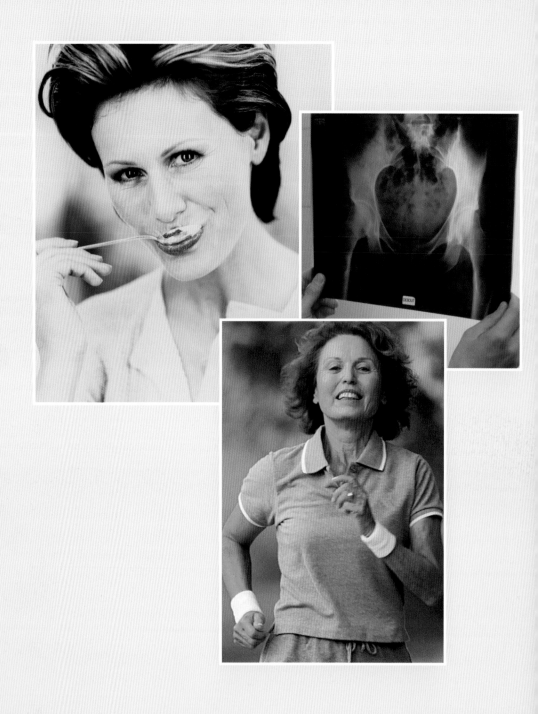

3

MAINTAINING
BONE HEALTH

Bone is made of living tissue that renews itself continuously throughout life. But from midlife onwards this process slows and the skeleton loses bone mineral. At menopause the decrease in oestrogen production can have a further marked effect on bone health, often leading to osteopenia and osteoporosis. This chapter looks at ways of assessing bone mineral density and ways to offset bone loss. It also reviews the changes we might experience in our joints and gives positive strategies for overcoming them.

HOW BONES ARE MADE

Bone, one of the heaviest organs in the body, is formed essentially in two components: one organic, composed of cells, vessels and nerves, and the other mineralized matrix, composed mainly of a water solution of protein (collagen) that becomes heavily embedded with crystals of calcium, known as hydroxyapatite crystals. The three main types of cells in bone are osteoblasts, osteoclasts and osteocytes (see box, right).

Osteoblasts produce the collagen and generate the matrix, which then is filled with hydroxyapatite – or calcium – crystals. The calcium is deposited in layers called lamellae, and these are crossed by minute canals known as Haversian canals or osteons. It is their densely packed arrangement that gives compact bone its great strength. During our life, our bone is also resorbed, or digested, by the osteoclasts, which break bone down, digesting the matrix.

Special multicellular bone units, which act like patrols and travel across the surfaces of our bones with the osteoclasts, digest small amounts of the matrix; these are then replaced by the newly formed bone from the osteoblasts, which in turn become trapped as osteocytes for a number of years. In this way, our complete skeleton is renewed every 7 to 10 years. These units also repair small cracks and defects that may appear in the bone, and they are responsible for remodelling the bone after a fracture.

BONES AND JOINTS FOR LIFE

During our early years, the deposition of bone far exceeds its resorption, resulting in growth and in mineralization of the existing bone. During adulthood, most people will achieve a stable balance, with the net amount of bone remaining constant. As we age, however, the balance shifts towards resorption, causing a reduction in the amount of bone and a loss of mineralization of the existing stock. The extremes of this process are called osteoporosis and osteomalacia respectively (see pages 68–72).

The reason this process is particularly important to women is that with menopause, the abrupt reduction in oestrogen levels results in an increased resorption of bone, which quickly outpaces the

Keeping Bones Strong

Calcium is key to bone strength, but how and when you take it is very important. Take calcium in small doses (400 mg per dose) with plenty of water throughout the day. If you take any more at one time it will be eliminated as a waste product. Take calcium with meals, but do not take it with any fibre or iron supplements, as these will hamper its absorption.

3 main cells in bone

Osteoblasts are cells that produce the protein collagen and generate the bone matrix. They also renew and repair bone.

Osteoclasts are cells that break down calcified bone matrix and are involved in the remodelling of bone during our growth years, in combined action with the osteoblasts. At menopause, osteoclast activity becomes greater than that of the osteoblasts.

Osteocytes are osteoblasts that have become incorporated into bone as mature bone cells.

formation of new bone and can lead to osteoporosis. An asymptomatic condition, osteoporosis causes no pain or any other known symptom until a fracture ensues. These fractures can cause serious loss of function in the wrist, severe chronic back pain and incapacity or great difficulty in walking and mobility, leading in many cases to death in later life. In fact, the number of deaths attributed to hip fractures in older people is very similar to that of heart attacks and cancer, with women being affected about 10 times more often than men.

QUALITY OF LIFE

The care of bones and joints has also been gaining increased attention as movement and activity become more and more valued as fundamental elements of our quality of life. In the younger postmenopausal population, trauma and fractures are the greatest cause of disability and death, while in the older group hip fractures are among the most frequent and seriously disabling conditions, often leading to loss of independence and even death. In the UK, hip fracture is the number one reason why older women lose their ability to live independently and need to be institutionalized.

In addition, joint problems such as osteoarthritis account for a substantial loss in quality of life, with a large associated economic and social cost for treatment. Arthritis is one of the most common diseases of this stage of life. It affects millions of adults and half of all people aged 65 and older. The three most common kinds of arthritis in older people are osteoarthritis, rheumatoid arthritis and gout. In fact, hip and knee replacements are among the most frequently performed operations in people over 50 years of age. Although the link between arthritis and gender is less clear, gender is certainly a factor in some rheumatic diseases. Lupus, rheumatoid arthritis and fibromyalgia are all more common among women. This indicates that hormones or other male-female differences may play a role in the development of these conditions.

THE RIGHT WAY FORWARD

Whereas some of these alterations are simply the result of aging and may be altogether unavoidable, much can be done to prevent and reduce the consequences of these problems. A healthy lifestyle, which includes a balanced diet, weight control and exercise, will substantially reduce the risk of fractures, falls and the worsening of arthritis. In addition, a few medical treatments are now available that may be very helpful in dealing with the causes and consequences of these conditions. However, these medical treatments tend to be expensive and long-lasting, and may have side effects, so individual needs and risks should always be discussed with your healthcare professional before you embark on any long-term therapy.

HOW AND WHY BONES CHANGE

The organization of our skeleton and muscles is a wonder of natural engineering. Few people ever question why our bones are in the core of our limbs, surrounded by soft tissue such as muscles, tendons and skin. But could it be the other way around? Insects and other invertebrates have shells and hard skins called exoskeletons, but they restrict the size to which these animals can grow. Our system, with the bone inside, obeys certain principles of engineering that humans have learned to use in large structures, such as suspension bridges and sailing boats. In these structures the compression forces act on a single supporting element that holds the weight through a series of more or less flexible ropes (the steel cables in suspension bridges and ropes in

sailing boats), which are under constant tension. This distribution of tasks – much like the tasks undertaken by our bones and joints – results in great strength and flexibility, and a relatively low overall weight.

EARLY DAYS

In the embryo, the first signs of the skeleton appear as cartilage buds around the fourth week of development, already in a position compatible with the limbs they will originate. This cartilage is a semi-rigid structure like those we have in our ear lobes and at the tip of our noses. However, by the ninth week, blood vessels from the surrounding tissue penetrate the cartilage and start the process that will

Hand bone development

The coloured x-rays below show bone growth in the human hand at different ages (left to right: one year old, three years old, 13 years old and 20 years old). The bones are shown in pink/blue. The infant and child hands show wide spaces of cartilage between each finger bone at each joint, where ossification will occur. Wrist bones appear absent in the one-year-old as they are made of cartilage, but they have begun to appear in the three-year-old. By 13 years, ossification has occurred widely – all wrist bones are seen and the spaces between finger joints have narrowed. In the 20-year-old hand, all bone joints have closed.

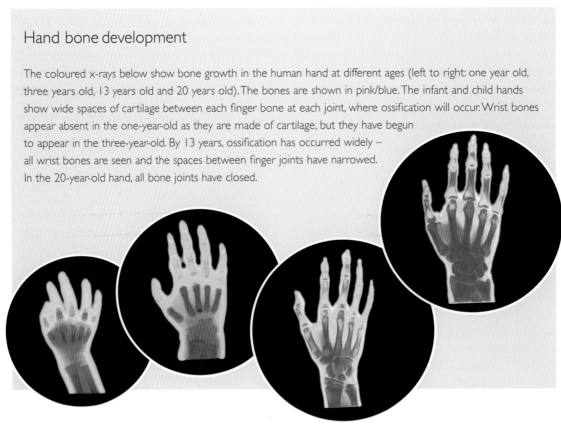

convert these buds into real bone. These blood vessels penetrate the buds through their mid-portions, and areas of a special calcified tissue start to appear, replacing the cartilage. Later on, other vessels penetrate the edges of the bones, close to the joints and form other centres of calcification. These centres of calcification grow continually and eventually get very close to each other, leaving only discs of cartilage that will continue to grow and will be responsible for our growth in height until the end of adolescence.

The cartilage in the tips of the bones forms an important cushioning system for our joints, which will allow for lubrication and good movement. Unlike bone, cartilage will never be replaced. Cartilage tissue has a poor capacity to recover from trauma and wear; later in life, as a result of wear and tear, thinning and loss of this cartilage may lead to a condition generally known as osteoarthritis (see page 79).

THE BONE CYCLE

From the moment bone starts being formed it will also be continually resorbed and rebuilt in a turnover process that goes on throughout our lives. This continuous maintenance system has several important implications. First, bone is the greatest deposit of calcium in our body, and calcium can be taken away from the bones to keep our blood levels constant. Small variations in blood calcium levels may lead to heart and muscular problems, because calcium is a fundamental element in the contracture of muscles. Second, as bone is constantly subject to traumas and small fractures, this system allows for continuous repair of micro-cracks that may occur under strenuous activity, as well as for the repair of major fractures that result from greater trauma or accidents. In any case, bone is one of the few tissues in the human body that is capable of fully regenerating, rather than forming a scar. Third, during the growth years, the deposition of calcium is greater than its absorption, with a resulting increase in the strength of the bones.

During adulthood, this process reaches a stable balance, which will tend to be lost as we age, when the resorption of bone becomes greater, leading sometimes to osteopenia (see page 72) and osteoporosis.

The Role of Hormones

Several hormones, vitamins and the blood levels of ions such as calcium and phosphate play a role. Sex hormones such as oestrogen and testosterone are thought to be the main hormones responsible for the closure of the growth plates of the long bones, and therefore the regulators of our growth. Whereas large amounts of growth hormone will stimulate our growth during childhood, the discharge of sex hormones during puberty will bring our growth to a halt. Later on in life, lowering levels of sex hormones will cause our bones to become thinner and weaker, leading to problems experienced particularly by women after menopause, largely due to the sharp fall in the levels of sex hormones. In men, although a similar pattern is observed, there is a much more gradual loss of sex hormones, resulting in a slower pace of loss.

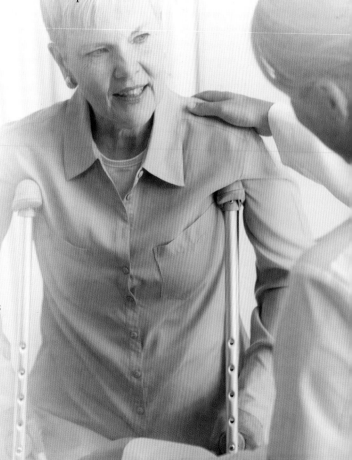

KEEPING TRACK OF BONE HEALTH

As a general rule, the health of bones runs parallel with the health of the rest of the body. To remain strong, bone needs a healthy diet, with plenty of calcium, vitamin D and other essential nutrients such as proteins and essential fatty acids. Vitamin D is usually absorbed in an inactive form and needs exposure to sunshine on the skin to become active. Therefore, regular exposure to sunshine, especially early in the morning, is also essential for healthy bones. Exercise is another essential element in bone health, and small changes in your daily activities can make a real difference to your general mobility and flexibility (see pages 130–151).

If you are deemed at risk for bone disease, your doctor should be able to advise a number of methods that can be used to assess bone quality and density. Some of the most popular methods include x-rays, DXA, ultrasound and CT-scans. Each has its advantages and limitations. It is important to discuss with your healthcare professional which method might be the best for you. It is sensible, too, to remember that there is a wide variety of causes for reduced bone density, which may or may not be treatable, and bone density should be adjusted for age and ethnic group.

X-RAYS
The oldest, and probably the simplest of all these methods, x-rays are based on the exposure of the body part to be examined to a penetrating radiation, which is then registered on a photographic film. The negative film is inspected for changes in shape, texture and density of the image. Because calcium does not allow the x-ray to pass through, the calcium in bone appears as white on the film; the more calcium a bone has, or the thicker it is, the whiter it will appear.

As early as the 1960s, it was recognized that older patients would have bones that were not as dense as those of younger patients – and it became apparent that they were weaker too. During the 1960s and 1970s, a number of experiments established that the

Calcium
The brightest of any natural substance, calcium 'obstructs' x-rays from reaching the photographic film and therefore appears white. So, the thinner the bone, the less white will appear on the x-ray plate.

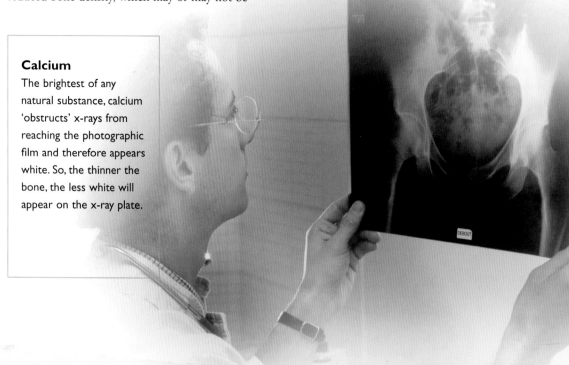

strength of a bone was directly related to the amount of calcium it contained. This finding helped to establish the importance of measuring bone mineral density (BMD), which accounts for about 70 percent of bone strength. However, in weaker bones it was still fairly difficult to determine the BMD, and in obese patients, who have a thicker cover of soft tissue, it was difficult to separate the image of bone from that of surrounding soft tissues.

Initially, most measurements were made in the wrist, but as most of the life-threatening fractures take place in the hip, a system with two different types of x-rays was developed to improve the quality of the measurements. It became known as dual-energy x-ray absorptiometry or DXA.

DUAL-ENERGY X-RAY ABSORPTIOMETRY

DXA was quickly accepted as the best method to determine BMD. However, its ability to observe the texture and shape of bone remains substantially inferior to that of x-rays, particularly with the development of more modern, computerized x-ray systems that allow a precise determination of densities. Several x-ray systems have been launched over the last decade, claiming to be more economical and as efficient as DXA, which uses a small amount of radiation to measure the most common fracture sites, such as the spine and the hip.

Smaller and less expensive DXA machines have been developed. Limited to scanning the wrist or heel, these machines are used in mobile units, making DXA more available to the general population. There is some controversy over the issue of which bone or bones should be scanned, as some evidence suggests that scans of specific areas are more sensitive to predict fractures of that particular site (hip scans are more sensitive than wrist scans to

WISE WOMAN
Bone markers

Substances associated with bone metabolism, bone markers can be measured in blood or urine samples. The concentration of bone breakdown products and calcium in the urine, for example, can give an initial estimate of the amount of bone absorption taking place.

predict fractures of the hip, for example). But these specific differences are relatively small, and if all fractures are considered, any site of cancellous or trabecular bone (see pages 69–70), such as the wrist, spine or hip, will have the power to predict fractures. Therefore, considering costs and benefits, many doctors will accept that for the majority of cases a scan of the wrist or the vertebrae is enough if those scans are more readily available.

ULTRASOUND

Ultrasound is based on sending a pulse of high-frequency sound through a bone, usually the calcaneus (the heel bone), and measuring the same sound with a microphone on the other side of the foot. It is claimed that the stiffness of bone determines how the sound vibrations are altered, and therefore weaker bones show a different sound. However, although it is inexpensive, noninvasive and relatively efficient, the results of ultrasound are far from perfect because the covering soft tissues, such as skin, fat and muscles, have a significant influence on how the sound is actually transmitted or echoed.

COMPUTERIZED TOMOGRAPHY (CT)

Developed for bones that are buried deeply, particularly the vertebrae, CT-scans can help determine the shape of the bone (in case of any malformation), identify fractures and measure BMD. CT-scans are based on a series of x-ray images taken from different directions, which are then handled by the computer to allow 2-D or 3-D reconstructions, according to different planes or points of view. CT-scans are efficient and comprehensive, but expensive, and they expose individuals to a higher dose of radiation than that used with DXA scanning, which is why most doctors do not recommend CT-scans for osteoporosis screening.

OSTEOPOROSIS

It is clear that the older we get the greater we are at risk of fractures related to a progressive weakening of the bones. Why precisely our bones get weaker is a complex issue, and medical science is still trying to understand all the processes involved. As usual in these situations, because progress is slow and discoveries come in small steps, by the end of the 20th century there was a great deal of confusion about terms, definitions and general orientation on research and treatment of bone weakness, particularly that associated with aging.

OSTEOPOROSIS DEFINED

In 1994, the World Health Organization (WHO) defined osteoporosis as a 'disease characterized by low bone mass and microarchitectural deterioration of bone tissue, leading to enhanced bone fragility and a consequent increase in fracture risk'. Whereas this definition has become almost universally accepted, there is still much discussion on what parameters should be used to characterize individuals as osteoporotic or normal. For the most part, bone mineral density (BMD) is the method of choice.

Once the bone density has been obtained, there is further discussion on what values should be accepted as 'normal'. T- and Z-scores are the most widely used values and rely on comparing the individual values of BMD with that of the standard population. The Z-score relies on comparison with an age-adjusted population, and the T-score relies on comparison with a standard healthy, young population, adjusted only for gender.

The WHO suggested the following guidelines for interpreting T-score results:
- Normal – BMD value no lower than a T-score of -1.
- Low bone mass (osteopenia) – BMD value with a T-score between -1 and -2.5.
- Osteoporosis – BMD value with a T-score of -2.5 or less.

However, the T-score presents potential for confusion. Which baseline population should we use as standard? Should it be from the same ethnic background? Should we standardize for geographic areas or countries? If we compare aging people with a standard young group, almost the entire population would show a severe decrease of bone density – should we then treat everybody?

These questions are not easy to answer and, before considering any prolonged drug treatment as

WISE WOMAN
Back pain

It is commonly thought that back pain is caused by osteoporosis, but it is generally accepted that the only clinical symptom of osteoporosis is a fracture. That is, patients don't feel their bones weakening at all until they break. Back pain and other forms of musculo-skeletal pain can be caused by a variety of conditions, but back pain related to osteoporosis will only accompany a fractured vertebra.

risk factors for osteoporosis

- ▶ Being older than 65
- ▶ Previous fracture
- ▶ Family history of osteoporosis
- ▶ Hyperparathyroidism
- ▶ Premature menopause
- ▶ History of frequent falls
- ▶ Amenorrhoea (lack of menstrual periods)
- ▶ Smoking
- ▶ Chronic use of corticosteroids or thyroid medication

a result of your T-score, you should discuss your score with your healthcare professional, who, taking into account other factors, such as your lifestyle, any medication you are taking and any relevant nutritional factors, will be able to help you devise a customized plan to prevent further loss and promote and maintain bone health.

OTHER CONTRIBUTING FACTORS

Women who have experienced premenopausal amenorrhoea (lack of menstrual periods) are particularly prone to osteoporosis. In cases of anorexia nervosa, for example, or in younger women who undergo extremely vigorous exercise regimes, the body responds by switching off oestrogen production, thereby leading to bone loss and increased risk of fracture.

All the elements that increase the likelihood of a fall – reduced vision and hearing, reduced muscular power and control, such as in Parkinson's and other diseases – will also increase the risk of fractures. Studies have shown that poor home conditions, such as low lighting, loose carpeting and slippery baths, also contribute to an increased risk of fractures. Finally, weather conditions, particularly icy roads and pavements, also contribute, with wrist fractures being far more common during the winter months.

It would make little difference treating a patient with drugs for long periods if these factors were not also addressed.

THE PATTERN OF OSTEOPOROTIC FRACTURES

The second part of the WHO definition of osteoporosis is the 'microarchitectural deterioration of bone tissue'. To understand this we need to look at the different types of bone. Whereas the long bones would be properly described as tubes of hard tissue resembling pipes, the bone closer to the joints and the irregular bones, such as vertebrae, look rather like hardened sponges, which are formed according to the shape of the joint itself or the necessary shape of the short bones. This bone is normally called trabecular or cancellous bone. The result of this appearance is that the surface of the bone is greatly increased per unit of volume.

Because the cells responsible for bone turnover normally resorb bone from the bone surfaces, the areas of trabecular bone are usually affected by osteoporosis at a much higher rate (as much as nine times higher) than the long tubular portions. This also explains the pattern of osteoporotic fractures, which affect primarily the areas of trabecular bone – most frequently in the wrist, neck of the femur and

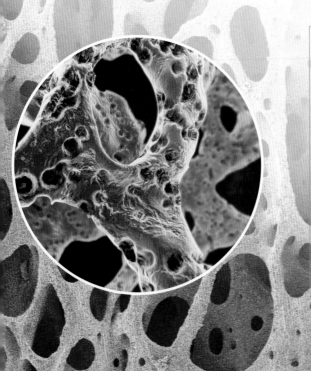

Changes in Bone Structure

HEALTHY BONE (background)
The strength of 'normal' bone comes from its tough, calcium-rich matrix. At menopause, oestrogen and progesterone levels fall, resulting in loss of bone mass.

OSTEOPOROTIC BONE (inset, left)
As bone disintegrates, tiny holes appear, leading to a weakened structure and less bone matrix in which calcium can be deposited.

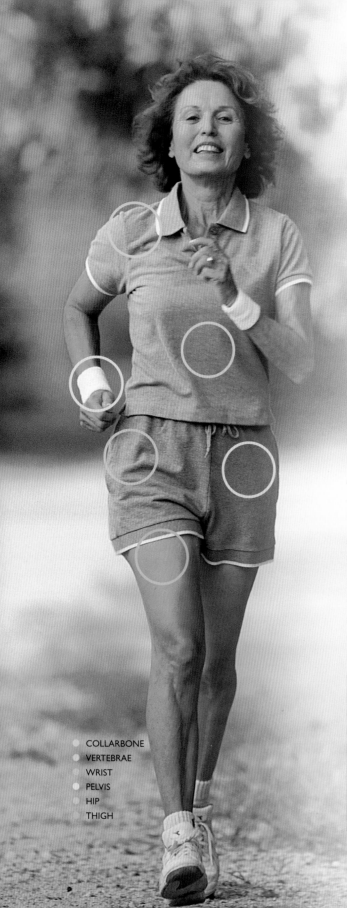

vertebrae – the cancellous-rich areas that also have a high load-bearing requirement.

Fractures After Menopause

The incidence of osteoporotic fractures has a very well-established pattern. Immediately after menopause there is a sharp increase in the incidence of wrist fractures, often resulting in some permanent loss of function of the wrist and hand, with frequent residual stiffness, pain or a combination of both. Wrist fractures are a major sign of osteoporosis, and patients who have an early fracture of the wrist, if left untreated, will have a risk several times higher than that of the general population of suffering a hip fracture in later life.

The precise incidence and patterns of vertebral fractures are still under investigation. It is thought that a number of such fractures go unnoticed and sometimes are diagnosed only by chance. Most of these fractures heal well and cause no permanent neurological problems, so individuals tend to dismiss them as just another episode of pain. However, these fractures can cause reduction in height and deformities in the backs of affected patients, resulting in the characteristic curved posture of elderly people (see box, right).

THE TOLL OF HIP FRACTURES

Between the ages of 70 and 75, the incidence of hip fractures starts to increase, with a sharp trend upwards around the age of 80, and a continuous increase afterwards. The approximate lifetime risk of a hip fracture in women is about 1 in 5, and this

COLLARBONE
VERTEBRAE
WRIST
PELVIS
HIP
THIGH

Common Fracture Sites

Osteoporotic fractures occur most commonly in the hip, wrist and vertebrae, because of the more porous and fragile structure of the bone found in these areas. Other common sites are the collarbone, pelvis and thigh.

Kyphosis

Also known as 'dowager's hump', or curvature of the spine, kyphosis results from the bones of the spine losing density, causing the vertebrae to collapse and the ribcage to tilt downwards. The illustrations below show the vertebrae in a normal spine (left) and an osteoporotic spine (right). In both cases, the fourth vertebra is shown in section to reveal the honeycombed internal bone structure. In the affected bone, we can see the loss of bone mass that weakens the internal bone structure, causing cracking and collapse of the vertebrae and cartilage degeneration (shown in red). The illustration on the right is an MRI-scan of the back of a 60-year-old with osteoporosis, in which vertebral collapse is clearly visible.

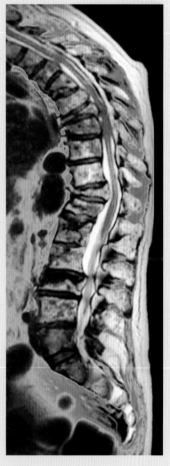

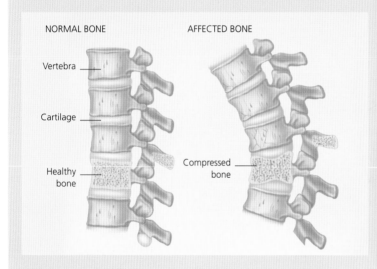

NORMAL BONE   AFFECTED BONE

Vertebra

Cartilage

Healthy bone   Compressed bone

figure increases with age; that is, about 1 in 3 women over the age of 80 will have a hip fracture. According to the European Parliament Osteoporosis Interest Group, there were 480,000 hip fractures in the European Union in 1999 – and the numbers are rising dramatically.

The consequences of a hip fracture are no less serious. According to a recent study on outcome following hip fractures, 120 days after a hip fracture around 20 percent of patients will have died and only 40 percent will be living in their own home, with the remaining 40 percent living in long-term care or permanent sheltered homes. In fact, the number of deaths resulting directly from hip fractures is currently approaching that caused by cancer and heart disease. This is why osteoporosis has recently been gaining so much notoriety and public concern.

However, along with an increased awareness of the problem, several treatments and prevention programmes have been proposed to reduce the risk and incidence of such fractures. They range from exercise regimes (see pages 130–151) to a healthy intake of substances such as calcium and vitamin D, and the specific use of drugs, such as those used in HT or bisphosphonates (see pages 76–78).

CAUSES OF BONE WEAKNESS

OSTEOPENIA

Referred to medically as any reduction in bone density perceptible on x-ray examinations, osteopenia is usually the result of a reduced amount of calcium being in the path of the x-rays. This term is generic, however, and applies to any cause of reduced calcium and may even be noticed on the x-rays of an obese person if the soft tissues also resorb a substantial amount of radiation, thereby reducing the contrast between bone and soft tissue.

In clinical practice, the most common cause of osteopenia is osteoporotic bone loss. According to current radiology practice, maybe 95 percent of all osteopenias perceived in x-ray examinations result from pre-osteoporotic loss. However, there are several other causes of osteopenia, such as osteomalacia, hyperparathyroidism and certain types of malignancy, such as multiple myeloma.

Disuse is another very common cause of osteopenia. In fact, when our limbs are immobilized, by being placed in a cast for the treatment of a fracture, for example, osteopenia will be noticed after periods as short as two weeks. The main difference between these cases and osteoporosis is that they are potentially reversible, while the alterations in bone caused by osteoporosis may not be.

OSTEOMALACIA

The term osteomalacia means 'soft bones' and is usually a consequence of a lack of vitamin D. This deficiency can be caused by several factors: for example, low levels of vitamin D in the diet, low levels of exposure to sunshine and other genetic forms of inadequate vitamin D metabolism. (This condition is usually similar to rickets, with the term 'rickets' commonly being used for children and osteomalacia for adults.)

Osteomalacia differs from osteoporosis because the organic matrix of bone, which is formed of collagen fibres and osteoid substance, is present but fails to become properly calcified. Also, osteomalacia can cause pain and discomfort. Whereas osteoporosis is accepted as being asymptomatic, the main symptoms of osteomalacia are aching, tender bones.

Osteomalacia is usually diagnosed through blood tests, including those for calcium levels. A small sample will occasionally be taken from the hipbone to confirm the diagnosis. Treatment aims to target the causes wherever possible – by raising the amount of vitamin D in the diet and increasing exposure to sunlight. Vitamin D injections may be needed, in which case calcium levels need to be monitored.

HYPERPARATHYROIDISM

The parathyroid glands regulate the calcium levels in our blood. Through the secretion of parathyroid hormone (PTH), these four small glands regulate the amount of calcium that is absorbed from our diet, the amount that is secreted by our kidneys, and the amount that is stored in our bones – with our bones storing many pounds of calcium that can be sent to other parts of our body at the request of the parathyroid glands. When one of these glands is overactive (hyperparathyroidism), a benign tumour develops, too much PTH is made and our bones constantly release calcium into the bloodstream. This loss causes our bones to lose density and hardness and leads to osteoporosis – a problem that is amplified in postmenopausal women, as the process is going on already.

A study of postmenopausal women with hyperparathyroidism at the University of Northern Sweden has shown that the body can restore bone density in postmenopausal women after the excess hormone is removed, but this is a very slow process and, depending on the amount of bone loss, the bones may never regain their 'normal' calcium levels and overall density. After surgery to remove the parathyroid tumour, most doctors recommend supplemental calcium, and further drug treatment (see pages 76–78) may be considered appropriate.

SELF-HELP FOR BONE HEALTH

There are several drug-free steps you can take to help prevent or reduce the rate of bone loss. Of course these will be related to your lifestyle and may include changing your diet, probably introducing supplements, following an efficient exercise programme that includes balance training, and avoiding situations that could lead to falls or fractures. These actions are very important because even if some of them do not reverse or completely stop the bone loss, they will certainly reduce the risk of fracture. A regular exercise programme, for instance, will reduce your fracture risk not only by reducing the rate of bone loss but, above all, by increasing your muscular control and balance, thereby avoiding falls.

The Importance of Calcium

Just as diet is very important in good general health, several dietary components can bring substantial benefit to your bones and joints. Calcium is perhaps the most important item in this regard, as it is the main constituent of hydroxyapatite, the mineral component of bone matrix, of which we have large quantities in our skeleton. Calcium is normally absorbed in our intestine and excessive amounts are eliminated by the kidneys. In addition to strength-

Carbonated Drinks

Studies have found that fizzy drinks – even sparkling mineral water – can increase the risk of osteoporosis and bone fractures by using up calcium, and it is estimated that just two cans of soft drinks per day can have an effect.

It was previously thought that the carbon dioxide (CO_2) that creates the fizziness in carbonated drinks was neutralized in the gut. However, recent research has found that the CO_2 can enter the bloodstream, where the body tries to neutralize it with alkaline calcium – taken from bone deposits.

A recent paper published in the journal *Osteoporosis International* reported that the acidity of the typical Western diet – low in fruits and vegetables and high in carbonated drinks and processed foods – may already have had a significant long-term impact on bone health. The report went on to state that, over a decade, a person who weighs between 63–70 kg (140–155 lb) could lose an additional 15 percent of their bone mass on the Western diet.

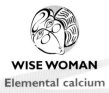

WISE WOMAN

Elemental calcium

It's important to remember when taking a calcium supplement that it should be elemental calcium. No supplement is 100 percent elemental – always read the label carefully to determine the elemental calcium content.

ening bones, calcium is extremely important for the contraction of muscles – including the cardiac muscle – and very consistent amounts and concentrations must be present in our bloodstream and muscle cells to allow them to contract and work properly. Low or high levels of calcium in the blood can quickly lead to disturbances in the cardiac rhythm and to spastic contractures of the muscles which, if left untreated, may prove fatal. (See page 110 for recommended daily intake and sources of calcium.)

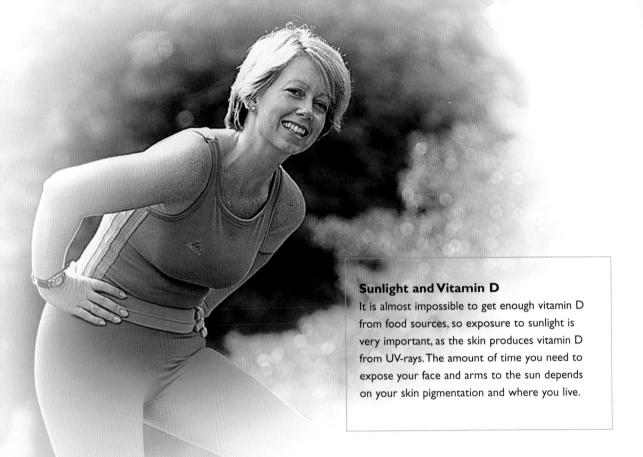

Sunlight and Vitamin D
It is almost impossible to get enough vitamin D from food sources, so exposure to sunlight is very important, as the skin produces vitamin D from UV-rays. The amount of time you need to expose your face and arms to the sun depends on your skin pigmentation and where you live.

Vitamin D

Vital in regulating the metabolism of calcium, vitamin D is also essential in the absorption of calcium in the bones. Most of our vitamin D is absorbed as a precursor, or pre-vitamin D, which is metabolized in our bodies, particularly in the kidneys, into the active or hormonal form. However, for this transformation to take place at a satisfactory rate, it is essential that the pre-vitamin D receives some radiation from sunshine in the form of ultraviolet rays. It is therefore important that we expose ourselves to a reasonable amount of sunshine, particularly in the early hours of the morning, when the most beneficial ultraviolet rays can filter through the atmosphere. People who live in areas with little sunshine – or whose culture prevents them from exposing their bodies – are prone to develop osteomalacia (see page 72) due to a lack of vitamin D.

In short, the main causes of vitamin D deficiency are: intake below recommended levels, limited exposure to sunlight, impairment of vitamin D conversion in the kidneys to its active hormone form and inadequate absorption of vitamin D from the digestive tract.

It is possible to take too much vitamin D, which may cause side effects and even toxicity. However, exposure to sunshine alone is very unlikely to result in vitamin D toxicity and so is diet alone, unless large amounts of cod-liver oil are consumed. Toxicity is much more likely to occur from a high intake of vitamin D in supplements, which is why it's important not to exceed the recommended dose. Excessive vitamin D can cause nausea, vomiting, poor appetite, constipation, weakness and weight loss. In very severe cases, it can also raise blood levels of calcium, causing mental status changes such as confusion. High blood levels of calcium can also cause heart rhythm abnormalities.

An ordinary multivitamin will provide you with the daily recommended intake of vitamin D (see page 111 for more information).

OTHER LIFESTYLE DECISIONS

Exercise is very important in keeping bones and joints healthy and supple. It is important to keep in mind that weight-bearing exercise – even in the simple form of walking – can help prevent bone loss and keep your muscles strong and your joints supple. Increased muscle strength and improved coordination can in their own right help to prevent falls and fractures.

The key is very simple: physical activity doesn't have to be a chore, and making seemingly tiny adjustments to your daily routine will help. At a minimum, every woman should endeavour to achieve 30 minutes of physical activity a day. Try getting off the bus a stop early and walking the rest of the way; always take the stairs instead of the lift and don't hold the bannister; carry your shopping home instead of taking the car. If it helps, plan your physical activity and make it a more social occasion. Make a regular date with a friend and go for a walk in the local park. The companionship and support may make it easier for you to stick to a new routine (see pages 130–151 for more information on exercise).

It Really Is Time to Make Changes ...

Like giving up smoking. In addition to causing disease in the respiratory system, smoking can also facilitate osteoporosis. Statistics from the U.S. Centers for Disease Control show that postmenopausal women who currently smoke have lower bone density than women who do not smoke. Also, women who currently smoke are at greater risk for hip fracture compared with non-smoking women. See pages 167–168 for strategies to help you kick the habit.

Drinking alcohol also has a negative impact on bone health. Alcohol interferes with the balance of calcium in several ways, but mainly by increasing the levels of parathyroid hormone, which reduce the body's calcium reserves. Alcohol intake also interferes with the production and absorption of vitamin D. In addition, chronic heavy drinking can cause hormone deficiencies in women and men.

7 ways to prevent falls

▶ Wear supportive shoes with low heels and rubber soles for maximum traction.
▶ Avoid slippery pavements and be cautious on steps and kerbs.
▶ Get your shopping delivered in bad weather.
▶ Keep your hands free when out and about – use a backpack or shoulder-bag.
▶ Keep rooms free of clutter, and keep electrical and telephone cords clear of walkways.
▶ Use carpet runners and tack rugs to the floor.
▶ Use a rubber bath mat in the bath or shower.

Alcoholic men tend to produce less testosterone, the sex hormone that is linked to the production of osteoblasts, the cells that stimulate bone formation. In women, chronic alcohol consumption often produces irregular menstrual cycles, reducing oestrogen levels and increasing osteoporosis risk. Also, levels of the 'stress hormone' cortisol – known to decrease bone formation and increase bone breakdown – tend to be elevated in alcoholics.

Finally, the effects of alcohol on balance and gait cause alcoholics to fall more frequently than non-alcoholics. Heavy alcohol consumption has been linked to an increase in the risk of fracture including the most serious – hip fracture. Vertebral fractures, which tend to be uncommon in those under 50 years of age, are more prevalent in those under the age of 50 who abuse alcohol (see pages 165–169 for information on kicking harmful habits).

DRUG TREATMENTS

Several drugs have been used in attempts to prevent bone loss and weakening as well as the fractures that happen as a consequence, but there are problems with this approach. First, most treatments need to be taken for a prolonged period, often several years, if they are to be effective. Second, the financial cost of these treatments is not small, and several health agencies have concluded that it is still less expensive to treat the eventual fractures than to try to prevent them with medications. This may sound cynical, but the truth is that the costs are measured not only in direct cost of the drug, but also in the side effects that they bring, such as increased risk of other serious diseases such as cancer and blood clots that form in the legs and sometimes reach the lungs.

Third, because we can only be sure of the long-term effect of these drugs after very long-term trials, most companies will market them before their very long-term effects and side effects are fully understood or appreciated.

This is not to say that drugs should not be taken at all, but the possible benefits must be carefully considered and weighed against the risk of side effects and the cost of the chosen treatments. It is a choice that should be carefully discussed with your healthcare professional in the light of factors such as personal or family history of breast cancer, blood clots, heart diseases and other conditions that may be favourably or adversely affected by these drugs.

HORMONE THERAPY

HT is based on the principle of restoring levels of sex hormones – particularly oestrogen – to those that were observed before menopause. Recent results from long-term trials conducted by the Women's Health Initiative (WHI) have put the good and bad effects of different forms of HT in perspective. One area of study was whether or not HT would enhance protection against heart disease and stroke and also against hip and vertebral fractures. The general conclusions were mixed. Long-term HT can reduce the risk of fractures (particularly those of the hip and vertebrae), but may increase the risk of breast cancer, stroke and blood clots, and does not reduce the risk of heart disease.

Again, the only way to make a sound decision is through a careful discussion of the pros and cons of your particular situation with your healthcare professional.

Selective estrogen receptor modulators (SERMs)

This family of drugs has oestrogen-like effects on some tissues and anti-oestrogen effects on others. One of the SERMs family, raloxifene (Evista), has been approved by the CSM for the treatment and prevention of osteoporosis. It has been developed to bind to the oestrogen receptors in some cell membranes, and in this way stimulate the cells just as oestrogen would, but without the side effects, since these drugs are not oestrogens. Raloxifene was designed to reproduce the effects of oestrogen on bones, but without oestrogen's effects on breast tissue or the uterus. Raloxifene has been shown to prevent bone loss, have beneficial effects on bone mass, and reduce the risk of spine fractures. It is taken as a tablet once a day. However, like any other drugs, raloxifene may also have side effects, which may include hot flushes, sweating, muscle soreness, weight gain, rashes, and clot formation in some blood vessels.

Calcitonin

(Miacalcic, Forcaltonin) is a hormone involved in calcium regulation and bone metabolism. It is naturally produced by certain cells in the thyroid gland and its main effect is to lower the levels of calcium and phosphate in the blood by stimulating calcium absorption by the bones. Calcitonin is obtained from other animal species such as salmon and pigs and is approved by the CSM for the treatment of osteoporosis for those at high risk for the disease and for whom a bisphosphonate is unsuitable. It is taken as a single daily nasal spray (or, rarely, as an injection under the skin).

Calcitonin has been shown to slow bone loss and increase spinal bone density. Some patients report that calcitonin also relieves pain from bone fractures. The effects of calcitonin on fracture risk are still unclear. Injected calcitonin does not affect other organs or systems in the body besides bone, but with time, most patients will develop an anaphylactic response to the drug.

Side effects may include flushing of the face and hands, increased urinary frequency, nausea and a rash. The only side effects reported with nasal calcitonin are a runny nose and other signs of nasal irritation.

Teriparatide

(Forteo) is a new drug recently introduced for the treatment of postmenopausal osteoporosis. It consists of a small fragment of parathyroid hormone and induces the formation of new bone, increasing bone mineral density and bone strength, therefore reducing the chance of getting a fracture (although it is too recent to have long-term studies available). Teriparatide can be used by postmenopausal women with osteoporosis who are at a high risk for having a fracture. It can also be used by those who have had a fracture related to osteoporosis, or who have multiple risk factors for fracture, or who cannot use other osteoporosis treatments. Teriparatide is easily self-administered by daily subcutaneous injections (similar to insulin injections), with a maximum duration of treatment of 18 months. In the UK it should only be prescribed by a specialist.

BISPHOSPHONATES

Bisphosphonates are substances similar to pyrophosphate, a naturally occurring compound that interferes with the regulation of calcium metabolism and can help to prevent bone breakdown. These substances had been known in the chemical industry for more than a century, but their capacity as drugs only started to be investigated in the 1960s. Several less common conditions such as Paget's disease and multiple myeloma (a form of bone cancer) were initially seen to benefit from these drugs. More recently, some of them have been licensed for use in osteoporosis.

The eight bisphosphonates currently licensed by the CSM for treatment of human disease are alendronate (Fosamax), etidronate (Didronel), pamidronate (Aredia), ibandronate (Bondronat), risedronate (Actonel), clodronate (Bonefos, Loron), tiludronate (Skelid) and zoledronic acid (Zometa). Whereas they have slightly different properties and may be tolerated differently by different individuals, they all work on the same principle: by inhibiting the osteoclasts – the cells that digest or resorb bones. The drugs of choice for prevention and treatment of osteoporosis are alendronate (Fosamax) or risedronate (Actonel). Etidronate (Didronel) may be considered if these drugs are not suitable or give side effects. Other bisphosphonates are used to treat Paget's disease of bone, high calcium levels found in cancer and bone pain due to secondary cancer.

As we have seen, during our lifetime bone undergoes a constant renovation process that includes the digestion of tiny amounts of bone that are then reconstructed by the osteoblasts; these eventually become embedded in the calcium and become osteocytes, the mature bone cells, in the process known as bone turnover. During menopause, the activity of the osteoblasts is decreased in relation to that of osteoclasts, resulting in more bone being removed than deposited again, a process that leads to an overall loss of bone mass.

Bisphosphonates are absorbed in the crystals of hydroxyapatite. These directly inhibit the action of osteoclasts and are not usually eliminated from the body. Whereas there is no evidence that bisphosphonates inhibit fracture healing, large doses of Etidronate have been shown to inhibit bone mineralization when used continually or in very high doses.

Bisphosphonate tablets should be taken on an empty stomach. Patients with kidney disease need to be particularly careful before embarking on a course of these drugs. If you decide to take bisphosphonates, it is also important to keep up a good intake of calcium and vitamin D (see page 111 for the recommended daily intake). However, calcium should not be taken at the same time as the bisphosphonates, as this will prevent the body from absorbing both.

The precise duration of treatment has not been firmly established. In standard osteoporosis dosing of alendronate or risedronate, the treatment usually continues for several years. With the less well studied bisphosphonates the duration of use may be considerably shorter as there is still some concern over the long-term effects, particularly if very high doses are taken and for a prolonged period of time.

STRONTIUM RANELATE

Recently licensed in the UK and other parts of Europe, strontium ranelate is the combination of the mineral strontium, similar to calcium, with ranelic acid. Strontium is normally stored in our bones and teeth, and the small amount found in the foods we eat is stored in our bones.

Strontium was tested as a treatment for osteoporosis in the 1950s without success. However, in the mid-1990s, new research showed that strontium ranelate increased bone formation. Renewed interest in this mineral as a treatment for osteoporosis led to several research studies. Recent reports from a three-year study show that strontium ranelate not only increases bone formation but also reduces bone breakdown. As a result, strontium ranelate reduced the risk of spine fractures in women with postmenopausal osteoporosis. However, studies have not yet shown a reduced risk of hip fracture.

JOINTS AND MENOPAUSE

Another important set of structures is the joints. We need them for flexibility – to move and reach, and to perform all sorts of activities that we take for granted. Supple joints are complex and specialized structures, and can last for several decades without problems. In fact the majority of people will reach old age without serious joint problems. However, a sizable proportion of the population will experience diseases and derangements of these mechanisms, which can be very limiting, painful and even crippling.

There are a number of diseases that, while not directly connected to menopause, often begin during the menopausal years, and some studies implicate the hormonal changes at menopause.

OSTEOARTHRITIS (OA)

One of the most common types of arthritis, OA is a degenerative disease characterized by the breakdown of the cartilage between the bones of one or more joints. Cartilage acts to 'cushion' the bones of the joints. Commonly affecting middle-aged and older people, OA generally affects hands and weight-bearing joints such as knees, hips, feet and the back.

Though not yet directly connected with menopause, it is recognized that OA often begins during the menopausal years. Up until the age of 50, men and women are affected by OA at approximately the same rate; after that age more women than men develop the disease and it tends to be more severe, affecting more joints.

Osteoarthritis is a very generic term and it must be further divided into primary and secondary osteoarthritis. Primary osteoarthritis is the type that occurs without a specific or known cause. It may be that some people have a genetic predisposition to OA, or have during their lives had some other undetected disease. Secondary osteoarthritis is the term used when a specific cause can be determined, such as infections, fractures across the joints and inflammations of the synovial membrane, as in rheumatoid arthritis and other diseases affecting joints.

The general process of OA often starts with a wearing of the cartilage, eventually leading to the exposure of subchondral bone and eventually bone erosion, which can lead to pain and stiffness in the affected joints. When examining x-rays of joints, the first visible sign is a reduction of the space between the two adjacent bones. With the progression of the condition, hardened lumps, or osteophytes, start to appear at the edge of the bones and the bone under the cartilage may become thicker, an action that is a precursor of bone erosion.

Treatment

The best way to prevent OA is to keep your joints supple through careful but almost continuous use. Movement is a key factor in promoting proper lubrication and nutrition of the cartilage. Low-impact exercises such as walking and swimming (see pages 138–142) are ideal to keep joints supple and healthy.

If things start to go wrong, however, there are very few treatments available. Because cartilage does

NORMAL JOINT   OSTEOARTHRITIS

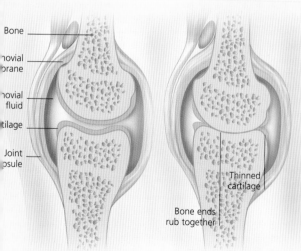

Bone

novial brane

novial fluid

tilage

Joint psule

Thinned cartilage

Bone ends rub together

not have blood vessels, its healing is difficult, and once areas of torn cartilage develop it may be impossible to recover them. Several treatments have been proposed, but few, if any, have conclusive large-scale results. The food supplements glucosamine and chondroitin sulphate (see box) have been found to be helpful, but it is important to be sure that the pain is caused by OA and not to stop taking any other drugs you may be on without discussing it with your doctor.

In some cases, it is possible to use surgery to replace cartilage, but the problem is where to take the cartilage from.

A variety of more aggressive surgical treatments are also available, such as joint fusion and joint replacement, but these should be reserved for the more advanced cases because they involve greater risks. Although individual needs should be discussed between the patient and the surgeon, it is usually accepted that joint replacements should be avoided before the age of 55 or 60 if possible.

RHEUMATOID ARTHRITIS (RA)

A chronic, progressive autoimmune disease, RA causes chronic inflammation of the joints and, in some cases, the tissue around them. The joints become painful, stiff, inflamed and swollen, with severe cases often leading to joint destruction. Because it is an autoimmune disease (in which antibodies are produced that attack the body's own tissue), RA can also affect many other organs.

The disease affects twice – maybe even three times – as many women as men, and several studies have pointed towards a relationship between RA in women and fluctuating levels of sex hormones. Interestingly, studies have shown that women who suffer from RA often feel their symptoms ease during pregnancy, when female sex hormone levels are high, while the highest incidence of RA occurs in women who are experiencing menopause, when levels of these hormones are decreasing.

Glucosamine and Chondroitin Sulphate

These substances are found naturally in the body, and some studies have suggested that patients with mild to moderate osteoarthritis and arthritis could prevent or delay the progression of the conditions by taking them. Both substances are available as dietary and nutritional supplements, but glucosamine is often extracted from animal tissue such as crab, lobster and shrimp shells and from cartilage such as shark cartilage. So it should not be taken by people with an allergy to shellfish.

The results of some medical trials have revealed that people on an increased intake of either supplement reported a reduction in pain similar to that obtained by people taking drugs such as ibuprofen and aspirin. The U.S. National Institute of Health (NIH) is currently conducting trials to assess the long-term benefits and problems that an increased intake of these substances may cause. Because they are sold as dietary supplements it is possible to obtain them without prescription, but their quality and purity are also uncontrolled. If you decide to take one of these you may be advised to look for more detailed information and discuss your plan with your doctor.

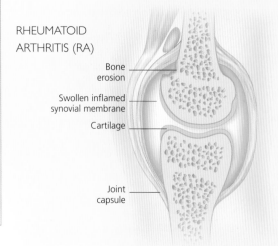

RHEUMATOID ARTHRITIS (RA)

Bone erosion

Swollen inflamed synovial membrane

Cartilage

Joint capsule

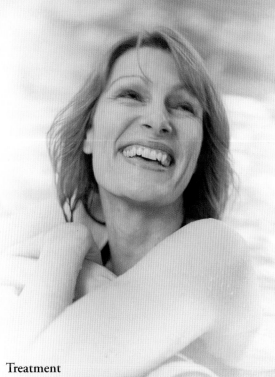

Treatment

As there is no known cure for RA, the emphasis is on alleviating symptoms, reducing pain and inflammation, and maximizing joint function. The optimum treatment seems to be a combination of medication, exercise and patient education.

FIBROMYALGIA

This chronic condition causes pain, stiffness and tenderness of muscles, tendons and joints. However, although it is one of the most common diseases affecting joints and muscles, its cause is currently unknown and it is not even fully accepted as a disorder by all members of the medical community. Fibromyalgia causes no inflammation; neither does it cause damage to internal body organs (unlike other rheumatic conditions). The pain in fibromyalgia is caused by an increased sensitivity to different sensory stimuli and an unusually low pain threshold that causes these patients severe – often debilitating – pain from ordinarily minor sources. This pain is usually felt in the upper back, neck, chest, shoulders, arms and buttocks.

Along with pain, increased levels of fatigue and lack of sleep as well as emotional and mental disturbances are reported in around 50 percent of those who experience fibromyalgia. Other symptoms include severe headaches and numbness of parts of the body.

Treatment

As the symptoms vary so much between patients, treatment is given on an individual basis through customized treatment programmes that combine medications with patient education, exercise and stress reduction techniques. A recent study has shown acupuncture to be useful in the treatment of fibromyalgia.

LUPUS

Known formally as systemic lupus erythematosus (SLE), lupus is another autoimmune disease in which the body's defence mechanism goes into overdrive and attacks its own tissues. The symptoms of lupus are many and varied, which can make it difficult to diagnose, but joint and muscle pain is a common complaint, and many people with lupus go on to develop arthritis. Lupus can be triggered at puberty, after childbirth, after a prolonged course of medication and at menopause.

Treatment

There is no known permanent cure for lupus. Again, the goal is to relieve symptoms, decrease inflammation and protect organs by lowering the level of autoimmune activity in the body. Many patients with mild symptoms may need no treatment or intermittent courses of anti-inflammatory drugs. Others with more severe symptoms may require high doses of corticosteroids and other drugs to suppress the immune system.

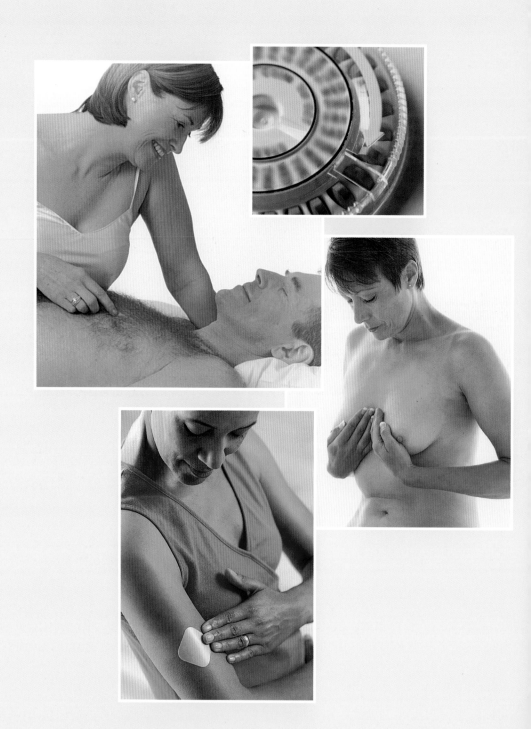

4

SEX AND SEXUALITY

As a major part of a woman's life, sexual desire and activity is often affected by menopause. Some women experience a decrease in libido and a falling off of sexual activity, while others report an increased interest in sex and greater sexual satisfaction. This chapter outlines the physical and hormonal changes that can bring about a loss of desire, and it provides techniques for ensuring a satisfying love life.

CHANGING
SEXUAL RESPONSES

Many women experience a loss of libido after and just before menopause, and there are a variety of reasons why this is so. Menopause is marked by the loss of a regular bleeding pattern and sometimes heavier bleeding, which is disturbing and can have a serious affect on libido and mood. Some couples dislike having sex while the woman is menstruating – particularly if bleeding is heavy – and this, plus an inability to predict the next period, may contribute to the overall stress. Other early menopausal symptoms, such as night sweats, or difficulty sleeping and the resulting irritability, can contribute further to a lowered libido. On top of all this, a woman may start to notice slight changes in her genital area – mild itching and less lubrication during sex are symptoms that come and go before the actual menopause. Because they come and go they can be confusing, and mood swings and lack of interest in sex are often cited as the causes rather than the result.

Physical Changes

As soon as the true menopause takes place and the ovaries have dramatically reduced their oestrogen output, the vagina and vulva start to alter. The vulval area becomes paler as the blood supply diminishes. The labia of the vulva become thinner and less plump, the mons pubis beneath the pubic hair gets smaller and a gradual loss of pubic hair begins. The clitoris gets smaller and the hood of the clitoris retracts, leaving this very sensitive area unusually exposed. This can sometimes be a cause of discomfort during sex as the clitoris is so sensitive that the pressure during intercourse becomes unpleasant. These changes can be reversed by oestrogen preparations taken by mouth or in the form of a local cream (see pages 172–185), and they may also be reversed using alternative replacement therapy (see pages 188–203) and by including more phytoestrogens (see pages 112–114) in your diet.

Changing position during sex and experimenting with different lubricants can also help. Keep in mind that certain medications, particularly antihistamines and antidepressants, can cause mucous membranes throughout the body to become dry.

Some women complain of loss of sensation all over their skin and especially around their nipples, worrying that sensitivity in previous erogenous zones is being lost. This may be helped by engaging in more concentrated foreplay, employing fantasy and sensate focus exercises, and performing the sexual enhancement exercises shown opposite.

Orgasm Potential

Many women find it easier and easier to reach orgasm with age. They have more confidence and a greater ability to guide or help their partners stimulate them, more experience knowing what position or technique works best, less and less distraction or worry, and less

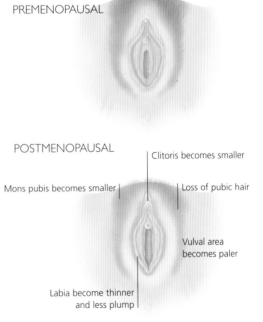

PREMENOPAUSAL

POSTMENOPAUSAL

Clitoris becomes smaller

Mons pubis becomes smaller

Loss of pubic hair

Vulval area becomes paler

Labia become thinner and less plump

inhibition. Unfortunately, some women find the physical changes in the vulval area make it more difficult to achieve orgasm. This is mainly because they are worried about discomfort or pain.

Vaginal oestrogen treatments and adequate lubrication will always help with this to some extent. However, it is not unusual for the actual sensation of orgasm to be less satisfying. There are oestrogen receptors in the muscles of the vaginal walls and those supporting the uterus. With less oestrogen around, these muscles get weaker and do not contract as strongly during orgasm. Mastering the pelvic floor exercises (see page 50) and having regular sex will help overcome or prevent this loss of powerful muscle contractions.

WISE WOMAN
The partner problem
•

The lack of a partner or having a partner who has lost either the ability to have sex or interest in it undoubtedly affects a woman's sexual function negatively. A woman whose partner is able to resume sexual activity, with the help of drug therapy after months or years without sexual intercourse, may experience severe vaginal discomfort due to lack of vaginal elasticity and lubrication.

SEXUAL ENHANCEMENT EXERCISES

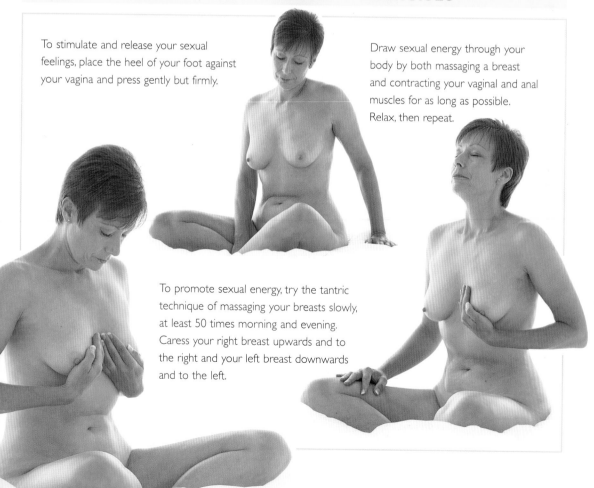

To stimulate and release your sexual feelings, place the heel of your foot against your vagina and press gently but firmly.

Draw sexual energy through your body by both massaging a breast and contracting your vaginal and anal muscles for as long as possible. Relax, then repeat.

To promote sexual energy, try the tantric technique of massaging your breasts slowly, at least 50 times morning and evening. Caress your right breast upwards and to the right and your left breast downwards and to the left.

ASSISTING DESIRE

When women complain of lack of libido and poor sexual response around menopause, it may be more a question of psychological factors than physical ones. Low self-esteem and poor body image can be far greater culprits here than hormones. Your mood, attitude to sex and level of attraction to your partner seem to have a greater effect on libido than any physical impediment.

It helps to think of sex as a good wine. Just like a good wine, sex can improve with age – although it will not be the same as it was. The fear that sex will not be what it was is one of the greatest inhibitors for perimenopausal and menopausal women and especially their partners (who are themselves, for the most part, older men).

In terms of sexual response, women are luckier than men. A woman's sex drive peaks at around 28 to 30 years and continues on a plateau until well into her 50s, 60s or even 70s. A man's sex drive starts to diminish from the age of about 19. However, many a woman's first reaction to her partner's inability to have an erection, or to keep one for as long as before, is to feel she herself is failing. It is somehow her fault; she no longer feels as attractive to her partner, believing he doesn't see her as sexy any more. But, unless there are other problems in the relationship, this is unlikely to be true. It is far more likely the man is worrying about his own erection and nothing else.

Rather than become discouraged, now can be the time for a woman to take charge subtly and show that she feels sexy; there is nothing more likely to

Employ a Sex Toy

A sex toy not only adds a new dimension to your lovemaking but can be a boon to a woman without a partner. Vibrators in particular are great for keeping arousal levels up. There are a plethora of models available in different sizes, shapes, textures, smells, colours and speeds. Some are used for clitoral stimulation, others are better for penetration, and some can be used to stimulate the vagina and clitoris at the same time. It's really a matter of what works for you! In the United States, 'female sexual arousal disorder' is a recognized medical condition, and a few years ago a tiny vacuum pump, the 'Eros clitoral therapy device', was licensed by the Federal Drug Administration for its treatment. The device works by increasing blood flow to the clitoris and thus helping reduced sensation, lubrication and the ability to orgasm.

Your choice of a sex toy depends on what you want out of it – is it something your partner will enjoy, too, or is it just for your own gratification? If you're uncertain what to buy, you could start out with erotic underwear or edible body paint, and see whether this improves your sex life.

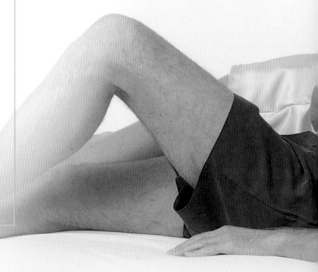

arouse and stimulate a man than showing him he is making his partner feel very sexy.

Get Lubricated

Of primary importance to arousal is the ability to become lubricated, as fear of painful sex will lead to a loss of desire. Lowered oestrogen levels can lead to reduced vaginal lubrication, and to loss of elasticity and thinning of vaginal wall tissue. This does not usually occur until a couple of years after menopause, and is helped dramatically by local oestrogen preparations or systemic oestrogen supplements – those taken orally or applied as a patch.

You can also use a nonhormonal vaginal lubricant or moisturizer. Many women find that applying a water-based lubricant such as KY Jelly is all they need, and rather than being a 'treatment' this becomes an enhancement of sexual pleasure. Vaginal moisturizers (Replens, KY Long-Lasting Vaginal Moisturizer) act directly on tissue to make it less dry.

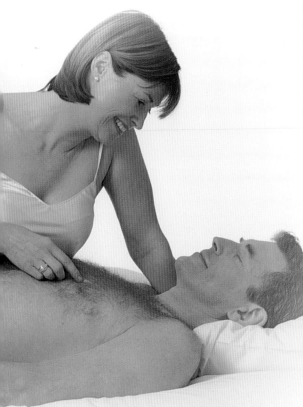

reasons for fantasizing

- ▶ Fantasies are safe ways to experiment with different types of sexual activity.
- ▶ A fantasy helps you more easily focus your body and mind on sexual sensations.
- ▶ Whether or not you share yours, a sexual fantasy can make sex more exciting.
- ▶ A fantasy can substitute for a partner and provide an escape from mundane experiences.
- ▶ The stronger your fantasy life and visualizations, the easier it will be to increase your arousal when you wish.

If you suffer from irritation and burning that also occurs outside of sexual activity, you may prefer to use one of these. Vaginal moisturizers also help to maintain an acidic vaginal environment and may help to prevent recurring vaginal infections.

Regular sexual stimulation, whether by thinking or reading about sex, masturbating or stimulation by a partner – or by having sex – all promote blood flow to the vagina and genital area and encourage the glands producing lubrication to continue to work and keep tissues in that area responsive longer. Time spent flirting, undressing each other, kissing and touching, will help to build arousal, which takes longer as you get older. The more time spent on these preliminary activities, the greater the chance for arousal and natural lubrication.

Think Sexy

For women, the brain is the most important organ of desire. If you are thinking about problems at work or at home you stand little chance of getting excited sexually. If you think about sex, however, your body starts to prepare you for action. To help preserve your sexuality, start thinking about sex, any time, anywhere – your early sexual experiences, your most exciting partner, the most risky sex, sex in a film…. Get your partner involved. Discuss what you would both like to try, things you used to do, what you might enjoy about different sexual techniques – even if you have only read about them. Try telling your partner what you enjoy most about foreplay, and show him or her how you like it done or share one of your fantasies.

By middle age most couples have developed a routine for sex; same night, same place, same position. Variety can be the spice in your sex life. If you normally have sex at night, have sex in the afternoon – and talk afterwards; don't go to sleep. Instead of in bed, try sex in the garden or in the bathroom, and remember there are 68 more positions than the missionary! Go somewhere

WISE WOMAN
Libido
•

Many medicines prescribed for general illness have an adverse effect on libido. If you are taking any prescribed medication, including pills for high blood pressure, depression or water retention, you should consult your doctor to check side effects and discuss alternative therapy. Antihistamine pills have a drying effect on all mucous membranes and may be a cause of your discomfort.

special or do something different with your partner, suggest skipping dessert in the restaurant and returning home for sex with coffee. Book secretly into a local hotel for a night and imagine you are having an illicit affair.

You may have to make some changes to your normal routine simply for comfort, so try some of the possibilities shown on pages 90–91.

Keep Your Hands in Touch
Because your skin will become less sensitive, touch and massage become more important, so take time to touch your partner all over and encourage him or her to do the same to you. Massage each other or share a shower, washing

SENSUAL MASSAGE

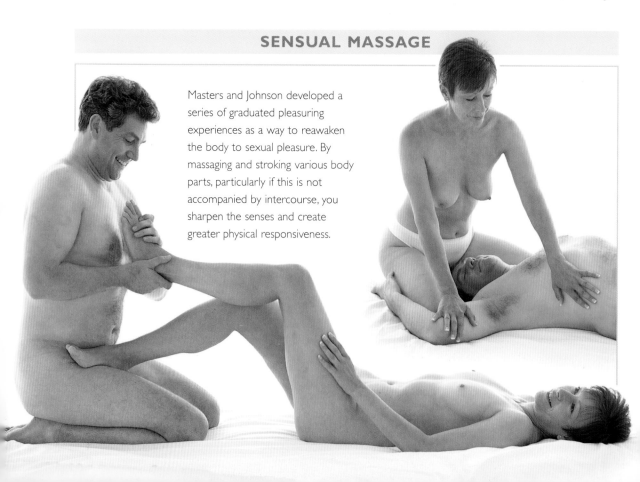

Masters and Johnson developed a series of graduated pleasuring experiences as a way to reawaken the body to sexual pleasure. By massaging and stroking various body parts, particularly if this is not accompanied by intercourse, you sharpen the senses and create greater physical responsiveness.

each other and taking care to touch the most sensitive areas. Wash your breasts with lots of soap while your partner watches and encourage him or her to help.

One way of maintaining desire is to try sensate focus exercises. You practice playful, non-goal-orientated touching and caressing, and explore each other's body and sensual responses while telling each other what you feel. You may well spend several weeks touching and caressing before attempting penetrative sex and orgasm, but couples who have had satisfying sex in the past and are trying to rekindle desire find that just a couple of sessions of teasing and touching without progressing to sex is often enough. Stopping and starting foreplay, and tempting without reward keep you thinking about sex, make your senses more acute, and your body more responsive.

Keep in Shape

Around menopause, it is more important than ever to exercise regularly. Exercise improves mood by stimulating the release of endorphins and serotonin and improves self-image by maintaining body shape and muscle tone. Any exercise will help to increase libido, but dancing is particularly good.

A firm pelvic musculature plays an essential part in assisting desire and enhancing love-making techniques. If pelvic floor exercises (see page 50) are done regularly, they help to focus your mind on genital sensations and will strengthen the vaginal muscles used to grip the penis during intercourse.

Now is the time to accentuate your shape and not to hide it. Just one new, well-fitting bra can change your figure and the way you think about yourself. Why not be adventurous and invest in lingerie that you find sexy? If you feel good about yourself and confident about the way you look, you will feel sexy and be more attractive.

Try Some Hormonal Help

Despite much research, a cream or pill with Viagra-like effects for women has not been forthcoming. Female sexual desire seems to depend more on being

▶ TESTOSTERONE AND DHEA

Studies have shown that testosterone improves sexual enjoyment and desire, and it is sometimes prescribed to women who complain of loss of libido. Although produced in small amounts by women, it is essentially a male sex hormone and as such can have side effects including increased facial hair and acne. To monitor for harmful effects, blood tests for liver function and lipid levels are done. Testosterone treatment is available as a patch, which has less side effects.

DHEA (Dehydroepiandrosterone) is a contro-versial prehormone produced by the adrenal glands. It is converted to male/female hormones in the body and can increase levels of oestrogen and testosterone, though it declines in production from age 25. It is feared that DHEA can speed the development of cancers dependent on the sex hormones. There is evidence that DHEA has a positive effect on mood, but no evidence that it improves libido. It is not used in clinical situations in the UK.

in the right mood for sex and physical stimulation than on localized effects. The old traditional remedy of champagne, music and candles is still recom-mended. However, some drugs and herbal medicines can have positive effects.

While not having any direct effect on desire and libido, oestrogen improves a depressed mood and maintains the vaginal tissues' elasticity and lubri-cation, thus making sex more enjoyable. Wild yam and red clover are claimed to act similarly.

Ginseng has been taken for generations and is prized for its aphrodisiac effects. It contains compounds similar in structure to human sex hormones and is believed to help hormonal imbalance. It is not, however, suitable for anyone with heart problems, high blood pressure or known oestrogen-dependent cancer.

VARIATIONS TO LOVEMAKING

TIMING AND POSITIONS

Sexual energy varies throughout the day and is often higher in the morning. Making love on arising may prove more pleasurable than at night.

Taking a greater role in initiating sexual behaviour and the positions used will have benefits for both you and your partner. By taking the lead, you'll remove from your partner some of the pressure to perform, particularly useful if he is finding it more difficult to attain and maintain an erection. You'll also be able to choose positions that are more comfortable for you.

FOREPLAY

Both to help you become sufficiently lubricated, and to help an older partner attain an erection, you might enjoy indulging in more prolonged and stronger foreplay. Lingering kisses and constant stroking or sensuous massage, and more tactile stimulation of breasts and clitoris (and penis) may be required to stoke the fires of desire.

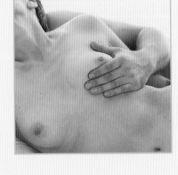

Woman on top positions

These allow you not only to control your partner's depth of penetration and the pace of his thrusting, but also make it easy for you to stimulate your clitoris with your fingers at the same time.

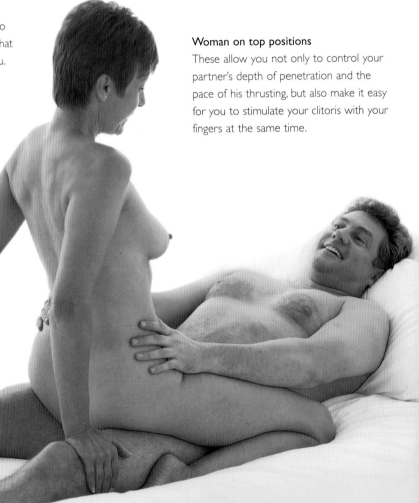

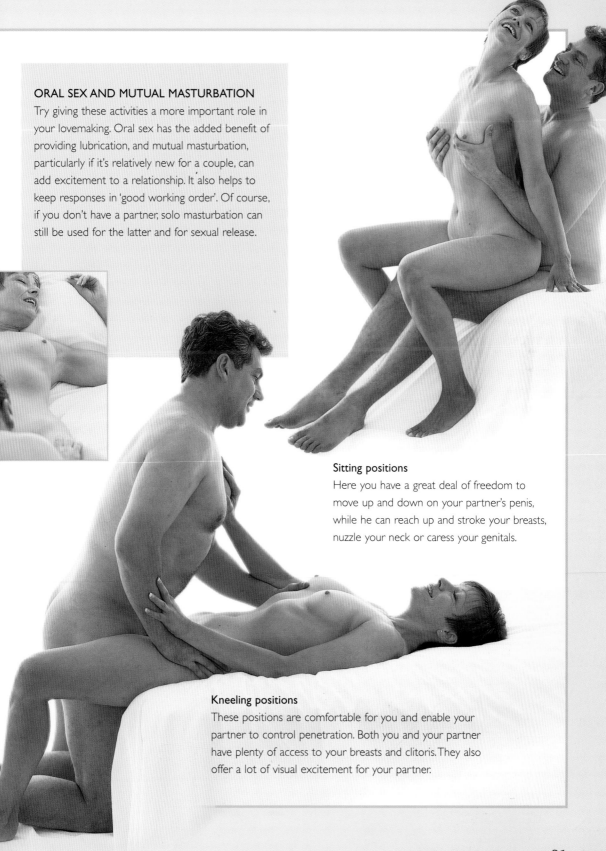

ORAL SEX AND MUTUAL MASTURBATION

Try giving these activities a more important role in your lovemaking. Oral sex has the added benefit of providing lubrication, and mutual masturbation, particularly if it's relatively new for a couple, can add excitement to a relationship. It also helps to keep responses in 'good working order'. Of course, if you don't have a partner, solo masturbation can still be used for the latter and for sexual release.

Sitting positions

Here you have a great deal of freedom to move up and down on your partner's penis, while he can reach up and stroke your breasts, nuzzle your neck or caress your genitals.

Kneeling positions

These positions are comfortable for you and enable your partner to control penetration. Both you and your partner have plenty of access to your breasts and clitoris. They also offer a lot of visual excitement for your partner.

SAFE SEX

Going through menopause does not protect you against STDs (sexually transmitted diseases) or a possible late pregnancy, so when it comes to sexual matters, it is important to play safe.

PROTECTING AGAINST INFECTION

Many women of menopausal age find themselves playing the dating game again and are at risk from a number of STDs – even if they have had a hysterectomy. Along with the sexual excitement that accompanies a new partner or partners, syphilis, chlamydia, gonorrhoea, hepatitis B and HIV may also be part of the relationship.

Genital warts and herpes are common STDs for women of menopausal age. Genital warts are caused by the human papilloma virus (HPV), the most common sexually transmitted infection in heterosexuals. External warts can appear on the skin of the genitals, or the virus can infect the cervix internally. Some strains of HPV can cause precancerous changes of the cervix, which, if not detected by a cervical smear, can lead to cervical cancer. Ask your partner if he or she has warts and look at his or her genital skin as much as is possible without ruining the sexual experience. Don't rely on a condom to protect you from vulval warts from your partner's external warts. If you see or feel something on your genital area that you think may be a wart, make sure you visit your gynaecologist.

Herpes is now most usually transmitted by oral sex. We have all been very well educated not to have sex if there is a genital blister or lesion. However, most people tend to ignore the innocuous 'cold sore' on their mouths and give each other genital herpes from their oral sores.

Women are more prone to contracting STDs (both man-to-woman and woman-to-woman) yet less likely to exhibit symptoms than men, so infections may not be diagnosed until serious problems develop. Menopause can make women particularly vulnerable because vaginal atrophy makes the delicate vaginal tissue more susceptible to tearing, allowing infection to take hold. See the box, opposite, on the guidelines that must be followed with all new partners or with a long-standing partner who you suspect is not monogamous.

PROTECTING AGAINST PREGNANCY

Most women over 40 are still potentially fertile and even after age 50 there is still a chance of conceiving. Generally a woman is considered sterile if she is over 48 and a year has passed since her last period, but to be safe it is recommended to allow another 12 months before stopping birth control. With the introduction of readily available birth control in the first half of the 20th century, the number of women between 45 and 59 with very young children halved within 40 years.

Women in perimenopause often think wrongly that they are too old to get pregnant. They frequently seek contraceptive advice after a 'scare' over a possible pregnancy. They often use contraception intermittently and stick with the same method just because they have been using it for years. Or, they may be embarking on a new relationship after a time with no partner, and they may have preconceived ideas about certain methods of birth control or be totally unaware of new advances and increasingly effective methods. One example is the 'morning-after' pill, which many older women view as something for young girls who have 'been careless' when, in fact, it is safe, effective and easily available for any age.

Female Sterilization

For women over 45, whose families are complete, sterilization offers permanent contraception. There are various techniques of blocking or cutting the fallopian tubes, including clipping them and cutting or cauterizing, and it is usually done under general

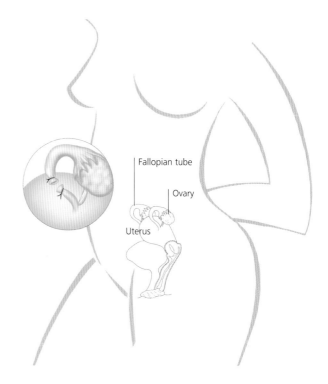

Fallopian tube

Ovary

Uterus

anaesthetic with a laparoscope. Sterilization does not alter menstruation or hormonal changes. The ovum is released as usual from the ovary and travels down the fallopian tube until it reaches the blocked portion, where it dies and is reabsorbed; this is then followed by normal menstruation. The sperm and ovum never join together and fertilization cannot take place. One method of sterilization involves inserting a tiny tube through the cervix and into the fallopian tubes, where a blocking device is deposited and remains. This does not involve cutting the abdomen or entering the abdominal cavity, and therefore lowers the risk of infection and later adhesions. Sterilization only fails if the surgery was not successful or if a clip used to block the tube falls off. This almost never happens and it is a very safe and reliable form of contraception. It is not considered a reversible method, and the decision to undergo sterilization involves pre-operation counselling to ensure that the couple understands this. Regardless of her age, doctors are very reluctant to perform sterilization on a woman who has never had children unless it is for medical reasons. One benefit of sterilization is that cutting or blocking the fallopian tubes seems to lower the risk of ovarian cancer but no one can explain why this should be.

Other methods of contraception, however, are equally effective as sterilization for older women because they are less fertile and tend to use contraception with greater care and compliance.

Combined Oral Contraceptive Pill (COC)

Providing there are no contraindications (see page 95) the combined oral contraceptive pill (oestrogen and progesterone) is considered safe until menopause. Older women using them experience certain non-contraceptive benefits, including a reduced risk of benign breast disease and ovarian, endometrial and colon cancers. They also reduce functional ovarian cysts. The pill has been shown to stabilize or even increase bone mass and so help to fight osteoporosis. It may also give some relief from the symptoms of menopause (see pages 30–59).

In the past it was believed that taking the pill meant you experienced an increased risk of breast cancer, cardiovascular disease and venous thromboembolism (VTE). Pills containing desogestrel and gestodene do have an increased risk of VTE, but others are safer in this respect.

The COC is available in patch form (Evra), and the big advantage – apart from not having to remember to take a pill every day – is that the dose is not altered if you have diarrhoea or bowel disturbance, and some drug interactions are avoided. Any women with abnormal vaginal bleeding should have this investigated by a doctor before starting a method of contraception that will mask it. The patch is not currently used in the UK except under exceptional circumstances.

A new COC, Yasmin, contains drospirenone, and is promoted as helping to reduce weight gain while taking the pill. It has a mild diuretic effect, which can be of help to women who find bloating and water retention a problem while taking the pill. But the difference is in ounces not pounds.

Progestogen Contraception – Pill, Implants, Ring and Injection

The progestogen, or progesterone, only pill (POP), also called the minipill, is less effective at preventing pregnancy than the COC, but in older women whose fertility is reduced it is very effective. However, it does not give very good control of the

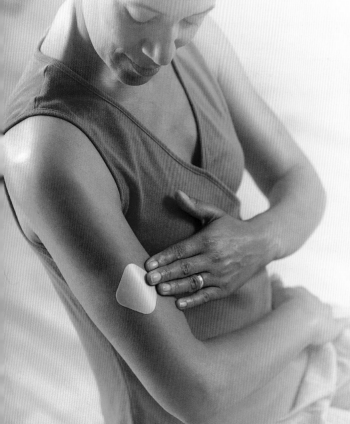

Wearable Contraception

The birth control patch is a sticky patch similar to the one used for HT; it can be placed on the upper arm, abdomen or buttock, and stays on for a week. The patch is changed once a week for three weeks, and then it is removed for seven days, just as the pill is stopped for a week.

menstrual cycle, and some women find the irregular periods and lack of bleeding unacceptable.

The injectable progestogen Depo-Provera is an injection given every three months. It usually stops all bleeding, but it can take up to 18 months after stopping to return to a normal cycle. It is not

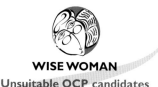
▶ THE PILL AND HT

The Combined Contraceptive Pill contains synthetic oestrogens, which prevent ovulation and give good control over the menstrual cycle. It has disadvantages in that it can create significant prothrombotic changes in the blood raising the risk of blood clots. It is a very effective contraceptive.

HT contains a lower dose of oestrogen and does not suppress ovulation, therefore the ovum can still be released and become fertilized. HT is only one sixth as strong as the COC. Because HT contains a much lower dose of oestrogen it can sometimes be prescribed to women who smoke, have a raised blood pressure or who have a history of migraine headaches.

The Vaginal Contraceptive Ring

Not yet approved for use in the UK, but used successfully in several other countries around the world, the NuvaRing is a synthetic ring that releases both oestrogen and progestogen and is the lowest dose formulation of oestrogen that provides contraception currently available. It is placed in the vagina, and stays there for three weeks and is then taken out for a week. Rarely, women prefer to take it out for intercourse and replace it within three hours, but it is designed to stay in and cannot usually be felt by either partner. It is extremely well tolerated and is the only contraceptive agent that caused no weight gain whatsoever. It has the lowest incidence of breakthrough bleeding and low typical use failure.

advised for use in women over 45 as it can lower oestrogen levels and lead to loss of bone density.

The progestogen implant Implanon contains the progestogen etonorgestrel and is inserted under the skin in a single flexible rod. It acts as a contraceptive for up to three years, after which it must be replaced.

As with other progestogen methods, the most common side effects are irregular periods, weight gain, headaches and breast tenderness, but the rod can be easily removed if the method proves unsuitable

Intrauterine Devices (IUDs)

This method has always been popular, especially with women who do not have a history of heavy periods. The device is inserted through the cervix during or just after a period when there is no danger of pregnancy and the cervix is softer. The copper T-shaped device can remain in situ for up to eight years, depending on the manufacturer, and a copper coil fitted to a woman over 40 may be left in place until menopause. It should be removed one or two years after menopause to ensure adequate

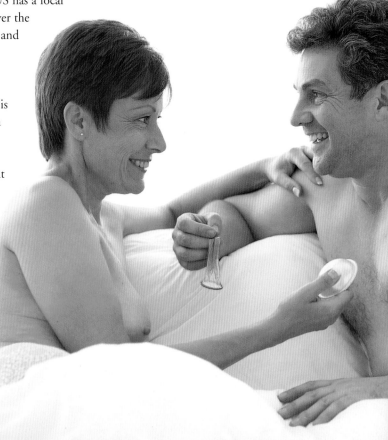

contraceptive protection. As with all intrauterine devices, it carries an increased risk of pelvic inflammatory disease because the threads attached to the IUD pierce the cervical mucus and provide a pathway for bacteria to enter the uterus. At the time of insertion, most doctors take swabs for infection and may recommend antibiotic treatment for a week if the tests show any infection. This risk is reduced in older couples who are more likely to be monogamous. The IUD has an unexpected advantage in reducing the risk of endometrial cancer by as much as 50 percent, probably due to encouraging phagocytes – the cells that clean up unwanted or defective cells.

The Intrauterine System (Mirena) is an IUD impregnated with progestogen. It is inserted in the same way as the IUD and needs to be replaced every five years. It is proving very popular with perimenopausal women whose periods start to get heavier and closer together. The IUS has a local action on the endometrium and over the first year menstruation gets lighter and less frequent, sometimes stopping almost entirely. It is 90 percent effective in reducing menorrhagia (abnormally heavy bleeding). This is unlike the normal IUD, which can make periods heavier. The IUS is being used by some doctors as the progestogen component of HT, but it is not yet licensed for use in this

▶ NONOXYNOL 9

It is true that Nonoxynol 9 is a good spermicide; it kills sperm efficiently. However, it is not true that it is a good microbicide, which means it does not protect against chlamydia or gonorrhoea, and offers no protection against HIV as was once thought.

It has also been found to be a possible irritant to vaginal tissue and if used twice or more in 24 hours can actually increase the risk of HIV transmission. Moreover, there is no evidence now that Nonoxynol 9 increases the efficacy of condoms. Therefore non-spermicidal condoms should be used.

The World Health Organization recommends that Nonoxynol 9 still be used with female barrier methods such as the diaphragm and cap.

way. A smaller IUS is being researched for use by older women.

BARRIER METHODS

In couples aged over 40, condoms have a better-than-average success rate, generally because the users have had plenty of practice using them. However, there is a danger with this method when peri-menopausal or menopausal women start to use lubricants or vaginal oestrogens, as many of these are oil-based and will damage the condom, leading to breaks and tears. Unfortunately it is easy to assume that something recommended to improve your sex life will not harm a contraceptive. This also applies to female condoms, which are like male condoms but larger and with a ring device to hold them in the vagina (see image on page 92).

The Diaphragm or Cap

These are soft latex domes with flexible metal rings that block the passage of sperm to the cervix and hold spermicide in place to kill the sperm. The devices must be inserted into the vagina before intercourse and left in place for at least six hours after. If left in for renewed lovemaking, extra spermicide must be applied after three hours.

They are not always ideal for menopausal women as the spermicide can disrupt an already vulnerable vaginal flora and make some women more prone to vaginal infections. Diaphragms or caps may also increase the chance of contracting cystitis or inflammation of the urethra.

As the vaginal walls become more lax, frequent review of the fit of the cap is recommended. If there is any evidence of a prolapse or of a bulge in the front wall of the vagina (cystocele), it may be better to try a cervical, or vault, cap, which stays in place by suction and sits higher in the vagina only covering the cervix.

Older women who are successful users of diaphragms or caps find that the spermicide often helps with lubrication, and if there are no suitable alternatives, spermicides can be used on their own by women over 50. They provide lubrication and the foam variety is not too messy. Another alternative is the contraceptive sponge; this is a sponge impregnated with spermicide, which you insert into the vagina before having sex, use once and throw away. It is not a highly effective method, but if used by older women its success rate immediately improves and some couples find it more acceptable than the condom.

Natural Family Planning

Also known as the rhythm method, this involves measuring the body temperature with a special thermometer at the same time every morning to detect a small rise in temperature at ovulation, and testing the consistency of the cervical mucus. It is very difficult to interpret around the time of menopause when cycles tend to become irregular and may be anovulatory. It is certainly not recommended as an effective method around this time unless there is no alternative for religious, moral or health reasons.

Emergency Contraception

Both the morning-after pill and IUDs are suitable for women over 45.

The morning-after pill can be taken up to 72 hours after unprotected intercourse and now can be taken as one dose (instead of the previously recommended two doses separated by 12 hours). Whether the two doses are separated or taken together, the blood levels are the same at 24 hours, but with the separated doses there is slightly less side effect of nausea. If vomiting does occur within two hours then another dose needs to be taken. The morning-after pill is available from healthcare professionals and over-the-counter from some pharmacies. It is never recommended as a routine form of contraception but for true emergencies it is an ideal and effective method. Reports of ectopic pregnancy following the morning-after pill are rare, but it is important that any user understands that if the next period is in any way unusual (too light, too heavy, too painful or too late) she should consult her doctor.

An IUD can be inserted up to five days after unprotected intercourse, but the sooner one is inserted the better. It will prevent implantation of the embryo if it was fertilized and needs a follow-up check. The advantage of an IUD is that it can be left in place to continue working as a contraceptive for ten years or more.

Diagnosing Menopause with Hormonal Contraception Use

There are no set rules, and certainly no simple test. If you are using the combined pill or equivalent then suspicion is aroused if you start to get symptoms of menopause such as hot flushes at the end of the pill-free week. If this happens more than once then you can have a blood test to measure levels of FSH (see pages 14–15). If this is normal then it is advisable to continue with the same contraception. If it is raised then you should switch to a non-hormonal method and repeat the FSH test in six weeks. If the second FSH test is high and you are over 50 years old, and have accompanying symptoms of menopause such as hot flushes, then it is highly suggestive of ovarian cessation.

If you are using the progesterone only pill, then you can measure FSH levels while taking this pill. If the first test is high it must be repeated six weeks later, and the same criteria will apply as above. For the injectable progestogen, FSH measurements are not helpful, and it is better to measure oestrogen levels pre-injection if you are worried about falling oestrogen levels.

STOPPING CONTRACEPTION

There is no definitive test for ovarian failure. Unless you've been sterilized or have had a surgically induced menopause, the Family Planning Association advice is that women under 50 years of age must wait for two years to pass after their last spontaneous menstrual period before regarding themselves as infertile. If they are more than 50 years old then one year following the last spontaneous menstrual bleed is considered adequate. Obviously, this an arbitrary cut-off age and you may feel happier allowing two years whatever your age.

A BABY AT YOUR AGE!

More and more women are choosing to delay having children. With adequate birth control available and better antenatal care, women are lucky enough to be able to plan their families … or can they? In many cases, older couples are having to resort to assisted fertilization in some form or other and to stressful and expensive procedures to become pregnant and maintain the pregnancy. Unfortunately, a woman's fertility starts to decline in her mid-20s, with fertility peaking around age 24, and a man's fertility also declines after age 30, albeit not as dramatically. So why wait? Financial security, the knowledge of a mature relationship, a new late relationship, change of heart, career satisfaction – any number of reasons. And now, women tend to be fitter and healthier into middle age so late pregnancy is a definite reality. It is said to be egg quality that is the limiting factor and not the uterus or health of the mother.

WHAT ARE THE RISKS?

These days, with good antenatal care, antenatal genetic testing and excellent special-care baby units, the chances that your baby will be healthy whatever your age are overwhelming. Nonetheless the hazards of childbearing still increase with age. The risk of a mother dying during pregnancy or childbirth is still four times higher for a woman of 45 than for a woman of 25. There is generally a much higher risk of complications, especially for a woman having her first child over 40. The incidence of miscarriage, high blood pressure, intrauterine growth retardation, caesarean section and early or preterm delivery all increase with age.

The risk of a temporary form of diabetes called gestational diabetes, which can affect both mother and unborn child, is nearly seven times higher in women in their 40s than in women in their 20s. Older women are more likely to weigh more for their height, which contributes to the risk of developing type 2 adult onset diabetes in the mother

and causing the unborn baby to become too large, leading to early delivery or caesarean.

In the general population, the risk of spontaneous miscarriage is about 15 percent, but in women over 40 it rises to about 50 percent. This is largely due to chromosomal abnormalities of the fetus, as older women are more likely to have abnormalities of their ova. The incidence of Down syndrome, which is the most common age-related chromosomal defect, is 1 in 365 at age 35 and increases to 1 in 32 at age 45. With blood tests, amniocentesis, chorionic villus sampling and genetic counselling, most known genetic problems can be identified in time for the parents to make an informed decision about the future of the pregnancy.

High blood pressure developing in pregnancy is associated with a condition called pre-eclampsia or toxaemia of pregnancy. This requires urgent treatment and may result in early delivery to save both mother and child, but the mother's blood pressure usually returns to normal after delivery.

ways to increase your chances

If you are over 45 and want to get pregnant you can lower the risks and increase the chances of becoming pregnant with a few simple tips. One doctor calls these her 'pregnancy prescriptions' and recommends them to any woman trying to conceive.

▶ Make sure you are taking folic acid every day to cut the risk of neural tube defects in the fetus.

▶ Watch your weight: less than 95 percent or more than 120 percent of your ideal body weight inhibits conception. However, excessive exercise can lower your chances of getting pregnant.

▶ Decrease or stop your intake of alcohol as even a moderate amount can affect fertility. Your chances of conception are reduced by nearly a fifth with just one drink a week and drop to half with five or six drinks – and don't forget alcohol is bad for sperm too. Caffeine has also been shown to affect conception rate and it is best to reduce or cut it out.

▶ Have sex every other day around the time of ovulation, and if you can't tell when this is, make sure you have sex when you most feel like it. Don't have sex every day as this lowers sperm counts, and don't use lubricants during sex as they can slow down or even kill sperm.

▶ Make sure you get plenty of sleep and buy your partner a pair of baggy boxer shorts to try and maximize sperm production.

▶ Cut out recreational drugs and check the side effects of any medication you are taking, especially tranquillizers, steroids and antihypertensives. This applies to herbal medicines too; St. John's wort has been shown to damage sperm and many herbs, including gingko and ginseng, can have adverse effects on conception and pregnancy.

▶ Both partners must stop smoking.

When statistics are corrected for weight we see that it is not mainly age that is the determining factor here. Older women have no greater chance of developing hypertension or of fetal death if their weight is in the normal range for a 25-year-old.

In the last 25 years the birth rate for twins in older women has more than doubled, particularly for women over 45. This is partly explained by the use of fertility drugs but that is not the whole story. The raised FSH around the time of menopause is likely to cause the ovaries to produce more than one egg per cycle.

Babies of women over 40 are more likely to be in the breech or horizontal position at term, perhaps because older women can be less active or because the uterine muscles are not as efficient. This means there is a much higher rate of delivery by caesarean section as well as forceps and vacuum extraction.

Don't be discouraged, however. The antenatal care now available is excellent, and even with these increased risks your chances of having a successful pregnancy and healthy baby when you're over 40 have never been better.

ASSISTED PREGNANCY

With reduced fertility and the biological clock ticking, it is not unusual for women over 40 to need some help in becoming pregnant. As their periods become erratic or scanty, their chances of ovulating decrease. A blood test to look for progesterone in the second half of the cycle will tell if a woman has ovulated or not.

If there are no apparent problems the first line of treatment will be a so-called fertility drug such as clomiphene citrate, which stimulates ovulation – sometimes with the release of multiple ova. Newer drugs include the gonadotrophin drugs (such as Ovitrelle) and urofollitropins (such as Puregon and Gonal-F), and a very recent synthetic follicle-stimulating hormone drug.

If stimulating ovulation is not enough, then there exists a whole science called Assisted Reproductive Technology (ART) to carry on when fertility drugs don't work, ranging from artificial insemination (AI) to the futuristic-sounding 'ovarian cryopreservation' (see pages 102–103).

With AI, the most straightforward procedure, the man's sperm is introduced into the vagina or at the cervix, or a specially washed specimen is placed through the cervix directly onto the uterus around the time of ovulation.

If the fallopian tubes are blocked or endometriosis is a problem, then in vitro fertilization (IVF) is an option. Here eggs are harvested from the mother, usually after fertility drugs have boosted ovulation so there is a choice of eggs, and fertilized with carefully selected sperm from the male partner. If possible, several eggs are fertilized in a glass petri dish (which is the origin of the term *in vitro* from the Latin for 'in glass'). Up to three embryos are then selected and introduced into the uterus by a thin tube inserted through the cervix, where it is hoped at least one will implant in the wall of the uterus and develop as it would in a conventional pregnancy. IVF is also useful if there is a problem with low sperm count, hostile cervical mucus or unexplained infertility.

Zygote intrafallopian transfer (ZIFT) differs in that the embryos from the petri dish are transferred directly into the fallopian tubes, where fertilization would normally take place.

Gamete intrafallopian transfer (GIFT) is a technique in which a mixture of sperm and ova are introduced into the fallopian tube, where it is hoped one sperm will fertilize one ovum without further assistance.

Intracytoplasmic sperm injection (ICSI) is used mainly when there is a problem with the sperm. The outer layer of the ovum is removed and using a needle several times finer than a human hair, a single sperm is injected into the ovum. The resulting embryo is then transferred to the uterus as with usual IVF treatment. As with all these techniques, a higher success rate is achieved in women under 35, but assisted pregnancies still help many older couples who have delayed or been unable to have children.

CONDITIONS THAT CAN AFFECT FERTILITY

Fibroids are benign tumours of muscle tissue in the uterus. They are usually harmless, but older women are more likely to have them and they can complicate pregnancy and affect conception. In some cases, it is advisable to have them removed before trying to get pregnant. After menopause, fibroids shrink on their own as the oestrogen they depend on diminishes. For some unknown reason, Afro-Caribbean women are far more likely to have fibroids than Caucasians.

Endometriosis is a painful condition where the tissue that normally lines the uterus is found in small patches attached to other organs. The most common sites affected are the bladder, fallopian tubes, ovaries and lining of the abdominal cavity. The displaced tissue responds to the menstrual cycle and may cause pain at the time of menstruation. A quarter of female infertility is due to endometriosis, and the risk of this affecting conception increases with age.

Previous abdominal surgery, infections in the fallopian tubes (pelvic inflammatory disease or PID), polycystic ovary disorder, thyroid disease, uterine polyps and previous damage to the cervix that may have affected mucus production can all inhibit conception.

UNWANTED PREGNANCY

This is an issue for many perimenopausal women. Believing they could not get pregnant even if they wanted to, women in this age group are often very lax about birth control. It is recommended to continue using birth control, both to prevent pregnancy and disease (see pages 92–98).

LOOKING TO THE FUTURE

In October 2004 it was reported that the first baby born to a woman whose ovarian tissue had been frozen, thawed and re-implanted, was delivered in Belgium. The report has met with some criticism, as it may not be certain that the egg came from frozen ovarian tissue and not the untouched ovary left after chemotherapy treatment. The writers of the report claim that 'ovarian cryopreservation' heralds a breakthrough in fertility treatment and shows the way forward to preserve ovaries against disease and aging.

FREEZING EGGS

Whereas we have been able to freeze and thaw sperm successfully for decades, a woman's eggs are harder to collect, and unfertilized eggs have proved very difficult to freeze. This has meant that eggs collected had to be fertilized before freezing. The process for collecting eggs for in vitro fertilization (IVF) takes time, as the woman must be given powerful hormones at a

WHO WILL THIS PROCEDURE HELP?

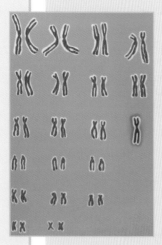

There are several diseases and various medical treatments that can destroy or severely damage ovarian tissue, such as Turner's syndrome, where only one X chromosome is present, and other genetic disorders where pieces of an X chromosome are missing. In these cases, the eggs in the ovaries die more quickly than normal, and women who experience these conditions will usually experience premature menopause.

Any treatment that damages or kills the eggs reduces fertility and hormone production and will lead to early menopause. The chemotherapy drugs cyclophosphamide and vinblastine and radiation treatment to the pelvic area all damage the eggs. The higher the dose of treatment and the older the woman, the more eggs will be lost and early menopause will be more likely.

Cryopreservation of ovarian tissue will mean that a woman can choose not to lose all her eggs due to a disease or medical treatment or simply from natural aging. Ovarian cryopreservation – also known as 'egg banking' – could also benefit women who delay child-bearing until their late 30s or early 40s, when conception rates are already less than 25 percent of women in their early 20s. The ovarian tissue could be collected and frozen in a woman's 20s and kept until later in life when she is ready to become pregnant.

There has been a great deal of controversy surrounding women who have assisted pregnancies and give birth in their late 50s or early 60s. The 'granny mothers', as they have been called, have been criticized for having babies they will be unable to take care of as they grow up.

specific time in the menstrual cycle for two to four weeks in order to stimulate the release of more eggs than usual. Some women may not be able to tolerate this hormone treatment or may have to undergo medical treatment for cancer or another condition before IVF can take place. Some cancers are sensitive to these hormones and the treatment is contraindicated. The woman who is at risk of losing her ovaries and fertility may not have a male partner at the time to fertilize the egg and, rather than find a sperm donor, may wish to keep unfertilized eggs until she has a partner. At the time of writing, only 23 pregnancies worldwide have been achieved using frozen eggs.

THE WAY FORWARD?

This new – and now apparently successful – technique of freezing ovarian tissue means that it may be possible to preserve fertility by removing an ovary through a laparoscope and storing slices of the frozen ovary containing thousands of immature eggs. The ovarian tissue is then thawed and returned to the abdomen near the opening of the fallopian tube or even elsewhere in the body and the eggs are aspirated and fertilized in the laboratory. In around four months, the ovary begins to function again, and normal ovulation and conception can occur.

In women undergoing chemotherapy, only one ovary is removed so that the remaining ovary can continue to produce essential hormones for as long as possible and has the chance to recover after treatment. It has been suggested that it would be surgically simpler to implant the thawed ovarian tissue into the forearm, but pregnancy would obviously only occur if the eggs were removed and IVF performed before implantation of an embryo into the uterus. A woman whose uterus has been removed may choose this option and find a surrogate mother for the pregnancy.

Children from frozen embryos – affectionately known as 'frosties' – are healthy and normal, with no increase in birth defects or developmental abnormalities. There is no reason to believe that those from frozen ovaries will be different in any way.

OVARIAN CRYOPRESERVATION

Several solutions have been identified that protect the cells during the freezing process; these are known as cryoprotectants, and they stop salts building up as water crystallizes during freezing. The cells are frozen to the temperature of liquid nitrogen and are kept frozen and stored in liquid nitrogen.

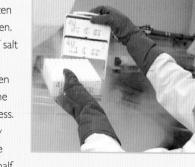

High concentrations of salt and the ice crystals themselves can damage and even kill the cells during both the freezing and thawing process. Freezing takes place slowly over several hours and the thawing takes only about half an hour.

Embryos have been successfully thawed after as long as 12 years. And pregnancy has occurred using an embryo frozen for nine years. We do not yet know how long ovarian tissue can be frozen and remain viable.

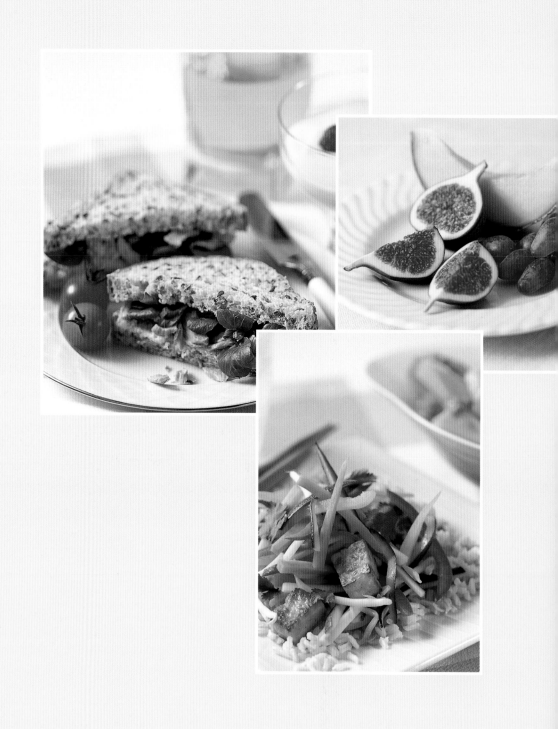

5

A NEW LOOK AT NUTRITION

*Throughout life you can do yourself a great deal of good by
following a healthy, balanced diet – but this is even more
essential at menopause. Eating the 'right' foods, those rich in
vital nutrients, has been proven to reduce the risk of
experiencing certain symptoms of menopause and helps
maintain a healthy weight. Here you'll discover your new
ideal diet and easy ways to make changes.*

NUTRITION AND MENOPAUSE

From the moment of conception and throughout life, the nutrition our bodies receives plays an important role in determining our health, vitality and well-being. In the short term, a healthy, balanced diet can help us look good, feel good and stay in shape. It can increase our resistance to colds and other infections, boost energy levels and improve physical and mental performance. In the long term, it will help protect against diseases such as heart disease, cancer, diabetes, cataracts and osteoporosis. During the menopausal years, choosing the right diet and incorporating certain foods, such as soya, into your diet can also help to alleviate many of the symptoms that commonly accompany menopause and reduce your risk of weight gain.

Interest in healthy eating and nutrition has never been greater; newspapers, magazines, friends and family all offer advice on what we should and shouldn't eat to stay healthy. With this abundance of often conflicting information, it can be difficult to know who to believe or what to eat. On top of this, it may seem as if nutrition experts are constantly changing their minds and moving the goal posts.

The truth of the matter is that the basic advice on what makes up a healthy, balanced diet has remained the same for several decades (see charts below).

GETTING THE BALANCE RIGHT

A healthy diet has several key ingredients but one of the most important is balance. Nutritionists divide foods into five main food groups. To ensure that you get all the nutrients your body needs, you should try to eat some food from each group each day.

Bread, Rice, Pasta, Noodles, Breakfast Cereals and Potatoes

With the current craze for low-carbohydrate diets, you may be forgiven for thinking it's best to avoid foods in this group. In fact, this couldn't be further from the truth. Most nutritionists agree that

---

Bread, rice, pasta, noodles, breakfast cereals and potatoes

5-12 SERVINGS A DAY

1 serving equals
▶ 1 slice bread
▶ 135 g breakfast cereal
▶ 1 medium-sized potato
▶ 100 g cooked pasta
▶ 100 g boiled rice

Fruits and vegetables

5-9 SERVINGS A DAY

1 serving equals
▶ 150 ml unsweetened fruit juice
▶ 1 slice melon or pineapple
▶ 1 apple, orange, peach or pear
▶ 2 kiwis, plums, satsumas or apricots
▶ 100 g strawberries, raspberries or grapes
▶ 1 tbsp dried fruits, e.g., raisins
▶ 135 g fruit salad or cooked or canned fruit
▶ 90 g cooked vegetables
▶ Large bowl salad

carbohydrates are an important part of a healthy, balanced diet. Carbohydrates provide protein, vitamins, minerals and dietary fibre, but their main job is to provide energy. One third of our total calories each day should be provided by foods from this group.

Aim to eat 6 to 11 servings of bread, pasta, rice, etc., a day. Choose complex carbohydrates such as whole grains, whole wheat bread, brown rice and fibre-rich cereals whenever possible. Diets that are rich in whole grain foods have been shown to offer a number of health benefits. One study found that women who ate three servings of whole grain foods a day were 30 percent less likely to suffer from coronary heart disease. Regular consumption of whole grains also appears to lower the risk of certain types of cancer, stroke and type 2 diabetes.

Fruits and Vegetables

Rich in vitamins and minerals, dietary fibre and phytochemicals (see box on page 109), fruits and vegetables offer a vast array of health benefits. The World Cancer Research Fund estimates that a diet rich in a variety of fruits and vegetables could prevent 20 percent of all cancers.

You should aim to eat 2 to 4 servings of fruits and 3 to 5 servings of vegetables a day. Frozen, canned and dried fruits and vegetables as well as fruit and vegetable juices all count. However, no single fruit or vegetable can provide all the vitamins or phytochemicals that contribute to staying healthy, so it's important to eat a variety to ensure you get all the ingredients you need.

Dairy Products (Milk, Yogurt and Cheese)

An important source of calcium, dairy products are essential for strong bones and teeth. Even after your

Dairy products

2-3 SERVINGS A DAY

I serving equals
- 200 ml skimmed or semi-skimmed milk
- 150 ml yogurt
- 100 g cottage cheese or 40 g hard, full-fat cheese, e.g., Cheddar

Meat and meat alternatives

2-3 SERVINGS A DAY

I serving equals
- 55–85 g cooked lean meat, chicken or fish
- 5 tbsp baked beans
- 2 tbsp nuts
- I egg

bones stop growing, calcium is important and particularly during menopause when the decline in oestrogen levels increases the loss of calcium from bone, making postmenopausal women more vulnerable to osteoporosis. Foods in this group can be high in fat, particularly saturated fat, so choose reduced fat and low-fat alternatives such as skimmed or semi-skimmed milk.

Aim to eat between 2 and 3 servings from this group a day, making sure you choose low- and reduced-fat varieties whenever possible.

Meat and Meat Alternatives (Fish, Eggs, Beans, Pulses, Nuts and Seeds)

Foods from this group provide protein, essential for the growth and repair of cells and for the production of enzymes, antibodies and hormones. Foods in this group also provide several important vitamins and minerals. Some of them, such as soya beans and products made from them, are rich in phyto-estrogens, which are particularly important for women going through menopause.

You should aim to eat 2 or 3 servings from this group a day. If you choose meat make sure it's lean, and trim away any visible fat before cooking. At least two servings a week should be fish – one of which should be an oil-rich variety such as salmon, mackerel or fresh tuna. Oil-rich fish are a good source of omega-3 fatty acids, which can help to reduce the risk of heart disease and stroke by helping to lower cholesterol levels in the blood and making the blood less sticky and likely to clot.

Foods Containing Fats or Sugars

Small amounts of fat are necessary in our diet to provide essential fatty acids and to allow the absorption of fat-soluble vitamins, but most of us eat far more than is good for us. A high-fat diet, particularly one that is rich in saturated fats – found in foods such as fatty cuts of meat and meat products, whole milk dairy products, butter and some types of margarine – increases the levels of cholesterol in the blood, and high cholesterol levels can lead to atherosclerosis and an increased risk of heart disease. Prior to menopause, women are protected against heart disease by the hormone oestrogen but as menopause progresses and oestrogen levels decline, the incidence of heart disease in women rapidly escalates.

Monounsaturated and polyunsaturated fats, found in oil-rich fish, olive oil, vegetable oils and nuts and seeds, do not have the capacity to raise blood cholesterol levels in the same way that saturated fats do. In addition, they provide essential fatty acids that help to make the blood less liable to clotting, thus reducing the risk of heart attacks and strokes. For more information on heart disease see pages 119–121.

Sugar provides 'empty' calories – calories that provide nothing else in the way of protein, fibre, vitamins or minerals – so it makes sense to cut down on sugar where you can.

Less fat and sugar doesn't have to mean less flavour. Making small changes, such as switching from whole milk to skimmed milk, choosing low-fat dairy products and lean meat, and using low-fat cooking methods such as grilling rather than frying, can make a real difference.

Total fat should provide no more than between 30–35 percent of your total calories each day. For a typical woman this represents 71 g per day. Saturated fat should provide no more than 10 percent of our total fat intake. For a typical woman this represents 21.5 g per day.

Water

Throughout menopause, as at other times, it is important to drink sufficient water.

Among other essential reasons, unless your body is properly hydrated, it will lack the resources to keep your vaginal tissue lubricated. An easy way to check to see if you're drinking enough fluid is to take a look at your urine; if you are drinking enough it should be a light yellow colour. If it's a dark yellow, you're not drinking enough.

▶ PHYTOCHEMICALS

Phytochemicals, or phytonutrients as they are sometimes called, are naturally occurring compounds that plants produce to protect themselves against bacteria, viruses and fungi. Although they are not nutrients in the true sense of the word because they're not essential in the diet, they are biologically active, and there is a growing amount of evidence to suggest that they can help protect against various types of cancer, heart disease and chronic degenerative diseases like cataracts and arthritis. A group of phytochemicals called phytoestrogens, found predominantly in soya beans and linseed, offer great benefits for menopausal women (for more information see pages 112–114).

Alcohol: Pros and Cons

If you haven't done so before, menopause is certainly a good time to re-evaluate your drinking habits. Throughout your life, your body has been less able to handle alcohol than a man's, and as you get older, your ability to tolerate alcohol decreases. You have less water in your body than a man, so you are less able to dilute alcohol; you also have fewer enzymes to digest it, and the differences in the type and amount of hormones means it is more harmful to your liver and increases the likelihood of strokes. Alcohol disrupts the calcium balance in your body, thus increasing your risk of suffering from osteoporosis.

Having more than one 'unit' a day (a half pint of beer, a small glass of wine or a single measure of spirits) is thought to increase your risk of cardiovascular diseases such as hypertension, stroke and coronary artery disease; falls and hip fractures; and breast cancer. Less serious but still troubling effects include hair and skin becoming dull in appearance, the triggering of hot flushes, insomnia and weight gain.

There are also some positive effects associated with alcohol. Women over 65 who consume no more than 75 ml per week were found to have a decreased risk of hip fractures, possibly because alcohol increases hormone concentrations, which inhibit bone loss. And in women over 50 with a higher than average risk of a heart attack, light to moderate alcohol intake appears to lower their chances of suffering one.

Women should not drink more than 14 units a week. This should be spread over the days and it is a good idea to have at least one alcohol-free day each week.

NUTRITIONAL SUPPLEMENTS

The jury is pretty much still out on whether nutritional supplements such as vitamins and minerals are helpful or necessary during menopause. While some experts believe they do have a role to play, others are less enthusiastic. What most experts do agree on is the fact that supplements are never a substitute for a healthy, balanced diet. As long as you take supplements sensibly, however, they can't make matters worse and may well be useful.

WHAT TO TAKE AND HOW TO TAKE THEM

Vitamin E

Some studies suggest that vitamin E may be helpful in protecting against heart disease by preventing LDL ('bad' cholesterol) from being deposited on the artery walls. Some women also find that vitamin E supplements help relieve hot flushes, vaginal dryness and breast tenderness, and contribute to the health of skin and nails.

Dose: 250 mg twice a day. Supplements containing natural vitamin E (d-alpha tocopherol) are more active.

Caution: Check with your doctor if you are taking anticoagulant drugs or are an insulin-dependent diabetic. The upper safe limit for short- and long-term use of vitamin E supplements is 800 mg a day.

Calcium

A good intake of calcium will help to reduce the risk of osteoporosis. The recommended daily allowance (RDA) for women over 19 years old is 700 mg a day. Many experts believe there should be an increase in the RDA for menopausal women, particularly for those who have chosen not to take HT. In North America the RDA for calcium for postmenopausal women is 1,200 mg per day.

Dose: The body can absorb calcium better if it's taken in smaller doses spread throughout the day rather than in a large dose taken once a day. Ideally, you shouldn't take more than 600 mg at any one time. Calcium supplements are best taken with food because the presence of other vitamins and minerals like magnesium will help to improve absorption. If you also take iron supplements, you should take them at a different time from your calcium supplements. Supplements containing calcium citrate or calcium malate are more easily absorbed by the body than those containing calcium carbonate.

Caution: The upper safe level for calcium supplements is 1,900 mg per day for short-term use and 1,500 mg per day for long-term use.

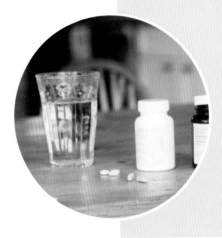

Magnesium

If you take a calcium supplement you should also take a magnesium supplement because an imbalance in calcium and magnesium can reduce the effectiveness of both. Some studies suggest that magnesium supplements may help to reduce the risk of heart disease and lower blood pressure.

Dose: The RDA of magnesium for women over 30 is 320 mg per day. You need to take magnesium and calcium in a ratio of 1:2, so if you take 250 mg of magnesium you need to take 500 mg of calcium. Magnesium supplements should be taken with food to optimize their absorption. Magnesium citrate is most easily absorbed by the body. Large doses of magnesium can cause diarrhoea and nausea – if this occurs try lowering the dose and taking magnesium gluconate, which has a gentler effect on the digestive tract.

Caution: If you have kidney disease seek medical advice before taking magnesium supplements. The upper safe level for supplements is 400 mg per day for short-term use and 300 mg per day for long-term use.

Vitamin D

Vitamin D is essential for the absorption of calcium. You can get vitamin D naturally if your skin is exposed to sun for 15–20 minutes a day. But if you take calcium supplements you should also take a vitamin D supplement. In one large study, postmenopausal women who took 800 I.U. of vitamin D a day (from a combination of food and supplements) had a 37 percent lower risk of developing hip fractures compared with their peers who took less than 200 I.U. a day.

Dose: Vitamin D supplements of 600 I.U. can be taken at any time of the day with or without food.

Caution: The upper safe level for vitamin D supplements is 2,000 I.U. per day for short-term use and 600 I.U. per day for long-term use. This allows for a contribution from sunlight.

Vitamin C and Flavonoids

Some studies suggest that taking vitamin C and flavonoids may reduce the heavy menstrual bleeding that often occurs near the time of menopause. Some people also find taking flavonoids helps hot flushes and mood swings.

Dose: 500 mg vitamin C along with 250 mg of flavonoids twice a day.

Caution: The upper safe level for vitamin C supplements is 3,000 mg per day for short-term use and 2,000 mg per day for long-term use. Women on the contraceptive mini-pill should not take excessively large doses of vitamin C at the same time of day, as this may reduce the pill's effectiveness.

Isoflavones

Current evidence suggests that the benefits of isoflavones are far greater if they are derived from natural foods rather than from concentrated supplements.

Dose: 50 mg per day, choose products containing genisten and daidzein.

Caution: Women who have had or are at a high risk for breast cancer should seek medical advice before taking isoflavone supplements.

PHYTOESTROGENS
A NATURAL ALTERNATIVE TO HT

Over 2,000 years ago, Hippocrates, the father of modern medicine, wrote: 'Let food be your medicine'. Today, many physicians, naturopaths and nutritionists are starting to understand that food can play a key role in preventing and managing many of the health problems associated with menopause. A growing body of evidence is emerging to suggest that a group of chemicals called phytoestrogens, found in foods like soya beans and linseed, can help to alleviate many of the symptoms associated with menopause as well as help to reduce the risk of osteoporosis and heart disease, which are dramatically increased at this time.

Phytoestrogens are also known as plant oestrogens, as they are found in several plants and plant foods, but not in any significant amounts in animal products such as meat or dairy foods. They have a similar structure to the hormone oestrogen and can bind to oestrogen receptor sites throughout the body, mimicking the effects of oestrogen.

There are three main groups of phytoestrogens: isoflavones, coumestans and lignans. The principal phytoestrogens found in the human diet are the isoflavones and lignans.

THE BENEFITS OF PHYTOESTROGENS

Oestrogen helps to regulate the body's temperature and when levels drop, the body has difficulty regulating its heating and cooling mechanisms. While 70–80 percent of women in the Western world experience hot flushes during menopause, only 18 percent of women in China, 14 percent of women in Singapore and less than 5 percent of women in Japan experience them. Many experts believe the fact that the typical Western diet provides around 1 mg of isoflavones a day, whereas the traditional Asian diet contains between 50 and 100 mg a day, may well be the reason why these rates differ so dramatically. Although many studies have shown that incorporating between 40 and 50 mg of isoflavones into the diet can reduce the frequency and severity of hot flushes, several of these studies have been criticized because there is a strong placebo effect. Phytoestrogen-rich diets typically

Phytoestrogen	Found in
Isoflavones	Soya beans and products made from soya beans, lentils, chickpeas, pinto beans, haricot beans, peanuts, millet
Coumestans	Sprouting beans e.g., alfalfa sprouts, mung bean sprouts, soya bean sprouts
Lignans	Linseed, rye bran, whole wheat, barley, sesame seeds, pumpkin seeds. Small amounts in most other cereals, fruits and vegetables

result in a 40–50 percent reduction in hot flushes, compared with a 25–35 percent reduction if nothing is taken, and an 80–90 percent reduction with HT. While the jury is still out on the subject of whether a phytoestrogen-rich diet can ease hot flushes, many women find it does help.

Easing Vaginal Dryness

The cells that cause the vagina to become moist and lubricated in response to sexual stimuli are stimulated by oestrogen, and when levels start to decline the number of these cells also starts to drop. Some studies have suggested that eating a diet rich in isoflavones can prevent the loss of these cells.

Increasing 'Good' Cholesterol

The risk of heart disease rises dramatically during menopause. Oestrogen helps to encourage the production of high density lipoproteins (HDL), which help to protect against heart disease. As oestrogen levels start to fall, this protective effect is lost. Studies have shown that postmenopausal women who supplemented their diets with soya protein experienced a 14 percent improvement in HDL cholesterol in just four weeks. The evidence suggesting that soya protein can help to prevent heart disease is so convincing that the Food and Drug Administration in the United States and the Joint Health Claims Initiative in the UK have authorized food manufacturers to include the following on their packaging: 'Including at least 25 g per day of soya protein as part of a diet low in saturated fat can help to reduce blood cholesterol'. This claim can be used on all foods that provide a minimum of 6.25 g of soya protein and retain its naturally occurring phytoestrogens.

WISE WOMAN
Linseed

•

Linseeds are rich in other phytoestrogens. Sprinkle them over breakfast cereals or stir them into yogurt. Alternatively, try adding them to baked goods such as breads and muffins; you can replace up to one fifth of the flour in a recipe with linseeds. You can also add them to stuffings or breadcrumb toppings. To allow your body to get the most benefit from the seeds, it's best if you grind them. You can do this in a coffee grinder or mini food processor.

Reducing the Incidence of Osteoporosis

The decline in oestrogen levels during menopause increases the rate of calcium loss from bone and as a result makes post-menopausal women more vulnerable to osteoporosis. Women whose diets are rich in phytoestrogens have a lower incidence of osteoporosis.

Moister, Thicker Skin

Oestrogen helps to keep the skin moist and helps to maintain its natural thickness. When levels drop the skin becomes thinner, rougher and less elastic. Some studies suggest that a diet rich in phytoestrogens can help to prevent these effects.

INCLUDING PHYTOESTROGENS IN YOUR DIET

Most of the clinical studies that have shown a benefit from a phytoestrogen-rich diet have used a diet that contains between 20 and 50 mg of isoflavones a day. An intake of 45 mg a day seems to be a level to aim for; this works out to 2 to 3 servings of isoflavone-rich foods a day. Don't be tempted, however, by the idea that 'if a little is good a large amount must be even better'. Studies have shown that as you increase your intake of phyto-estrogens, the proportion that your body absorbs decreases. This built-in safety mechanism means there is very little danger in overdosing from food. The same is not true with supplements, however, and some adverse side effects have been noted in people taking high doses of isoflavone supplements.

There may also be photoestrogens in your diet that, although natural, are not necessarily good for you. Chief among these is coffee, including decaffeinated coffee, which can interfere with progesterone, resulting in migraines (see page 43).

FOODS RICH IN PHYTOESTROGENS

Green soya beans (edamame)
Fresh soya beans in pods are harvested when they are young and tender. When steamed and salted they make a delicious snack. Green soya beans are available from Chinese supermarkets.
▶ 20 mg isoflavones per 100 g

Canned soya beans
These can be added to salads or casseroles or puréed with olive olive, lemon juice and garlic to make a dip similar to hummus.
▶ 80 mg isoflavones per 100 g

Tofu or bean curd
Made from puréed, pressed soya beans, tofu is low in fat and is a good source of protein. There are three basic types: firm, soft and silken. Firm tofu has a texture similar to cheese; it can be marinated and used to make kebabs or cut into cubes and added to stir-fries. Soft tofu is used in recipes that call for blended tofu or in Oriental soups. Silken tofu has a texture similar to set yogurt; it can be used to make dips, salad dressings, sauces or desserts.
▶ 11–30 mg isoflavones
   per 100 g

Textured vegetable protein (TVP)
This is a meat substitute made from soya-bean flour. It is low in fat and rich in protein. It is available as dehydrated chunks, as a ground

beef substitute or incorporated into prepared foods such as burgers or sausages. The ground beef substitute can be used in dishes such as spaghetti sauce or lasagne.
▶ 114–245 mg per 100 g
   (dry weight)

Soya milk
This is available unsweetened or sweetened and in a variety of flavours. Look for one with added calcium. Soya milk is cholesterol-free and available in low-fat varieties. It is also lactose-free. Soya milk can be used in the same way as cow's milk, as a drink, on cereals, in cooking or to make smoothies.
▶ A 250 ml glass provides
   10–20 mg isoflavones

Tempeh
A thin cake made from fermented soya beans, it has a mushroomy, slightly smoky flavour. It can be grilled and used as a meat substitute or added to stews, casseroles or pasta sauces.
▶ 35–191 mg isoflavones
   per 100 g

Isolated soya protein
This powder can be mixed into drinks and sauces or added to baked goods such as bread.
▶ 46–100 mg isoflavones
   per 100 g

Soya flour
Made from ground, roasted soya beans, it comes in full-fat or low-fat versions. It can be used as a substitute for white flour in recipes such as muffins and cakes. It has quite a strong flavour, so it is best mixed with another type of flour; try substituting 20–30 percent wheat flour with soya flour.
▶ 188–276 mg isoflavones
   per100 g

Miso
Made from fermented soya beans, miso is used mainly as a seasoning or condiment. It is very salty and should be used sparingly.
▶ 8–28 mg isoflavones per
   15 ml (1 level tbsp)

Soya desserts
There are many different types including yogurts and ice creams. Isoflavone content will vary according to brand.
▶ Soya ice cream – 4–5 mg
   isolfavones per100 g
▶ Soya custard – 5 mg isoflavones
   per 100 ml
▶ Soya yogurt – 16 mg
   isoflavones per100 ml

Soya and Linseed bread
▶ contains around 7 mg
   isoflavones per slice.
NB Soy sauce, soya oil and soya margarine contain no isoflavones.

MENOPAUSE SUPERFOODS

Superfoods are natural plant foods that have a higher than average nutritional profile. They can be used to supply specific individual nutrients (such as iodine from kelp or dulse seaweed) or blended to deliver a full complement of essential nutrients, including minerals, vitamins, trace elements and micronutrients such as superoxide dismutase (SOD), Coenzyme Q_{10} and various antioxidizing agents. Following is a list of commonly available superfoods and their nutritional benefits. All these superfoods are said to have revitalizing, rejuvenating and cleansing effects on the entire system, and are invaluable in helping us maintain our energy levels and vital physiological functions well into old age.

SPIRULINA
Perhaps the best known of the fresh water algae varieties (which also includes chlorella and blue-green algae), spirulina is an extremely rich source of many essential nutrients, including beta-carotene (vitamin A precursor), selenium (thought to be vital in the protection against arthritis), vitamin B_{12} and the highest natural source of complete protein known (75 percent). It is usually grown in high altitude lakes and is one of the purest foods available.

WHEAT GRASS
A good example of how sprouting a seed or grain can increase its nutritional value (see box on page 116), wheat grass is a potent source of vitamins, minerals and chlorophyll, and it is also mildly cleansing and detoxifying. Usually grown from the

spelt wheat variety, which incurs far fewer allergic reactions, wheat grass is often quite safe even for people with known wheat intolerance.

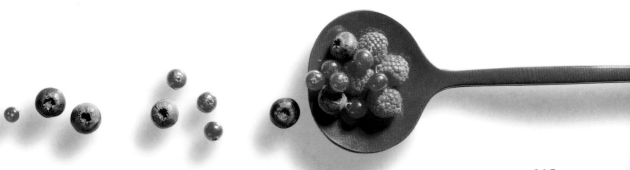

SEA VEGETABLES
The sea itself is a rich source of minerals, which is one reason why sea salt has health-enhancing properties. It is not merely sodium chloride, but should in its original form also contain most, if not all, of the minerals and trace elements necessary for life. Unfortunately, our oceans are becoming an ever more polluted environment, and what was once a vital source of nutritional products now carries unacceptable risks. However, it is still possible to find relatively unpolluted sources of sea vegetables. One of the best is Scandinavian purple dulse. The iodine and other minerals in sea vegetables can support the thyroid and boost a flagging metabolism.

BILBERRY AND OTHER BERRIES
Berries are extremely important foods. There was a time when these fruits would have been staple foods and would have been foraged wild in the woods. They are chiefly known for having strong immune-enhancing properties due to high levels of biofla-vonoids, plant chemicals that have a variety of actions including acting as antioxidants, and helping the body to eliminate free radicals and repair cell

damage. Some, such as bilberry, have other important properties. Bilberry tones and supports the pancreas and adrenals, and therefore assists in the regulation of blood sugar and the maintenance of energy levels. It is also said to be powerfully restorative to failing eyesight.

MACA

This superfood from Peru is actually a tuber, similar to the potato. It has a sweet taste and is perfect for those who have problems maintaining stable blood sugar levels, including diabetics, as it satisfies the craving for sweet things as well as actually helping to regulate blood sugar. In fact it is beneficial to the entire endocrine, or hormonal, system. Like the herb ginseng, it is adaptogenic and helps to impart stamina and resistance, and like ginseng it also has a reputation as a sexual tonic, used to increase fertility, but also in later life to restore a flagging libido, for both men and women.

HOW AND WHEN TO TAKE THEM

Superfoods are often available in powdered form, and can be mixed into drinks, such as fruit smoothies, where the taste of the fruits can help to disguise the occasionally unfamiliar taste. To make a 'superfood fruit smoothie', take some soft fruits – half a banana, some fresh berries, a slice or two of pineapple, or some papaya or mango – and one cup of fresh-pressed apple juice, and place in a blender. Add your favourite superfood or superfood blend, following the package instructions for the dosage, blend and drink.

The best time to consume this drink is in the morning, before breakfast or even occasionally instead of breakfast if you are on a cleansing diet. Apart from being nourishing in their own right, some fruits (like pineapple, mango and papaya) help in the assimilation of nutrients by supplying extra enzymes that strengthen digestion.

Sprouting Beans, Seeds and Pulses

A great way to eat beans, seeds and pulses is to sprout them yourself. Certain nutrients, especially vitamins, can be increased up to fivefold by sprouting, and bean or seed sprouts are also true living foods, with a huge potential in terms of raw vital energy.

To sprout your own beans you will need a seed sprouter, a series of stacking trays – made from clear perspex or glass – with drainage holes and a base tray to catch the water as it drains through. These, along with the seeds themselves, can be bought from health-food shops.

Sprinkle a handful of seeds into each of the trays. You can use one type of seed or pulse per tray, or mix them. Stack the trays one on top of the other, and pour on the water, which will then filter through the layers into the base tray (remember to empty the base tray afterwards). Place the trays on a windowsill in your kitchen, or anywhere that allows them to receive abundant natural light.

Water twice daily, and you should see the first shoots coming up within two or three days.

You can also use a standard jar to sprout your seeds. Cover the bottom of the jar with seeds or pulses, and then use an elastic band to secure a piece of fine cotton muslin or cheesecloth over the top of the jar. The water can be poured in through the cotton, and then out again by inverting the jar, leaving the seeds moist. Water and drain twice daily and soon your jar will be full of lively seedlings.

KEY NUTRIENTS FOR BONE HEALTH

The decline in oestrogen levels that accompanies menopause accelerates the loss of calcium from bone, greatly increasing the risk of osteoporosis. You can help to reduce this risk by making sure your diet contains enough calcium and other key nutrients.

CALCIUM

Our bones are made of a thick outer shell and a strong inner mesh filled with collagen, calcium and other minerals. Calcium is responsible for making the bones rigid and strong. Bones are living tissue, and old bone is constantly being removed and new bone put in its place; calcium gets deposited and withdrawn from the skeleton every day in a process known as remodelling. After menopause, calcium is lost from the bone at a greater rate than it can be deposited, which can result in the bones becoming fragile and susceptible to fracture. In addition to this, since oestrogen assists the absorption of calcium from food, once oestrogen levels begin to fall, the body becomes less efficient at absorbing calcium.

Although the most important time to ensure a good calcium intake is while bones are still growing, calcium is important even after the bones have stopped growing, and particularly around menopause. The recommended daily allowance (RDA) for calcium for premenopausal women is 1,000 mg per day, for perimenopausal women the RDA is 1,200 mg per day and for postmenopausal women the RDA is 1,400 mg per day (for more information see page 110). To meet the RDA of 1,200 mg, you need to eat three servings from the dairy food group each day (see page 107).

If you don't like or can't eat dairy products, make sure you include other good sources of calcium in your diet (see box on page 118). Some brands of mineral water have high calcium contents and can contribute significant amounts of calcium to the

4 calcium depleters

Protein: Intakes in excess of 100 g per day increase excretion of calcium in the urine, which is one reason why many nutritionists are reluctant to recommended high protein/low carbohydrate weight-reducing diets.

Salt: A high sodium intake can cause leaching of calcium from the bones. As a general guide, if a food contains more than 0.5 g of sodium per 100 g or per serving it is high in salt; if it contains 0.1 g or less it is low in sodium.

Alcohol: More than 2–3 units of alcohol a day can damage osteoblasts, the cells that make new bone.

Carbonated drinks: Phosphate, in the form of phosphoric acid, is used as a preservative in most canned soft drinks. Phosphorus is necessary for proper bone formation but it is needed in balance with calcium. Too much of either one can hinder absorption of the other. When phosphorus levels exceed calcium levels in the blood, the body responds by stimulating bone breakdown to release calcium into the blood.

The calcium content of foods

Food	Calcium
100 g tofu	480 mg
100 g sardines, canned in tomato sauce	460 mg
100 g canned salmon (eaten with bones)	300 mg
200 ml skimmed milk	249 mg
200 ml semi-skimmed milk	248 mg
200 ml whole milk	237 mg
small pot (150 g) low-fat yogurt	225 mg
35 g Cheddar cheese	216 mg
35 g reduced fat Cheddar cheese	252 mg
100 g watercress	170 mg
50 g almonds	120 mg
100 g dried apricots	92 mg
115 g baked beans	59 mg
85 g steamed broccoli	34 mg
1 orange	58 mg

Bottled waters (1 litre)	
San Pellegrino	208 mg
Badoit	190 mg
Ashe Park	122 mg
Vittel	91 mg

diet, particularly for women who won't or don't drink milk or eat dairy products. If you live in a hard-water area, tap water also contains useful amounts of calcium; your local water supplier (you'll find their details on your water bill) should be able to give you an idea of exactly how much calcium your tap water contains. In some hard-water areas water can contain as much as 250 mg calcium per litre. In addition to eating a calcium-rich diet, many experts recommend that postmenopausal women take a calcium supplement (for more information about supplements see pages 110–111).

VITAMIN D

Essential for the absorption of calcium, Vitamin D is formed by the action of sunlight on the skin. There are very few dietary sources of vitamin D: oil-rich fish such as herring and mackerel, eggs, fortified margarines and some breakfast cereals. For most women, the main source of vitamin D is the sun. All it takes is about 15–20 minutes of direct sunlight on your hands, arms or face a few times a week for the body to make enough vitamin D to last you through the winter months. The RDA for men and women under 50 is 5 mg per day, but this is based on the absence of adequate exposure to the sun. It's assumed that people in that age group can otherwise achieve all the vitamin D they need from sunlight. After the age of 50 there is an RDA of 10 micrograms a day; this can be achieved only by taking vitamin D supplements.

MAGNESIUM

Needed to convert vitamin D into the active form that the body can use, magnesium may have an important role to play in helping to keep our bones healthy. Good sources of magnesium include Brazil nuts, sunflower and sesame seeds, bananas, pine nuts, cashews and dark green, leafy vegetables such as spinach.

VITAMIN K

This nutrient helps the body to make use of calcium; it improves calcium binding. Recent studies have found that women who have a good intake of vitamin K have denser bones and fewer hip fractures. Foods rich in vitamin K include kale, broccoli and spinach.

BORON

This mineral increases calcium uptake and has mild oestrogenic properties. Boron-rich foods include fruits (like apples, peaches and pears), peas, beans, lentils and sesame seeds.

PROTECTING YOUR HEART THROUGH DIET

Heart disease is the number one cause of death in women over the age of 45. Before menopause, oestrogen encourages the body to produce high-density lipoproteins (HDLs) or 'good' cholesterol, which protects the heart. Once oestrogen levels begin to decline, this protection wears off. While a high cholesterol level is only one of a number of factors known to increase the risk of heart disease (other factors include smoking, sedentary lifestyle, high blood pressure and a family history of heart disease), unlike some of the other factors, we can take positive steps to reduce our cholesterol levels.

'GOOD' AND 'BAD' CHOLESTEROL

Not all cholesterol is bad; it plays a vital role in the functioning of every cell within the body and is essential for the manufacture of certain hormones and other important compounds such as bile, which is necessary for digestion. Cholesterol is transported around the body in the blood and combined with protein in special packages called lipoproteins. Low-density lipoproteins (LDLs) carry cholesterol from the liver to the cells, while high-density lipoproteins (HDLs) carry the cholesterol that isn't needed by the cells back to the liver where it can be excreted. When the liver makes too much cholesterol, LDL cholesterol is deposited on the walls of the blood vessels, in exactly the same way that your pipes can become clogged with lime-scale. This build-up of cholesterol leads to narrowing of the arteries, a condition called atherosclerosis, which restricts the flow of blood to the heart. If the arteries then become blocked by a blood clot, the heart becomes starved of oxygen and damaged. HDL cholesterol, on the other hand, helps to remove cholesterol from the arteries.

The food you choose affects not only LDL and HDL cholesterol levels but also the likelihood of LDL cholesterol becoming oxidized. Oxidation

ways to keep your heart healthy

- ▶ Take regular physical activity. Brisk walking, swimming or cycling will help to increase levels of HDL cholesterol. Exercise also will help to protect your heart in other ways – it will give your heart muscle a good workout, reduce blood pressure, and help you control your weight and deal with stress.
- ▶ Keep your weight within the ideal range. People who are overweight are more likely to have high cholesterol levels. Regular exercise plus a low-fat diet will help you maintain a healthy weight.
- ▶ If you smoke – give up. Smoking reduces levels of HDL cholesterol; it also increases blood pressure and makes the blood more likely to clot.

changes the structure of the cholesterol, making it more likely to stick to the blood vessel walls, and studies suggest that LDL cholesterol that has been oxidized is much more readily deposited in the arteries. Certain foods can also make the blood less sticky and less likely to clot, so that the chances of arteries becoming blocked are reduced.

While medical experts have known about the link between high blood cholesterol levels and heart disease for many years, recent studies suggest that cholesterol is not the only factor involved. High levels of a substance called homocysteine in the blood have also been shown to increase the risk of heart disease and stroke. Homocysteine is an amino acid (a building block of protein) normally found in your body, but if blood contains too much

YOUR CARDIO-PROTECTIVE DIET

EAT MORE

Fruits and vegetables
Both are rich in protective compounds that act as powerful antioxidants, helping to prevent the oxidation of LDL cholesterol and reduce the chance of it being deposited in the arteries.
- Aim to eat at least 5 servings of fruits and vegetables a day.

Soluble fibre
Oats, oat bran, dried peas and beans and apples contain soluble fibre that dissolves in the stomach to produce a gum-like gel that soaks up LDL cholesterol, dragging it out of the body.
- Choose porridge, muesli or other oat-based cereals for breakfast, or sprinkle a tablespoon of oat bran over your regular cereal.

Nuts
Rich in monounsaturated fats and other heart-friendly compounds, nuts help reduce harmful LDL cholesterol and increase protective HDL cholesterol. A recent study found that people who consume small amounts of peanuts, other nuts or peanut butter five or more times a week reduced their risk of heart disease by 50 percent. All types of nuts offer health benefits but it's worth remembering that they are also high in calories – so don't overindulge.

- Try spreading peanut butter on your toast in the morning or adding a few chopped nuts to savoury dishes like stir fries.

Soya
Studies have shown that including 25 g of soya protein in your diet a day can help reduce harmful LDL cholesterol.
- Add soya milk to your cereal in the morning and choose soya yogurts. 25 g of soya protein is equivalent to 600 ml of soya milk.

Alcohol
Studies have shown that for women who have passed menopause, alcohol in moderation (1 unit a day of red wine, spirits or beer) can increase HDL cholesterol and reduce the risk of heart disease by up to 30 percent (see also page 109). Red wine is also rich in a group of phytochemicals called flavonoids, which help to prevent the oxidation of LDL cholesterol. Other good sources of flavonoids include tea, grapes, onions and apples.

Cholesterol-lowering spreads and foods
There are several margarines, spreads, low-fat olive oils, cream cheeses, yogurts, cereal bars and other products on the market that contain a special type of fat that

blocks the absorption of cholesterol. These products have been shown to reduce total cholesterol and LDL cholesterol, and clinical trials have shown that consuming 2–3 servings a day can result in a 10–15 percent drop in LDL cholesterol within three week. Check the dairy and snack food aisles at your local grocery store fo the range of products available in your area.

Oil-rich fish
Fresh tuna, fresh or canned salmon and sardines are rich in omega-3 fatty acids, which help to prevent heart attacks by making the blood less sticky and likely to clot, and by encouraging the muscles lining the walls of the blood vessels to become more flexible, improving the flow of blood to the heart.
- Try to eat at least 2 portions of fish a week, one of which shoulc be an oil-rich variety.

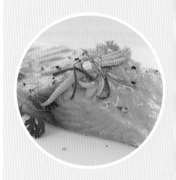

EAT LESS

Saturated 'animal' fats

Although some of the cholesterol in our body is absorbed from the food we eat, the vast majority is made by the liver. One of the factors known to encourage the liver to produce more cholesterol is a diet that is high in saturated fat – the type of fat found in full-fat dairy products and fatty cuts of meat. A diet high in saturated fat will increase levels of LDL cholesterol.

▶ Saturated fats are mainly found in animal foods such as butter, cream, lard, full-fat dairy products, fatty cuts of meat, clarified butter, pies and pastries. Palm oil and coconut oil are also high in saturated fat.

Trans fats

Small amounts of these substances occur naturally in meat and dairy products. They are also produced during the process of hydrogenation used to convert unsaturated oils to semi-solid fats in the manufacture of margarine. Trans fats are believed to have an effect similar to saturated fats on blood cholesterol and may also reduce the protective HDL cholesterol.

▶ Trans fats are mainly found in food containing hydrogenated vegetable oil, such as some types of biscuits, cakes, pastry, margarine and some prepared or frozen meals and fast foods.

homocysteine, it can trigger changes in the arteries that can lead to thrombosis (formation of a blood clot). Why some people have more homocysteine in their blood than others isn't clear. One theory is that it could be caused by an inherited condition that causes an imbalance in the system that controls homocysteine levels. Diet is also believed to be a factor. Many people with high homocysteine levels also have low blood levels of folic acid and vitamins B_6 and B_{12}. Persistently raised homocysteine levels can be reduced by taking supplements of folic acid (for more information on supplements see pages 110–111) Good sources of folic acid include green vegetables such as broccoli and cabbage, liver, dried peas and beans, eggs, whole grain cereal products, brewer's yeast, orange juice and wheat germ.

WISE WOMAN
Fats

Polyunsaturated fats, such as corn oil and sunflower oil, can help lower LDL cholesterol, but if you eat too much they will also lower your protective HDL cholesterol.

Monounsaturated fats, such as olive oil, walnut oil and rapeseed oil, can help to lower the LDL cholesterol but have no effect on HDL cholesterol.

MANAGING YOUR WEIGHT DURING MENOPAUSE

Although weight gain is not an inevitable consequence of menopause, most women find they need to work harder to control their weight at this time. It is often said that HT causes weight gain, but there's no real evidence to support this. In fact, one study found that women taking HT gained less weight than those who didn't. Some types of HT may cause fluid retention and bloating, which can make it feel as if you've gained weight, and some types can increase appetite, but if this happens, simply ask your doctor to prescribe another type. What does happen during menopause is that declining oestrogen levels trigger a change in body shape, and fat starts to accumulate around your middle rather than on your hips and buttocks; this can also make it feel as if you've gained weight.

Although the metabolic rate slows down as we get older, the effect is very modest and not enough to explain the weight gain that many women experience. A more likely explanation is that some of the other changes that can occur at this time may affect eating habits. It only takes a slight shift in the energy balance equation (see box, opposite) for your weight to start climbing. While it's important to come to terms with the fact that your body shape will change with age and some weight gain is usual, it's advisable not to let things get out of control. Obesity increases the risk of heart disease, certain types of cancer, osteoarthritis and high blood pressure. If you do find your weight creeping up, the sooner you address the problem the better. But don't panic; there's no need to resort to crash diets or fads. However tempting their claims may seem, they aren't usually helpful in terms of achieving long-term weight loss. Crash diets encourage a pattern of yo-yo dieting that can be damaging for both your health and your self-esteem. A much safer and more effective way to lose weight is to make small changes to your eating habits, which will lead to a reduction in energy intake, and combine these with increased activity levels, which will result in increased energy expenditure.

Fat Distribution

PREMENOPAUSAL   POSTMENOPAUSAL

TRIM THE FAT

The basis of any diet designed to help you lose weight is to reduce the number of calories that you consume. Gram for gram, fat contains twice as many calories as protein or carbohydrates, which explains why foods that contain a lot of fat also contain a lot of calories. Whatever type of fat you eat – whether it's healthy olive oil or less healthy cream and butter – they contain the same number of calories per ounce. It's because fat is so highly calorific that many diets focus on cutting out as much fat as possible. Although very low-fat diets can be an effective way to lose weight, many people find them boring and difficult to follow for long periods of time. Studies show that moderate-fat diets (diets in which 30 percent of total calories come from fat) are much easier to follow and more likely to produce long-term weight loss. For someone following a 1,400-calorie-a-day diet, this works out at around 47 g of fat per day.

COUNT YOUR CALORIES

A woman's energy requirement varies according to her age, level of activity and weight. The estimated average energy requirement for women aged between 19 and 50 years is 1,940 Cals; for women over 50 the figure is 1,900 Cals. To lose 1 kg a week, you need to reduce your energy intake by around 500 Cals a day, which means that most women should be able to lose weight on around 1,400 Cals per day. It's important to spread your calorie allowance throughout the day; eating little and often is the best way to keep blood sugar levels stable and avoid hunger. Aim for a balance of 300 calories at breakfast, 400 calories for lunch, 500 calories for your evening meal plus 2 snacks of around 80 calories each and a daily allowance of 200 ml skimmed milk for use in hot drinks.

One way to eat less is to add more fluids to your meal. One study showed that people ate fewer calories when they included soup in their meals, because they felt fuller sooner.

The Energy Balance Equation

Our weight is a reflection of the balance between the energy (calories) we consume and the energy we use. Our energy intake is determined by the amount and type of food we eat. Our energy expenditure is determined by a combination of our resting metabolic rate (RMR) and the amount of calories we burn in day-to-day activities.

The resting metabolic rate is the amount of energy our body needs just to keep it ticking over, like the fuel used by a car when the engine is idling but the car isn't moving. Even if we stayed in bed all day, we'd still need to use large amounts of energy just to maintain our body's normal functions. In most people, RMR accounts for between half and three-quarters of the energy required each day. The other component of our metabolic rate is the amount of energy we expend in exercise and everyday activity.

If our energy intake equals our energy expenditure, our body weight will remain stable, but if our intake exceeds our expenditure, the excess energy is stored in the body as fat.

Eating just a small amount in excess of your needs will result in a slow but steady weight gain. To lose weight, you simply need to tip the balance so that you use more calories than you consume; in this situation the body will draw on fat reserves to provide the energy it needs. You can do this by restricting the number of calories you eat or by increasing the amount of calories you use, but without a doubt the best way is by a combination of both – diet and exercise.

✗ High-glycaemic-index foods (GI greater than 50)

Glucose
Honey
Refined sugar
Muesli
Whole wheat cereals
Cornflakes
White bread
French bread
Waffles
Doughnuts
Crispbread

Bagels
Rice cakes
Rice
Biscuits
Parsnips
Potatoes
Chips
Crisps
Melon
Mango
Banana

Pumpkin
Pineapple
Chocolates/sweets
Ice cream
Soft drinks

CHOOSE YOUR CARBS CAREFULLY

With all the hype about low-carbohydrate/high-protein diets you may wonder if cutting out carbs is a good way to control weight. Although low-carbohydrate diets do help some people lose weight, many health experts have genuine concerns about the effects of these diets on our long-term health. One concern is that very-high-protein diets could damage the kidneys and cause leaching of calcium from the bones, increasing the risk of osteoporosis. There are, however, elements of these diets that may be worth incorporating into more traditional weight-reducing diets. Rather than cutting out carbs, think about the type of carbs you choose.

The glycaemic index (GI) is a system of ranking carbohydrates according to how quickly they are converted to glucose. Foods with a high GI are quickly broken down into glucose. In response, the body produces the hormone insulin to transport the sugar out of the bloodstream. The problem is that too much insulin encourages the body to store fat, and a growing amount of research suggests that eating a diet that contains a lot of high-glycaemic foods (GI greater than 50) results in increased insulin levels, heightened hunger and weight gain. Foods with a low GI (50 and below) are absorbed more slowly into the bloodstream. Basing your diet around low GI carbs may help you control hunger and weight gain.

UP YOUR PROTEIN INTAKE

Many nutritionists are now beginning to take on board the idea of upping the protein content of the diet slightly. Protein-rich foods such as meat, cheese and eggs are known to be more satiating than carbohydrates. In other words, a protein-rich meal will help you to feel full for longer and so reduce the risk of snacking in between meals. However, it's important to eat only until you are full. Many people gain weight simply because their portions are too big.

Many high-protein foods are also high in saturated fat, the type of fat that increases the risk of heart disease, so if you do want to step up your protein, it's best to select low-fat proteins such as lean meat, lower-fat cheeses and reduced-fat dairy products.

INCREASE YOUR EXERCISE

A combination of diet and exercise is by far the best way to lose weight. Exercise burns calories but it also helps develop muscle tissue. Muscle is metabolically

✔ Low-glycaemic-index foods (GI less than 50)

Fructose
Grapes
Oranges
Apples
Pears
Cherries
Fruit juice
Apricots (fresh and dried)
Milk
Yogurt
Nuts

Pasta
Whole grain bread
Oats
Bran
Carrots
Tomatoes
Broccoli
Watercress
Courgettes
Most beans (including
    baked beans)

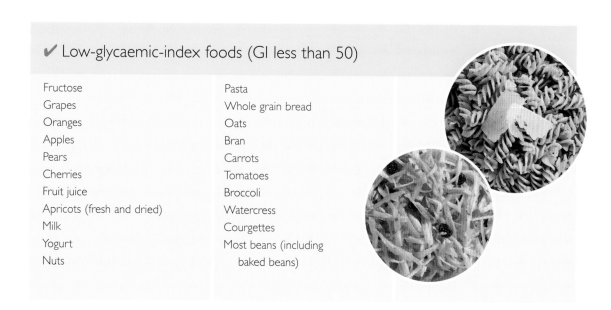

more active than fat (i.e., it uses more calories) so, in other words, the more muscle you have the more calories your body burns. Exercise will also help to improve your body's shape and tone (see also pages 130–151).

UNDERSTANDING YOUR RELATIONSHIP WITH FOOD

We all eat for a variety of reasons, and very often it's out of habit or to satisfy emotional needs rather than in response to hunger. Often we're unaware of these external cues that cause us to eat when we're not really hungry. Some people find it useful to keep a food diary to identify these external cues. Buy a notebook and divide the pages into columns, recording the date, where you were, who you were with (or what you were doing), how you felt, what you ate, and how hungry you really were at the time. Keep a record of everything you eat and drink and how you feel for a month. At the end of the month review your diary and make a list of all the triggers that prompt you to eat when you're not really hungry.

Once you've identified these trigger factors you will be closer to being able to think about solutions and ways to avoid those situations in future. Using

a technique that psychologists call behaviour modification, you can work out strategies that will help you avoid or change the way you behave when faced with these triggers.

If, for instance, you find that when you get home from work you're so hungry that you end up eating a family-sized pack of cheesy snacks while preparing dinner, plan ahead. Have a healthy snack such as a banana or yogurt before you leave the office so you won't be so hungry when you get home.

If your diary reveals that you use food as a way of making yourself feel better when you're unhappy or depressed, make a list of non-food related activities that will help lift your spirits when you're feeling low. Rent a DVD, have a manicure or take a long leisurely bath rather than reaching for a chocolate bar.

We all know that when it comes to losing weight there are no easy answers or quick-fix cures. Old habits are hard to break, and it's not easy to change ingrained behaviour patterns overnight. But by using behaviour modification techniques, you can teach your body to respond differently to external cues.

PLAN YOUR MENU

You can eat well without giving up the pleasure of taste. This day's meal plan gives you an idea of the types of food you should try to incorporate into your diet to give you a wide range of beneficial nutrients and maximize your energy throughout the day.

BREAKFAST
Cranberry juice contains a natural antibiotic that prevents the bacteria that cause cystitis from sticking to the walls of the bladder.
Muesli with linseed and blueberries makes a healthy, high-fibre breakfast rich in phytochemicals. Serve with soya milk fortified with extra calcium to help keep bones healthy.
Soya and linseed bread provides phytoestrogens, dietary fibre and a range of B vitamins. Serve with reduced-sugar marmalade or jam.

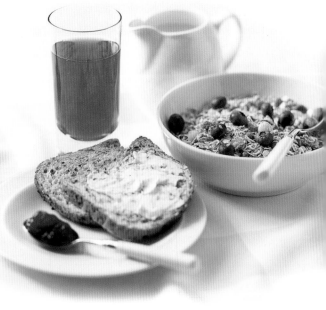

LUNCH
A salmon and watercress sandwich contains some great nutrients. Tinned salmon is a good source of omega-3 fats (mash the small soft bones in with the flesh to boost the calcium content).

Watercress contains 12 times more vitamin C than lettuce and more iron than spinach. It's also rich in several B vitamins, betacarotene, magnesium, potassium and a host of phytochemicals.
Soya yogurt will help to reduce your LDL cholesterol.
A glass of apple juice will boost your daily fruit intake.

MID-MORNING
Banana and soya milk smoothie
- If you use really ripe bananas you shouldn't need to add any other sweetener. Peel, slice and freeze the bananas before you use them: they will help to thicken the drink.

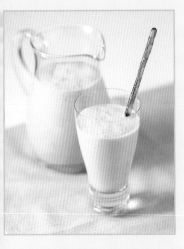

AFTERNOON
Fresh fruit or soya-enriched cereal bar
- Not all cereal bars are as healthy as they look or as low in calories as you might imagine. Choose a bar that contains 150 calories or less and avoid bars that list hydrogenated or trans fats in their ingredients.
- Choosing fruit as a between-meal snack will help you reach your target of at least 2 fruits a day.

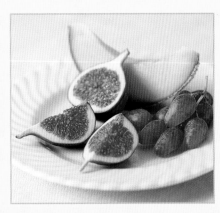

DINNER
Tofu and vegetable stir-fry with brown rice is a tasty meal that's low in fat and rich in protein and phytoestrogens. Stir-frying vegetables such as carrots and peppers in a little olive oil will help to improve the absorption into the blood of some of the vitamins and phytochemicals.

Tropical fruit salad provides a wide range of vitamins, minerals and phytochemicals. Try to eat a spectrum of colours to obtain a mix of different vitamins and minerals.

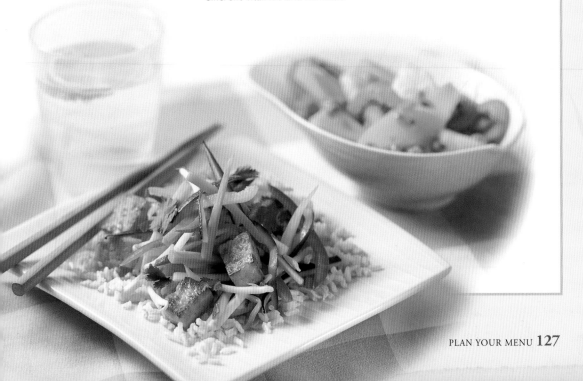

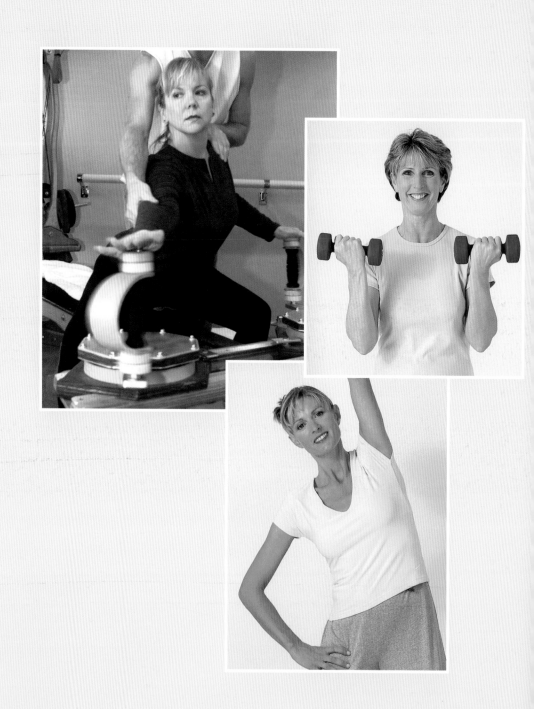

6

REVIEWING YOUR
EXERCISE ROUTINES

*Physical activity is good for you in so many ways. It boosts
your heart-rate, improves blood circulation and increases your
lung capacity. But exercise does more than that – it can
actually make you feel happier. This chapter looks at a
number of different exercise possibilities, their advantages and
disadvantages, and how, by adopting some simple exercise
strategies, you can look forward to becoming healthier, happier
and more active.*

WHAT EXERCISE IS RIGHT FOR ME?

We all know that exercise is good for our health and helps us live longer and better. However, as we go through life's different stages, the type and amount of exercise we need may change considerably. As we age, exercise bestows important benefits, and the older we get the more essential these benefits become to our quality of life. Though some exercises are more beneficial than others, the truth is that *any* exercise you do in addition to your normal level of activity will benefit your health in a very short time.

Apart from the physical benefits of exercise, such as lowering blood pressure and cholesterol levels and helping to control weight, if you exercise regularly you are also less likely to suffer from mental health problems, such as depression, as exercise helps individuals retain a sense of well-being and alertness. Exercise can work as a painkiller and a mood enhancer because it causes the body to release chemicals called endorphins, which not only block pain signals but also affect parts of the hypothalamus, the area of the brain responsible for determining mood.

ASSESSING YOUR FITNESS

The most important thing to do before starting any new exercise regimen is to assess your fitness. You have to determine how much your metabolism needs to increase to allow you to perform the desired activity, and there are several ways in which physical activity can be measured. Our muscles work like furnaces; they burn sugar to generate the energy (calories) necessary for exercise. In order to increase activity, you must increase the calories produced. To achieve a higher level of burning, muscles require more oxygen, which is transported by blood. The first mechanism to boost the amount of oxygen is an increase in pulse rate and breathing frequency, which in turn increases the blood supply and the availability of oxygen to the muscles, while also carrying away CO_2 and lactic acid.

Walk the Walk and Talk the Talk

A quick and easy way of assessing your fitness is the 'walk test'. Find a route, such as a path or sports track, that you know is about 800 m (half a mile) long. Walk the course as briskly as you can without stopping but without getting too breathless. Use a watch to time yourself – it shouldn't take more than 20 minutes, but if it does, don't worry, this is simply a starting point from which you can gauge your progress. After you have begun regular exercise, repeat the walk test periodically to check how much you have improved, and try to keep a note of your findings.

Then you need to know the level of intensity of the activity you are engaging in. The easiest way to do this is by doing the 'talk test', which breaks down

5 reasons to exercise regularly

▶ Exercise will help to reduce the risk of heart attack and other cardiovascular diseases by increasing heart and respiratory capacity.

▶ It will help to prevent osteoporosis by keeping bones strong and healthy.

▶ It will help lubricate cartilage, keeping it supple and reducing the risk of joint problems.

▶ It will keep the muscles around your joints stronger for longer, helping to prevent falls and other injuries.

▶ Should an accident happen, exercise will help to make any injury less severe and quicken its healing.

into three stages:

Light activity, in which you can perform an activity while singing, and in which you would be unlikely to perceive any increase in heart or breathing rate. Most people can carry out light housework and light gardening with this sort of approach.

Moderate activity, in which you can perform the proposed exercise and still talk comfortably while doing it; you will probably perceive a slight increase in heart and breathing rate. The level of workout required to reach this stage will vary considerably from one person to another, according to age and fitness level. However, most people will manage walking and climbing a moderate number of steps in this category.

Vigorous activity, in which a person becomes too out of breath to carry on a conversation. Most people will feel this way after a period of jogging or participating in other sports, particularly those that require almost continuous energy expenditure such as dancing, racket sports and cycling.

Your Maximum Heart-Rate

Another common way of measuring the level of activity is to determine your maximum heart-rate, or MHR. As mentioned earlier, the first mechanism that our bodies will use to compensate for the additional oxygen they need is to raise the heart-rate – increasing the speed with which the blood circulates and boosting the exchanges in the tissues, particularly in the muscles, so that the blood brings more oxygen and glucose and carries away CO_2 and lactic acid.

However, in order for the heartbeat to be effective, the cavity of the heart needs to fill up with the blood that is to be sent through the body, and that takes time. If the heart starts beating too fast, less blood will be sent by each stroke and the whole

WISE WOMAN
Lactic acid

If the amount of oxygen in the blood reduces, the cells start to produce lactic acid, which is a result of incomplete breakdown of the glucose molecule. Too much lactic acid can lead to muscle spasms or 'the burn', conditions commonly felt after participating in some sports.

mechanism may start to fail. In addition, it is necessary for electric pulses to travel through the heart, and after each pulse the contracting cells need to recover; this process imposes a limit on the speed at which our hearts can beat. The maximum heart-rate is therefore the rate at which the circulation of blood would be maximized with the heart continuing to beat at a sustainable pace.

Finding Your MHR

You can determine your MHR by subtracting your age from 220. So, if you are aged 56, your MHR should be 220 – 56; that is, 164. Once you have that, you can further determine the different levels of exertion you need to achieve. So, for moderate physical activity, your heart-rate should be between 50 and 70 percent of your maximum heart rate or, in our current example, between 82 and 115 heart beats per minute (bpm) for the duration of the exercise.

If you want your physical activity to be classed as vigorous-intense, your target heart-rate should be between 70 and 85 percent of your maximum heart-rate. In our example, the heart-rate of a 56-year-old would have to be between 115 and 139 beats per minute (bpm; see chart on page 132).

The simplest way to check your heart-rate is to take your pulse. To find your pulse, place your index and middle fingers just below the base of your thumb. Once you feel the radial artery, count the number of pulses per minute, or count for 15 seconds and multiply by 4.

It is unwise to

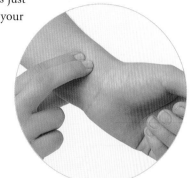

increase your heart-rate beyond 85 percent of your maximum estimated rate for a number of reasons. First, you will not increase the effectiveness of your exercise; second, you will substantially reduce the time during which you will tolerate doing the exercise; and third, you may increase your risk of heart problems such as ischaemic episodes and arrhythmias during exercise.

Putting Your MHR to Use

Sticking to your target heart-rate is very effective and probably one of the best ways to help you optimize your exercise for your aims. If, for example, you want to lose weight, it is probably much more efficient to keep going for a longer time in the moderate zone than to push for a few minutes in the vigorous zone. If, on the other hand, your aim is to increase your capacity and tolerance for exercise, you should remain for as long as possible in your 'vigorous' zone. As you increase your stamina and capacity, your basic heart-rate figures will not change. Instead, what you should notice is that it

takes longer and more energetic exercising to reach the desired heart-rate.

The Bottom Line

The American Heart Association (AHA) has published a paper that claims that if you think you are exercising enough you probably are. Basically, the AHA found that if a person perceives that the exercise she is doing is substantial, that amount of exercise is likely to reduce her risk of a heart attack even if it doesn't reach the formal recommended levels. So, simply by engaging in any exercise that you feel comfortable with means that you are probably reducing your risk.

EXERCISE SAFELY

Assuming that you accept that exercise is good for you and that you are keen to review your exercise routine, the next question is: what exercise programme is good for me? A good programme should include exercises to increase your respiratory capacity, your muscle strength, your balance and

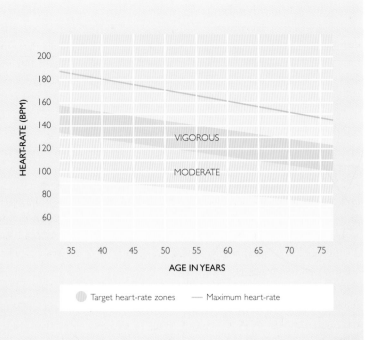

Heart-rate target zone

Use a watch or pulse monitor to check your heart-rate, and aim to exercise at a level that keeps your pulse within your 'target zone'. This should be between 50 and 70 percent of your maximum heart-rate (MHR) for moderate exercise, and 70–85 percent of your MHR for vigorous exercise. You can calculate your MHR by deducting your age from 220 (see example on page 131).

To find your target zone, look up your age on the chart and see where it crosses the orange bands.

HEART-RATE (BPM)

200
180
160
140
120
100
80
60

VIGOROUS

MODERATE

35   40   45   50   55   60   65   70   75

AGE IN YEARS

Target heart-rate zones   — Maximum heart-rate

your flexibility. Most important, it should be safe and pleasurable. The sheer variety of possible combinations should ensure that you find some physical activity to suit your interests. However, safety is paramount.

Listen to Your Body

It has been said that the greatest risk associated with exercise is actually not doing it at all. We've all heard of someone who had a heart attack in the gym or while jogging, and that is often used as an excuse for not exercising. However, according to the U.S. Centers for Disease Control (CDC), sudden deaths due to underlying cardiovascular disease are extremely rare, particularly among individuals participating in moderate-intensity physical activity. Obviously, people who have had a major cardio-vascular event should have a clinical examination before starting exercise, and should undertake an exercise programme tailored for their abilities.

When you exercise, keep yourself well hydrated by drinking relatively small amounts of water regularly; this will keep you comfortable and increase your awareness of the activity you are engaged in. On very hot days and after very strenuous exercise, there is an increased risk of overheating. Symptoms include excessive sweating, tiredness and dizziness. Almost invariably, over-heating responds to prompt treatment; move to a cooler place and get out of the sun.

In any case, the sensible advice is that if at any time during exercise you feel strange, particularly if you feel any chest pain, you should stop your exercise immediately and seek medical attention. Likewise, if you feel dizzy or breathless beyond what you would expect from the level of exercise you are doing, stop immediately and seek medical attention. However, even if you suffer from a pre-existing condition, your doctor should be able to help you tailor an appropriate exercise programme for you.

The key to exercising safely is to be realistic about the exercise you do, adjusting it for your age and level of fitness. For most adults, exercising for more than an hour a day will not increase their cardio-

Health Checklist

The American Heart Association (AHA) proposes the following checklist to help determine whether you should consult your doctor before starting an exercise programme. If any of the following apply to you, talk to your doctor first:

- You have a heart condition and your doctor recommends only medically supervised physical activity.
- During or right after exercise you frequently have pains or pressure in the left or mid-chest area, left side of the neck, shoulder or arm.
- You have developed chest pain within the last month.
- You tend to lose consciousness or fall over because of dizziness.
- You feel extremely breathless after mild exertion.
- You are on medication for your blood pressure or a heart condition.
- You have bone or joint problems that could be made worse by the proposed physical activity.
- You have a medical condition or other physical reason not mentioned here that might need special attention in an exercise programme (for example, insulin-dependent diabetes).
- You are middle-aged or older, have not been physically active, and plan a relatively vigorous exercise programme.

vascular performance but may increase the risk of complications, including injuries. Injuries are perhaps the most common risk with exercise, but serious injuries tend to be rare, and most minor injuries can be treated quite simply with one or two days of rest.

The Right Gear

To avoid injury and make exercise more enjoyable, wear clothing that is appropriate for the activity. When exercising outdoors on cold days, wear several thin layers so that you can discard items of clothing as you warm up.

Wear appropriate shoes that provide support for the ankles and cushion the feet. Ideally, wear shoes designed specifically for your chosen activity.

T'ai Chi

Often described as 'meditation in motion', t'ai chi's fluid and gentle movements help combat stress and fatigue and improve balance, flexibility, muscle tone and general health. It's best to find a well-qualified teacher when beginning to learn t'ai chi, but once learned its effects can be very life-enhancing

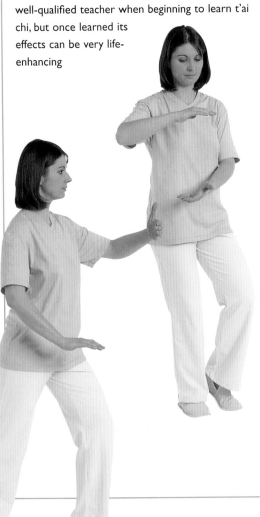

WHAT EXERCISE IS GOOD FOR ME?

In reality, the best exercise for you is the one that you like to do – an activity you associate with pleasure, to which you would like to return regularly, or a sport you would like to develop or keep up.

If you are new to exercise, build up slowly and steadily. A healthy level of exercise will make you feel breathless but still able to talk. Start your exercise session with a warm-up routine and finish with a cool-down (see pages 136–137). The time you spend warming up will depend on the type of activity you plan to do, but in general a warm-up should last about 10 minutes, and include some aerobic activities to raise your heart and breathing rates, followed by some stretches to increase the flexibility and suppleness of your joints and muscles.

A cool-down is similar to a warm-up, but will take about half the time, during which you gradually reduce the intensity of your activity. By doing a cool-down routine you allow your heart and breathing rates to slow down gently, and the stretches will help to prevent any post-exercise aching and stiffness – particularly important for those new to exercise.

Even if you don't have much time to devote to exercise, it's still worth doing a warm-up and cool-down, as they will get your heart and lungs working harder and limber up the joints and muscles so that you feel more fit. They will also reduce the risk of injury, such as strained joints or muscles.

WHAT YOUR CHANGING BODY REQUIRES

From the physical point of view there are essentially four reasons to exercise:

- To increase your cardio-respiratory capacity.
- To increase your muscle strength.
- To increase your flexibility.
- To increase your balance.

Any exercise or physical activity will to some extent achieve all of these goals, but some more than others. The different types of exercise are usually divided into categories, the most frequent being: aerobic exercises, anaerobic or strengthening exercises, stretching or flexibility exercises and balance exercises.

The earlier in life we start these exercises the longer and later we are likely to reap the rewards. However, the good news is that it is never too late to initiate or regain an active lifestyle. No matter how long you have been out of shape, how old you are or how unfit you feel, research shows that changing your lifestyle by incorporating regular, moderate-intensity exercise, can make you healthier and enhance your quality of life.

HOW MUCH EXERCISE IS ENOUGH?

There is no precise answer to this question – but if you are inactive, doing anything is better than nothing! Adults should strive to take on some physical activity of moderate-intensity for at least 30 minutes on five or more days a week. In addition, most adults will benefit from vigorous-intensity physical activity for 20 or more minutes on three or more days a week. If you want to exceed a moderate level of fitness, you need to exercise three or four times a week for 30 to 60 minutes at 50–80 percent of your maximum capacity.

Variety Is Key

Different types of exercise will develop different aspects of your body's abilities. Some exercises, such as walking and swimming, are thought to be particularly good because they exercise almost every muscle in a balanced manner while helping to increase your cardiovascular capacity.

Exercises that rely on repeated movements with weights or against resistance are called strengthening exercises, and they will increase your muscle mass, but in a more localized way. So if you do, for instance, movements with your right arm, only the muscles in that region will be affected and there is relatively little benefit for your cardiovascular capacity. However, if your muscles are stronger you will benefit in the long run because your capacity to exercise will be increased. Flexibility can be increased by stretching exercises, which should also be part of a well-balanced programme, usually before and after the main part of your routine. Finally, many people may benefit from specific exercises for balance, and these are particularly important for women as they age, as balance exercises will help to prevent falls.

7 things exercise does for you

- ▶ It gives you more energy.
- ▶ It helps you to sleep.
- ▶ It helps counter anxiety and depression.
- ▶ It helps you to relax.
- ▶ It helps you cope with stress.
- ▶ It improves your self-image.
- ▶ It gives you an opportunity to socialize and meet new friends.

WARM-UP AND COOL-DOWN EXERCISES

Warm up your muscles and mobilize your joints. A warm-up will enable you to stretch out any lingering aches and pains before your main exercise routine. When you cool down, gradually reduce the amount of effort you put in and come to a gentle stop. You may want to finish with a few minutes of contemplative deep breathing.

1 At the start of your warm-up put on some lively music and begin with a march to mobilize your arms and legs. March gently on the spot, lifting the opposite arm to the lifted knee. March for two minutes.

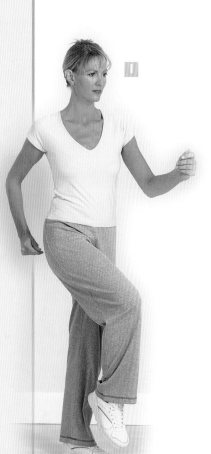

3 The hamstrings, found along the backs of the thighs, are among the most neglected muscles in the body. Stand straight, with your feet hip-width apart. Transfer your weight onto one leg, then slide your other foot forward, keeping it flat on the floor. Put your hands at the top of your standing leg and bend the knee as you bend forward from the hips until you feel a stretch in the straight leg. Hold for a few seconds before repeating with the other leg.

2 Mobile ankles ensure good balance by enabling the joints to respond better on uneven surfaces. Stand straight, hands on hips. Transfer your weight onto one leg and put your other heel forward. Then pick up your foot by bending at the knee, and put your toes to the floor. Repeat six times and then repeat with the other foot.

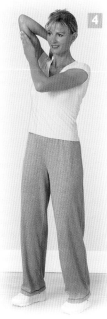

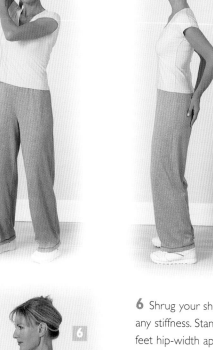

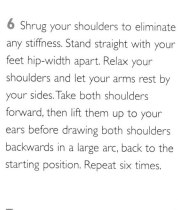

4 Get your triceps, found along the backs of your arms, moving to keep your shoulders supple. Stand tall and put one hand on your shoulder, as shown. With your other hand, ease your raised arm up until you feel a stretch. Aim to get the fingertips of your raised arm between your shoulder blades. Hold for a few seconds and repeat with the other arm.

5 Open your chest and stretch your chest and torso muscles. Place your hands on your buttocks, stand tall, lift your chest and take both elbows back until you feel a stretch across your chest. Hold for a few seconds.

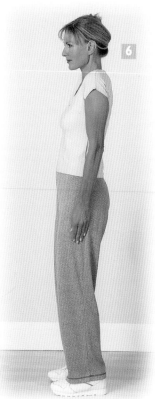

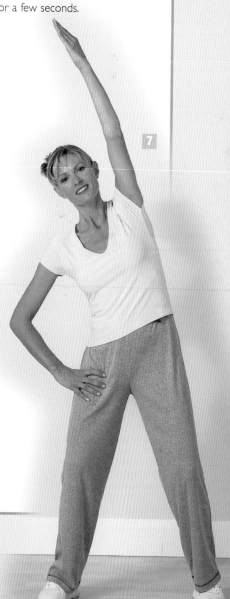

6 Shrug your shoulders to eliminate any stiffness. Stand straight with your feet hip-width apart. Relax your shoulders and let your arms rest by your sides. Take both shoulders forward, then lift them up to your ears before drawing both shoulders backwards in a large arc, back to the starting position. Repeat six times.

7 Stretch the muscles in the sides of your torso. Stand straight with your feet shoulder-width apart. Place one hand on your hip and lift the other hand up to the side. Lengthen your spine, then extend your arm and torso upwards and bend to the side until you feel a gentle stretch down the side of your body. Don't over-stretch. Hold for a few seconds before repeating on the other side.

AEROBIC EXERCISE

Also known as cardiovascular fitness, aerobic exercise increases stamina. It ensures that the heart, lungs and circulation are working efficiently. Sustained, moderate, stamina-building exercises burn fat and, when combined with a weight reduction diet, will help you shed surplus weight. While all aspects of fitness are important, improving your stamina will have the most direct and immediate effect on your health.

THE HEART OF THE MATTER

If performed regularly, stamina-building exercises will make your heart muscles stronger, enabling more blood to be pumped around your body per heartbeat. Because the heart is working more efficiently, it beats less often, and people on a regular exercise routine notice that their pulse becomes slower, even at rest, and that after exercise it reverts to its normal pace more quickly.

Regular stamina-building exercise also expands lung capacity, allowing more oxygen in and removing waste carbon dioxide (CO_2) more efficiently, meaning that you do not get out of breath as quickly. Also, fresh, oxygenated blood reaches the rest of the body's muscles, organs and tissues more efficiently.

To achieve these benefits the heart, lungs and circulation must work harder over a period of regular exercise until they – and you – are fitter than when you started out. The American College of Sports Medicine suggests guidelines for a healthy aerobic routine. They state that we should exercise between three and five days each week, with a warm-up period of 5 to 10 minutes before the more intense aerobic activity. The main routine should keep you within your desired intensity zone for 30 to 45 minutes. After that, the intensity of your workout should be gradually decreased, with a stretching routine and cool-down in the last 5 to 10 minutes. If weight loss is a major goal, your aerobic activity should last for at least 30 minutes five days a week.

Of course, doing aerobic exercises will also increase your muscle mass to a certain extent because your muscles will be moving against some resistance – provided by gravity, water (if swimming) or even your own muscular balance. Many of our muscles act in pairs, working in different directions. The extensors and flexors of the wrist are good examples. Both sets of muscles are acting all the time to provide a smooth and controlled range of movements: the flexors have to counteract the stabilizing force of the extensors when flexing the hand, for example, with similar mechanisms happening across the body. As long as both muscles are worked equally, they will mutually resist each other's pull and maintain a balance.

Exercise Choices

Cycling, dancing, step aerobics – there are many stamina-building exercises that are effective as long as they are sustained for 20 minutes or longer, or until mild fatigue sets in. You can also combine a range of aerobic exercises into a routine to do at home. However, one of the easiest exercises to adopt is walking.

WALKING

A low-impact, weight-bearing exercise, brisk walking compares favourably with other cardiovascular fitness activities such as jogging or aerobics. Basically, if you have been doing nothing at all, gradually building a walking programme will guarantee you benefits. Also, if you have been advised by your doctor to take more exercise or you are recovering from illness, walking could be perfect for you.

The Benefits

Apart from strengthening your heart, walking can boost the amount of HDL cholesterol in your blood, lower blood pressure, and make blood less sticky and thus less likely to clot. Walking has an effect on the likelihood of stroke. Another benefit is that it can help postpone and possibly even prevent the development of diabetes in people who are overweight. Walking also strengthens muscles and bones, making you more flexible, and boosts your immune system to fight off disease. There is even research that suggests walking can have a positive effect in dispelling depression. It can be done any time, anywhere, and does not require any special gear other than a comfortable pair of shoes and comfortable clothes, suitable for the climate.

Walking also has the advantage of variety; anywhere from hills to fields to round the local running track is suitable.

Fitness Walking

The rules for fitness walking are no different from those for any other sport: you should try to achieve a pace that will accelerate your heartbeat and respiration. Fitness walking will work most muscles in the body, with special emphasis on the lower limb muscle groups, which include the quadriceps, hamstrings, calf muscles and glutei. For all variations, good posture should be maintained. Look straight ahead with your chin level. Your arms should move in a natural rhythm, either swinging at your sides or bent at angles up to 90 degrees. Warm up and stretch before your fitness walk and cool down afterwards – and, above all, enjoy!

As you get fitter you will find that you perceive your level of exertion as moderate even though you are now working harder. This shows that your heart, lungs, blood circulation and muscles are adapting to the exercise by becoming stronger and more effective. Perhaps surprisingly you may find that you perspire more freely, too, but this is perfectly natural. It shows that your body temperature-

WISE WOMAN
Benefits of walking

According to research, if everyone in the UK walked briskly for at least 30 minutes a day, the incidence of chronic disease could be cut by 30 to 40 percent.

regulating system is now working more efficiently to dissipate the heat you generate when exercising.

The walking programme on pages 140–141 will help you build up your stamina over 12 weeks. If you follow the programme at the end of this time – no matter what level you started from – you will notice a difference in your fitness, general health and well-being.

Jogging

As you progress through your walking programme, you may be tempted to try jogging. There is good evidence that jogging stimulates bone mineral density (see pages 66–72), especially in the spine and hips, strengthens your muscles, reduces the risk of heart disease and helps you lose weight. The usual recommendation is to jog for 20–30 minutes three times a week, but studies suggest that you can get just as much benefit from shorter periods of jogging – or intermittent jogging and walking. Again, you

3 classifications of walking

Strolling Walking at the rate of about 3 mph with arms swinging loosely at sides.

Brisk walking Walking at a rate of about 4 mph with energetic arm motion.

Race walking Walking at a rate of 5 mph with quicker steps and arms at a 90-degree angle.

BEGINNER WALKING PROGRAMME

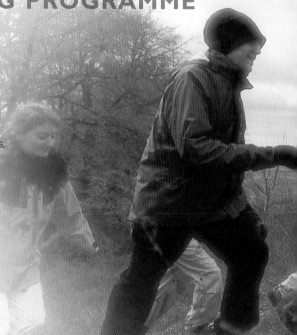

The best way to get the most from walking as an exercise is to walk every day and to increase the frequency, duration, length and intensity of your walk gradually. Keep in mind that 'lifestyle' walking, such as going to the shops, can count towards your daily and weekly targets. So, if you are going to your aerobics class, don't get in the car – get walking!

If you haven't done any exercise, or less than 30 minutes per week, in the past three months, if you are not used to walking, or if you are overweight, this is the programme for you. It aims to get you walking regularly and to get you to a level at which you can walk for 30 minutes at a moderate to brisk pace and not feel breathless, at least five times a week.

WEEK 1

DAY 1 Walk around your local streets or park for about 20 minutes. You can rest after 10 minutes or split your walk into two 10-minute sessions, if you prefer. Try to walk at a 'light-to-moderate' level, or at about 55–65 percent of your maximum heart-rate (see pages 131–132).

DAY 2 Repeat the walk you did on Day 1, thinking about your posture and technique, not worrying too much about speed.

DAY 3 If you found days 1 and 2 tiring, just walk for 10 minutes at a moderate pace. If days 1 and 2 were manageable, explore your neighbourhood for 30 minutes.

DAY 4 Walk for 10 minutes at a moderate pace. Also, using a map and looking at the areas you have explored so far, devise a set route that you can do at any time. It should be 1.5–3 km (1–2 miles) in length with good, even surfaces that will be walkable in all weathers. If possible, make it a route that begins and ends at your front door, and try to incorporate some quiet streets and green spaces.

DAY 5 Try out your set route, timing yourself as you go. Walk at about 55–65 percent of your maximum heart-rate. Note your time.

DAY 6 Walk for 10 minutes at a moderate pace.

DAY 7 Walk your set route at a light-to-moderate level at about 55–65 percent of your maximum heart-rate, and time yourself.

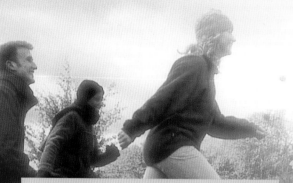

Don't Go Solo!
Make walking a social time – take family or friends; it's not only *you* who needs to walk more, motivate others to join in.

WEEK 2

Walk for 10 minutes at a moderate pace every day this week.

Also, walk your set route at least twice at a light-to-moderate level, increasing your heart-rate to 60–75 percent of your maximum heart-rate. Note your time and try to reduce it – even by a few seconds.

At some point this week, fit in another walk lasting 40 minutes to 1 hour at a light-to-moderate level. Try to make it different from your set route.

WEEKS 6–11

At a minimum, walk for 10 minutes at a moderate pace every day.

Walk your set route twice a week, timing yourself each time and keeping to your improved pace. Start looking at ways of extending your set route for future weeks.

Each week, complete at least one additional longer walk lasting about 1 hour. During this session and your set walk, try to make yourself slightly out of breath for at least 20 minutes, walking at a moderate-to-hard level.

WEEKS 3–5

At a minimum, walk for 10 minutes at a moderate pace every day.

Walk your set route at least once a week. Aim to improve your time by a minute by week 5. While you are walking your set route, spend 5–10 minutes at a 'moderate-to-hard' level, or at about 70 to 75 percent of your maximum heart-rate. This should make you slightly out of breath.

Take two longer walks of between 45 minutes and 1 hour during these three weeks. Try to walk at a slightly out-of-breath pace for at least 20 minutes of the walk.

WEEKS 12+

Walking should now be an integral part of your life. You should be able to walk 1.6 km (1 mile) without becoming exhausted and in less than 18 minutes. If you find this a struggle, continue with the programme for weeks 6–11 until you find it more comfortable.

Start to look at ways of increasing the intensity of your walking – use your arms more, incorporate hills into your set route. Gradually start to lengthen the time you walk and the distance you cover, trying to walk at a moderate-to-hard level for periods of 15 to 25 minutes in any one walk.

ways to stay fit

- Visit a fitness instructor. He or she will devise a programme that's just right for you.
- Join a gym or fitness centre. If variety is what you like, get down to the gym and give some machines a try.
- Exercise in water. Great for all-round fitness, water-based exercise builds muscle strength while also aiding stamina and suppleness.
- Try an exercise DVD or video if you want to start off exercising at home.
- Start a walking club. Encourage other members to take turns organizing walks in different areas.
- Take up a new sport or become re-involved with a sport you used to play.
- Dance the night away. Energizing and fun, all kinds of dance from belly to ballroom, if done on a regular basis, will bring results.

don't have to do this as a structured 'training routine'. You could take a brisk walk/jog to the shops or when you walk the dog. Make sure you warm up before setting out for a jog; it's just as important to loosen your muscles and joints for this type of exercise as for any other. Also, if you have any concerns over your health and fitness for moderate-intensity exercise, if you have arthritis, leg or back pain of any kind, cardiovascular problems or asthma, talk to your doctor before taking up jogging, or stick instead to brisk walking (see box, page 139).

SWIMMING

An excellent aerobic exercise, swimming makes use of almost every muscle in your body. Whereas most mammals swim by instinct, humans need to learn how to swim, so if you have not yet learned and want to start, ask about coaching at your local pool.

Water is a perfect medium for all-round fitness. Because water offers resistance, all water-based exercise builds muscle strength and endurance while aiding stamina and suppleness. Water's buoyancy also reduces impact on the joints, so exercise in water is particularly suitable for overweight people and those with bone or joint problems.

The Right Technique

The most important factor in making swimming an effective exercise is to develop a rhythm or cadence. This is important both for efficiency and endurance. Splashing a lot of water is often an indicator of poor technique and is likely to exhaust you more quickly. You should also be aware of different swimming strokes and, if possible, use a variety, both to add interest and to use different muscle groups. Front crawl is the most popular and the fastest, but endurance is important, so consider breast-, side- and backstroke as well.

Go to your local pool and ask about aquaerobics classes. These low-impact exercises use the resistance of the water to develop endurance, muscle strength, flexibility and balance. You may find it enjoyable to be part of a group exercising in a structured class rather than routinely swimming lengths. You could also try an inexpensive flotation belt, which will allow you to jog in the water. It's a great way to exercise and keep cool.

STAMINA-BUILDING MACHINES

The range of stamina machines available for exercise in the home runs from simple pedal devices to complete mini-gyms. They are known as cardiovascular machines because they are particularly good for the heart and blood vessels. You can choose a treadmill or exercise bike, a climber, a cross-country machine, or a variety of rowers, step or skiing machines.

Machines are available from sports shops and by mail order. Before you buy the machine, decide what you want to achieve and, if possible, try out different types at your local gym until you find one that suits your needs and gives you room for improvement. Sales staff in specialized shops should be able to give you advice and recommend the best machines for you.

Improve Your Moves

The advantage of the more advanced machines is that they can be adjusted to increase the effort involved and so will continue to challenge you as your fitness improves. In the case of stationary bikes, you can increase the amount of friction being applied to the wheel, making it more strenuous to pedal. With treadmills and climbers, the front of the device can often be raised so that you are, in effect, walking or jogging up an increasingly steep incline.

Machines that incorporate a flywheel are usually more expensive but less strenuous than those involving a hydraulic system. These machines allow you to keep going for longer before tiring.

Electronic Gadgets

Top-of-the-range machines usually include computers to monitor both your physical output and your improving fitness levels, thus helping you to fine-tune your exercise programme. They often include gadgets to measure the theoretical distance you have travelled, for example, or the number of calories burned while exercising.

These devices can greatly add to the overall cost and are a worthwhile investment only if you require this level of expertise – and know how to use this information in your fitness programme.

Which Machines Are Most Effective?

In terms of aerobic work there's not a great deal of difference between the machines, as they all achieve the same goals and depend on the amount of effort you put in. But stamina-building machines also provide muscle-toning benefits. For example, step machines, treadmills and stationary bicycles tone the muscles of the legs and buttocks. However, they do little to strengthen the upper body, so, if you are using one, make sure that your fitness routine does not neglect other key areas of the body.

Rowing and cross-country skiing machines are probably the most effective for stamina-building because they exercise the upper body – particularly the arms, chest and abdomen – as well as the legs, and so provide a complete fitness workout.

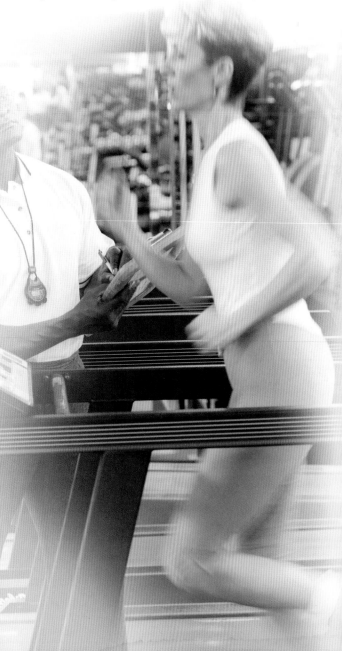

Stay Balanced

If you concentrate your efforts on the treadmill or exercise bike, you do run the risk of developing powerful leg and buttock muscles but weak shoulders, chest and arms. Make sure your routine includes resistance exercises for your upper body.

BEGINNER YOGA PROGRAMME

Gentle, slow-paced stretching and bending poses make yoga an excellent therapy at menopause, bringing energy and balance. There are many more poses than we can address here, but this flowing sequence is a good place for you to start, and may encourage you to practise regularly and even find an instructor who can take your understanding of yoga further.

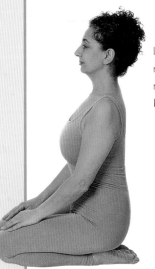

1 Begin by sitting on your lower legs, back straight but relaxed. Try to clear your mind of cluttering thoughts. Inhale, exhale.

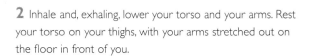

2 Inhale and, exhaling, lower your torso and your arms. Rest your torso on your thighs, with your arms stretched out on the floor in front of you.

3 Inhaling, come up onto your hands and knees. Exhale. Inhaling, keeping your toes tucked under, move forwards to take the weight of your body on your hands and toes. Exhaling, lower your pelvis towards the floor.

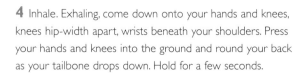

4 Inhale. Exhaling, come down onto your hands and knees, knees hip-width apart, wrists beneath your shoulders. Press your hands and knees into the ground and round your back as your tailbone drops down. Hold for a few seconds.

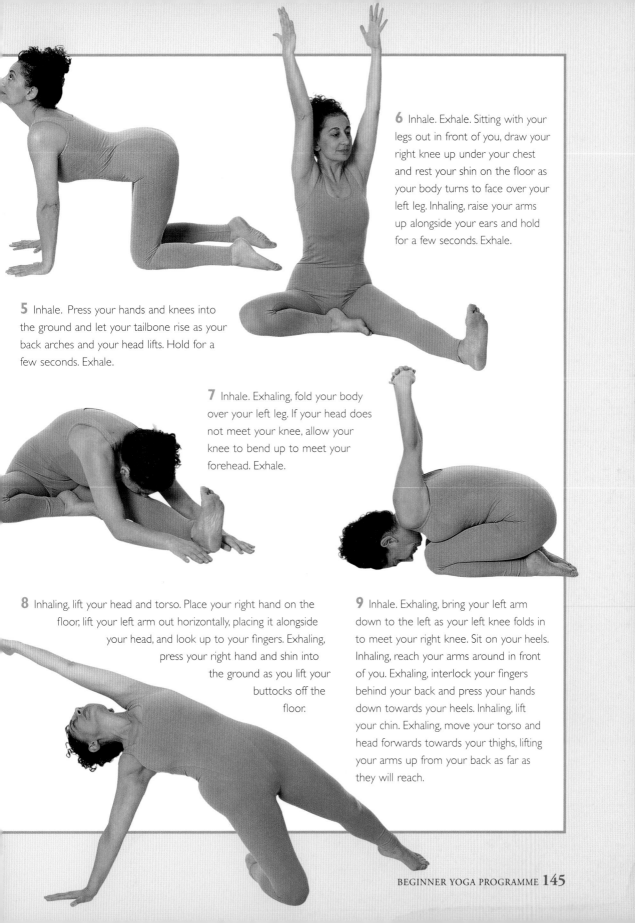

6 Inhale. Exhale. Sitting with your legs out in front of you, draw your right knee up under your chest and rest your shin on the floor as your body turns to face over your left leg. Inhaling, raise your arms up alongside your ears and hold for a few seconds. Exhale.

5 Inhale. Press your hands and knees into the ground and let your tailbone rise as your back arches and your head lifts. Hold for a few seconds. Exhale.

7 Inhale. Exhaling, fold your body over your left leg. If your head does not meet your knee, allow your knee to bend up to meet your forehead. Exhale.

8 Inhaling, lift your head and torso. Place your right hand on the floor, lift your left arm out horizontally, placing it alongside your head, and look up to your fingers. Exhaling, press your right hand and shin into the ground as you lift your buttocks off the floor.

9 Inhale. Exhaling, bring your left arm down to the left as your left knee folds in to meet your right knee. Sit on your heels. Inhaling, reach your arms around in front of you. Exhaling, interlock your fingers behind your back and press your hands down towards your heels. Inhaling, lift your chin. Exhaling, move your torso and head forwards towards your thighs, lifting your arms up from your back as far as they will reach.

INCREASING MUSCLE STRENGTH AND ENDURANCE

As well as building your stamina with aerobic exercise, it's important to build muscle strength and endurance, in order to improve your overall fitness and to tone and condition your muscles for all the small tasks that you do every day.

STRENGTH OR ENDURANCE?

Strength is the ability to lift, lower, push or carry an object of such mass and weight that the effort involved can only be sustained for a short time. You need muscle strength to lift a heavy suitcase into your car or to unscrew the tight lid of a jar. Endurance, on the other hand, is the ability to sustain a level of activity for an extended period. You need it for jobs such as carrying heavy shopping or digging in the garden. Improving muscle strength and endurance will provide you with important health benefits as well as enhancing your quality of life.

Just as aerobic exercise boosts the heart and lungs, so strength training can build up the muscles. Unless a muscle is regularly used, its tone diminishes and it becomes weaker. Unfit muscles are prone to injury, tire easily and limit the amount of activity your body can cope with. It really is worth spending time working on your muscles.

Strength, anaerobic or weight-bearing exercises are a part of a complete routine. Although they will not increase your cardio-respiratory capacity on their own, they will increase your muscle power. This is particularly important because muscle strength will increase your capacity for aerobic exercise, reduce your body fat and increase your lean body mass – which in turn will help you to burn calories more efficiently.

BENEFITS TO WOMEN

Stronger muscles benefit women just as much – if not more than – men, particularly after menopause, because:
- When bone is stressed appropriately through

Gyrotonics

This holistic exercise system is becoming popular worldwide. Created by a former ballet dancer, it incorporates elements of dance, yoga, t'ai chi and swimming, and its pulleys, weights and wheels stretch and strengthen muscles while also mobilizing and stimulating joints. It is taught on a one-to-one basis, and a qualified teacher will help you design a programme specifically for your needs.

muscle movement, it tends to get stronger. Strength or high-impact exercises are the most efficient exercises with which to increase your bone mass or reduce the amount of bone lost.

- After menopause there is a tendency to lose muscle mass, and with less muscle, your body becomes less efficient at burning calories. This change can result in a tendency to gain weight.
- Strength training decreases your risk of falls and increases your stability. This is especially important for older women as it may help to maintain independence.
- Stronger and more efficient muscles protect you from injury during normal daily activities, in particular when performing other forms of aerobic exercise. Exercises to strengthen your trunk will build up muscles in your abdomen and back, helping in turn to prevent low back pain and improve posture.

Just as with aerobic exercise, there is a variety of strength-training routines that you can tailor to your needs. Widely practiced in gyms and health clubs, strength training can be done with free weights or weight-training machines that offer resistance through a system of weights and pulleys. Women of all ages can weight train, and you do not have to be strong to benefit. And don't worry, you are not going to develop huge, bulging muscles – this is about building strength, not bulk. The important thing is to get your programme right. Talk to an instructor at your local gym about structuring a programme that would be suitable for you. Find out how all the machines work. Most gyms have free introductory sessions, so look around until you find one that seems right.

How Often Should I Practise?

When you start to train, 'how often' should be one of your first questions, as with strength training, there is such a thing as too much!

Because strength exercises can be used to target different muscle groups, you could have a session of strengthening exercises every day: you may choose to concentrate on your arms one day, work your legs

on the next day and focus on your trunk on the third day. However, for best results, after a good exercise session you should rest the muscles exercised for two days. Your muscles need this time to respond to the stimulus and build up additional mass. So for instance, if you chose to exercise your arms on a Wednesday it is probably best to wait at least until Friday to re-exercise them. Therefore, three times a week is the maximum frequency.

What Programme Should I Follow?

In general, your programme should be well balanced, exercising the muscles of your trunk (or core muscles), the upper limb and neck muscles, and the lower limb and leg muscles, either in the same session or in alternate sessions.

The trunk muscles are your abdominal and back muscles. They are important because they help to support your body for everything else that you do. If you want to walk, swim, cycle or do any other activity, strong trunk muscles will increase your capacity and reduce pains and strains, including lower back pain.

It's important to note that muscles work in pairs and need to be balanced. For every muscle that contracts, there's an opposing muscle that relaxes;

and when you want to move back in the opposite direction, the contracting muscle relaxes and the relaxing muscle contracts. If opposing muscles lose their balance they can pull your body out of alignment. So, if you have strong stomach muscles but weak back muscles, for example, you may experience lower back problems.

A complete routine would include abdominal curls for your abdominal muscles, upright rowing for your upper trunk and arms, squats for your pelvis and thighs, bicep and tricep curls and grip strengthening for your arms, followed by quadriceps, hamstring and calf muscle strengthening.

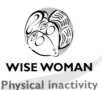

popular resistance aids

▶ Dumbbells can be used singly or in pairs and come in fixed sizes or adjustable types, to which additional weight can be added.

▶ Barbells strengthen the support muscles as well as the main muscle groups.

▶ Ankle and wrist weights increase the amount of resistance used when performing standard strength exercises.

▶ Elastic training bands increase the amount of resistance used in some very straightforward exercises you can do at home.

▶ Gym machines are easy to use and simple to adjust when you want to increase the amount of effort involved. Use the full range of machines to exercise all muscles adequately and decrease the risk of imbalance.

What Weight Is Right?

Use a weight that you can handle safely and comfortably. Start with one that will allow you to complete 12–15 repetitions fairly easily. When you become comfortable with a weight, increase the amount of weight progressively by small increments of 0.2 kg (½ lb) at a time. Too much weight will just tire or injure your muscles; too little will mean that your muscles are not properly challenged.

Bear in mind that strengthening exercises will not increase your physical capacity very much by themselves, so it is essential to alternate them with aerobic sessions. Also, even more than with aerobic activities, it is essential to warm up and stretch before you start your strength exercises and to stretch again at the end. Unless you are also doing isometric exercises, your muscle fibres will tend to shorten during the repeated movements against resistance.

If you want to learn more about using weights, visit your local gym, where an instructor should be able to help you design a strength programme. If you want to start doing resistance-type exercises at home, see pages 150–151 for some suggested muscle-toners.

Check Your Technique

Good posture or 'technique' is essential for strength training, so make sure your chosen weight does not compromise it. If your posture becomes poor – because you are using too heavy a weight or standing incorrectly – you may instead increase the risk of injury and reduce the benefits of the training. Again, talk your gym instructor about your technique to make sure you are not doing more harm than good.

BALANCE AND FLEXIBILITY EXERCISES

As we age, it becomes more and more important to maintain good balance. Your ability to maintain your balance depends on the information your brain receives from three sources – your inner ear, your eyes and the pressure sensors in your muscles and joints. Messages sent back from your brain enable your muscles to make tiny but constant adjustments to your posture, and it's important to have at least some part of your exercise routine devoted to training your muscles to respond automatically to your brain's signals – and keep you balanced.

Although older people have a higher risk of falling, falls can happen to any of us at any time – in the snow and even on the proverbial banana skin. So, if you haven't already started to practise, menopause, with its increased risk of osteopenia, osteoporosis and fracture, is a good time to train your balance. The flamingo stand is an easy way to start, and you can review your progress weekly. You may eventually want to test your balance further by raising both your arms out to the sides. When you feel confident with this, try the single leg squat, in which you stand in an upright position and raise one leg behind you, bringing it parallel to the floor. Keeping your standing leg slightly bent, when you feel reasonably well balanced, squat down by bending your standing leg. When you have gone as low as you can, return to the start position and repeat with your other leg.

If you need to, hold on to a table, wall, heavy chair or kitchen worktop with one hand when you start doing the exercises. When you feel more certain of your balance, try balancing yourself by placing only a fingertip on the surface, and then try the exercises without holding on at all. Ask a friend or family member to watch you in case you're unsteady. Finally, once you're steady on your feet without holding on, try doing these exercises with your eyes closed.

Flexibility exercises such as stretching, Pilates, gyrotonics and yoga (see pages 144–145) also improve balance and coordination.

These examples are by no means exhaustive or complete, but are examples of the types of exercises that will most benefit you at this time.

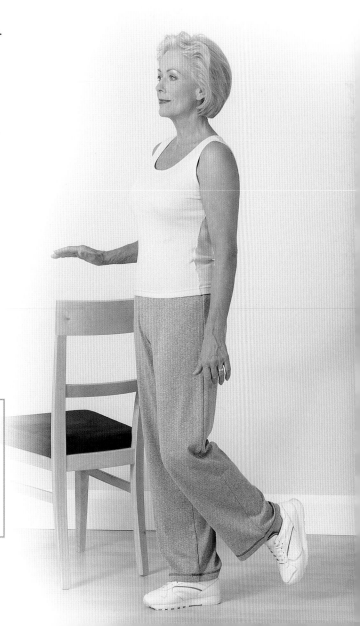

Flamingo Stand
Test your balance by seeing how long you can stand on one leg. Follow your improvement week by week until you can hold the flamingo stand for 30 seconds.

MUSCLE-TONING EXERCISES

These exercises will help to keep your muscles in good shape so that they can work more efficiently and you can do everyday tasks for much longer.

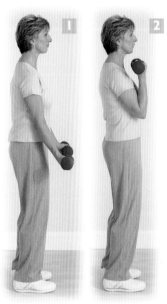
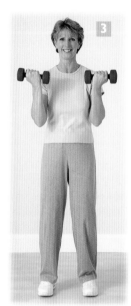

1–3 Arm curls using weights will not only strengthen the muscles at the fronts of your arms, but may help to increase bone mineral density in your wrists – one of the areas most prone to fracture. Be sure that the weights you use are right for you. Use a light weight to begin with and progress by increasing the weight. Stand straight, with your feet hip-width apart and your knees slightly bent. Holding the weights in an underhand grip with your palms facing forward, press your shoulders back and down and lengthen your arms, then curl your arms upwards towards your shoulders. Count to 3 as you lift, hold and count to 3 as you lower. Rest, then repeat 6 times.

TONING WITH AN EXERCISE BALL
Effective and fun, the exercise ball was developed as a tool to help patients recover from injury, but it was soon realized that the ball is useful for all over fitness. Because it is an unstable base on which to work, using a ball recruits many more muscles than those used when you are standing squarely on two feet. You can lift the ball, lie on the ball, sit on the ball – even stand on the ball – there are dozens of progressive exercises to learn, and it's great for people of all fitness levels.

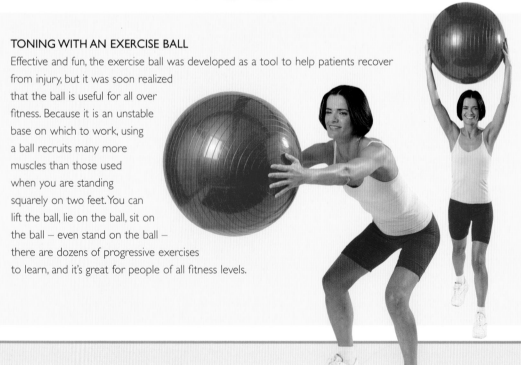

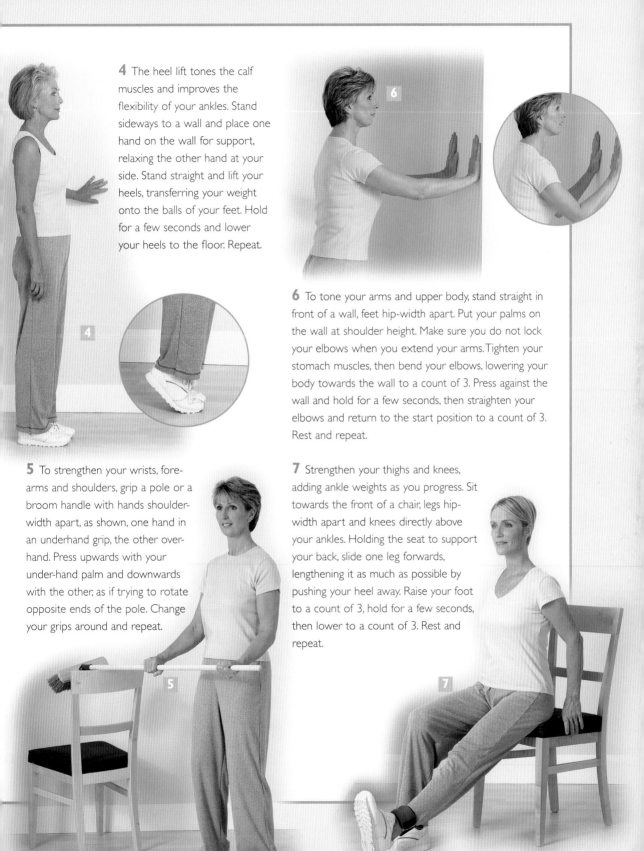

4 The heel lift tones the calf muscles and improves the flexibility of your ankles. Stand sideways to a wall and place one hand on the wall for support, relaxing the other hand at your side. Stand straight and lift your heels, transferring your weight onto the balls of your feet. Hold for a few seconds and lower your heels to the floor. Repeat.

6 To tone your arms and upper body, stand straight in front of a wall, feet hip-width apart. Put your palms on the wall at shoulder height. Make sure you do not lock your elbows when you extend your arms. Tighten your stomach muscles, then bend your elbows, lowering your body towards the wall to a count of 3. Press against the wall and hold for a few seconds, then straighten your elbows and return to the start position to a count of 3. Rest and repeat.

5 To strengthen your wrists, forearms and shoulders, grip a pole or a broom handle with hands shoulder-width apart, as shown, one hand in an underhand grip, the other overhand. Press upwards with your under-hand palm and downwards with the other, as if trying to rotate opposite ends of the pole. Change your grips around and repeat.

7 Strengthen your thighs and knees, adding ankle weights as you progress. Sit towards the front of a chair, legs hip-width apart and knees directly above your ankles. Holding the seat to support your back, slide one leg forwards, lengthening it as much as possible by pushing your heel away. Raise your foot to a count of 3, hold for a few seconds, then lower to a count of 3. Rest and repeat.

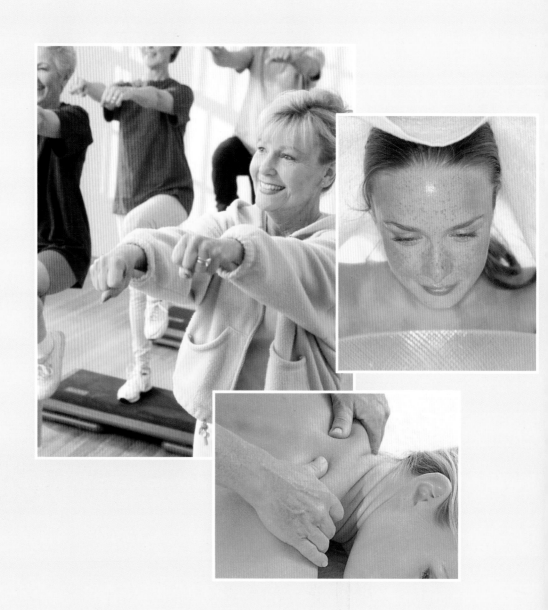

7

A SUPPORTIVE
LIFESTYLE

How we live our lives can affect our experience of menopause. There are things that are within our powers to adopt, adapt or avoid, which can have positive or negative influences on our well-being. This chapter shows women how to review their lifestyle choices and change them for the better.

PSYCHOLOGICAL EFFECTS OF MENOPAUSE

The major impact of menopause is experienced not just on the body but also on the mind and the feelings. In terms of human dynamic, it is a life phase representing a major psychological shift for women. It can seem that one minute you are young and attractive, with the future before you, and suddenly your choices are severely limited, to a point where you become 'invisible'. Finding that others see you so differently provides a shock, especially since the personality within your body continues to feel exactly the same to you – the human being.

Although menopause seems a natural psychological milestone that warrants some grieving (for your former life), it's good to know that there are additional, wonderful advantages. Fifteen percent of all women feel no unpleasant symptoms at all during menopause, and of the remaining 85 percent, the vast majority feel relatively minor side effects that do eventually end. Many women feel a new sense of empowerment. Always remember that the first female British prime minister didn't manage it until she was 54!

PARTLY PHYSICAL, PARTLY EMOTIONAL

It is difficult to separate the effects of menopause on the body from its effects on the brain. That's because they are completely connected. Just as you may have noticed distinct and regular mood swings during your menstrual cycle, during the menopause transition years life may seem one big mood swing – often in what feels like the wrong direction. It's important to understand that your body and mind are going through hormone withdrawal. In this sense you are similar to a reforming drug addict. Your body feels deprived of the oestrogen that has been racing around your tissues for the past 40

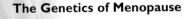

The Genetics of Menopause

Your genetic inheritance will predispose you to experience the change of life in a certain way. Many people think this means they can therefore do nothing to change a long-standing, fixed pattern, which can be particularly depressing because it makes them feel helpless. In fact it's not true. If you know you are likely to have a particular experience you can do a lot to prepare for it. It's always a good idea to gain as much information about your inheritance as possible. Forewarned is forearmed!

years, regulating your body's functions and rhythms. So it's not surprising that you experience a different relationship with your body and emotions.

On top of that, everything else in your life may influence how you experience this major transition. Moods, hormones, sex life, expectations of menopause, all of these connect to influence your physical changes. You can make them worse. You can also make them better.

GENES

We cannot escape from the structure laid down by our genes. But by understanding what our genes may predetermine for us, we can do a great deal to mitigate their effects. So, how could you apply preventive measures to menopause? Start off by taking an instant family history. How did the women in both your mother's and your father's family experience menopause? Did they sail through it without noticing? Or did they have a tough time? The odds are that their experiences will partly foreshadow yours.

You can get further clues of what to expect from menopause by looking back at your own monthly fluctuations during the menstrual cycle. If you have had a child, another clue can be found in how you reacted after childbirth. Women with depressions at key hormonal lows are likely to get depressed when menopause arrives. These predispositions can be indicators. If the indications are negative, work out (in advance) what preventive action you might take – such as hormones, natural treatment, support in the home, or letting your friends and family in on what is happening to you. You can eat differently, reduce stress levels, work on your marriage or your relationship, even arrange rapid medication if that is appropriate.

Sleeping Together ... Or Not

This can be a difficult and emotionally painful consequence of the physical changes. If you share a bed, you may get too hot, too restless or too sleepless. It may make sense to get twin beds or even separate rooms, but emotionally it still may feel like something is ending. Your intimacy is threatened. In order to feel better with a new separateness at night, perhaps you and your partner could agree to sleep apart only on the understanding that you enjoy regular cuddles or even that you start the night off together.

It's also important to see separate rooms in a positive light. It's puzzling that they have received such bad press. As long as you make sure that other aspects of your intimacy continue as you would like, separate rooms can be a lifesaver. You may end up feeling so much better as a result that you wonder why you didn't do it years ago!

HOW MENOPAUSE FEELS

It's normal to feel some sadness for the past and fear for the future. What is important is the way you deal with these feelings and what you make of them.

Negative Feelings

You may feel a loss of sexual attractiveness and therefore a fear that you might be abandoned. Unfortunately, judging from the way some men cope with the anxieties in their own midlife crises, this does sometimes happen. And it is of course the cause of great sorrow. But for every man who leaves his partner at this age there are many others who stay. Plus, there truly is life after the event. Many women who end their marriage in their fifties, perhaps having stayed with a partner to bring up children, have discovered that they fall in love again and experience a new relationship filled with teenage sensation but governed by mature expectation. Many women describe this as the best thing that has

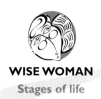

WISE WOMAN
Stages of life

•

We live in such a youth-orientated culture that we expect to feel, look and behave the same forever. Remember: midlife brings crises for both sexes. You lose a former youthfulness, you change, and you then experience another sense of youthfulness, but it's a different one. Be patient with yourself, and ask your family to be patient with you too. Research shows that we can carry on learning and remembering until we die. It's just that we take longer doing it. This does not *mean we are somehow losing intelligence – it just means we are slower. So be patient – and be kind to yourself.*

ever happened to them. It's a myth to think that because your periods have ended you are no longer attractive. You are as attractive as you feel, and you can work on those feelings. Invest in new clothes and make-up and make an effort to socialize.

Also, because you sometimes don't feel so well, you may fear a chronic illness. The years of menopause are times when your body reminds you to take it seriously. This fear can be allayed by following every avenue to good health. If you haven't eaten very well in the past, now is the time to learn a new regimen. If you haven't done much exercise, this is the time to begin. Pilates, yoga, walking and swimming are all activities that promote the production of endorphins. And exercise does more than improve your health; it also increases your sense of well-being.

Another fear may be that, because you are more frequently tired, you can't cope and are 'losing it'. Studies of menopausal women worldwide show that fatigue is their number one complaint. Making new sleeping arrangements (see box on page 155) and/or going onto hormone therapy or alternative health supplements will help. Once you stop feeling tired the depression will be likely to lift.

It can also be tough coping with the way Western society sees older people, especially women. Some women report feeling invisible. Whereas previously men might have eyed them in public, they now have a sense that younger men and women look right through them. This can be difficult, especially if you have been previously considered very attractive. You perhaps have relied on your outer appearance to carry you through social situations. When this has gone, what can you do? You may not be able to get your outer 'visibility' back unless you go to extremes and opt for expensive cosmetic surgery. But you can develop your personality to be more outgoing, funny and sympathetic. You can develop a new look. You can learn wonderful listening skills and you can flirt. Some older women positively relish being older and feeling sexier.

Accentuate the Positives!

For most women, the physical change is gradual. Many women don't understand that even when the ovaries finally stop manufacturing oestrogen the

5 **ways** to help others understand

▶ Tell your partner what to expect. If he doesn't know that there is a reason for your irritability he will understandably get increasingly upset.

▶ Explain that your moods will be a bit like your premenstrual syndrome used to be, only the fluctuation is different, and that once these hormonal fluctuations have settled down they won't return.

▶ Explain that tiredness is not laziness.

▶ Let him know that memory loss is not deliberate.

▶ When you feel fragile try something light-hearted like hanging up an origami paper model as a warning sign to treat you with care!

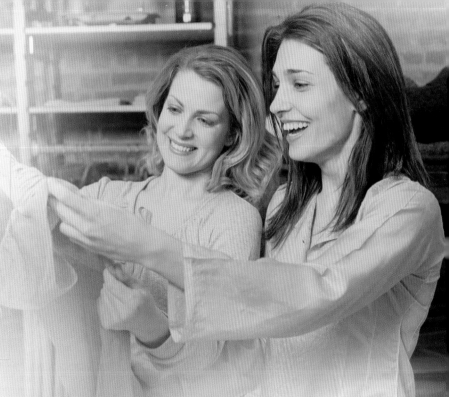

A New You?

There are so many ways in which you can work on how you feel. Pamper yourself a little and think about what could make you feel more positive. It might be a new hobby or pastime, or it could be treating yourself to a new outfit or a change of look. A facial, new make-up, hair style – or colour – don't feel you can't experiment.

adrenal gland carries on for five to ten years longer and, among other hormones, churns out testosterone. This means that without the mitigating effect of oestrogen you may actually feel sexier, more energetic and more effective.

Another thing that no one tells you is that although some of the sexual instinct dies down, this turns out not to matter so much because you are now able to see life without so many ups and downs.

It's also important to remember that good relationships keep going because partners love each other. In fact, a relationship that is strong in later life feels doubly reassuring because it has survived a stormy passage.

If sex becomes any kind of physical problem various forms of HT or alternative therapies such as black cohosh or dong quai (see page 195) are life-savers for enhancing your libido. However, not every woman likes the fact that her body is geared up for sex. You need to want to remain sexy, otherwise the sex act becomes unpleasant. A few women actually prefer to do without sex but feel guilty about this desire. If they have a partner who thinks sex must be a constant factor in the relationship, then clearly this raises a problem. Usually when such a situation arises, it indicates that something has never felt satisfactory in the relationship. But if you do want sex there's no reason why it shouldn't continue for as long as you remain healthy and fit.

The wonderful thing about not having periods any more is that you no longer get monthly fluctuations of mood, especially premenstrual syndrome! Your life returns to an even keel, and this can be wonderful for all relationships – personal or otherwise. Living without PMS is fantastic. It's a great time to try something new: starting a business, travelling, going into politics. It can be as if your life has been put on hold from your early teens to your mid-fifties and then you suddenly get it back again.

TAKING CONTROL OF STRESS

A variety of events and circumstances can disrupt emotional equilibrium at any time in our lives. Problems at work, financial concerns, worries about our children and relationship difficulties can all put us under stress. However, around menopause, we may be affected by particular stressors, including reaching the end of the fertile period of life and experiencing physical changes, should they occur. In addition, this is the time when children may leave home, and also the time when aging parents may become unwell and dependent.

In order to preserve emotional health during menopause, we have to manage our various stresses and the changes inherent in the process and beyond.

STRESS

We all experience stress. It may be that a certain amount of stress, for example in a work setting, helps us to function and even to perform better. However, being placed under too much stress and having problems coping with it can have detrimental effects on both our physical and our emotional well-being. As it's impossible to avoid stress altogether, it's important to make regular relaxation routines a part of your daily life. If stress becomes overwhelming, however, there are many ways in which you can counteract it (see page 162).

Am I Under Too Much Stress?

When your mind and body are struggling to cope with the levels of stress in your life, they may show it in a number of ways. Do any of the symptoms described in the box on the right apply to you? Some of these symptoms are emotional and may be helped by relaxation techniques. Others are physical. While they may be normal in response to a particular situation, you need to take action if these situations become more frequent or interfere with your life, or if they occur when you are experiencing only minor stresses. A person's behaviour often changes in response to excess stress, particularly in social situations. This may be more obvious to close friends and family than to the individual.

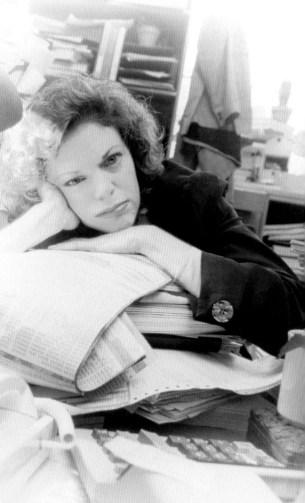

Learn to Delegate

You don't have to be superwoman all the time. Find ways to prioritize and delegate – at work and at home – and allow yourself to accept offers of help in the way they are intended.

The Next Step

If you are suffering from the symptoms of excess stress, you need to try to reduce your stress levels. In the following pages we mention various ways of managing such stress. However, it is important to be prepared to seek help if you need it, whether it be from friends, family, your healthcare professional or a support organization. Excess stress can manifest itself as very real physical symptoms. It is often hard to tell the difference between physical symptoms caused by stress and those that reflect an underlying medical condition. Therefore, you may need to see your healthcare professional, who will be able to suggest tests if they are needed and help you decide what to do next in terms of stress management.

Seeking Help

If you feel stress is affecting your health and you need help, your family doctor is likely to be your first stop. He or she will be able to help you think about the next step, which may involve counselling or some other form of therapy.

Counselling may be beneficial when looking for causes of stress, for dealing with particular issues and for developing strategies to cope with stress. Stress management programmes are also widely used to reduce stress. Cognitive therapy may be an option if you need help in changing negative perceptions that are contributing to your anxieties. Sometimes medication is appropriate. There are also a number of voluntary organizations that offer a listening ear and give support.

Relaxation Exercises

There are many relaxation exercises you can do; paced respiration (see page 32), yoga, including the child's pose (see page 36), deep abdominal breathing (see page 40) and meditation (see page 42) are all effective methods. A wide variety of relaxation tapes and classes are also available to help you enjoy relaxation. Aromatherapy is also a useful and pleasurable way to lift the spirits (see pages 160–161).

Signs of stress

Emotional symptoms

- Feeling tense and under pressure
- Having problems relaxing
- Being moody and irritable
- Complaining frequently
- Feeling afraid
- Being tearful
- Overreacting to minor irritations
- Losing your temper
- Having problems coping
- Having trouble concentrating
- Having difficulty making decisions
- Wanting to run away from situations
- Feeling the need to check things repeatedly, such as whether you locked the door.
- Feeling down and unable to enjoy things; stress and anxiety often accompany depression.

Physical symptoms

- Sweating
- Muscle tension
- Rapid heart beat
- Rapid breathing
- Trembling
- Nausea
- Dry mouth

Other physical features of excess stress may be constant or occur repeatedly over a long period:

- Frequent headaches
- Tiredness and lack of energy
- Problems sleeping
- Loss of appetite or an increase in appetite
- Aches and pains
- Flare-ups of certain other conditions, such as dandruff or irritable bowel syndrome.

Social symptoms

People under pressure may:

- Avoid social occasions and eventually become withdrawn.
- Smoke more or drink more alcohol.

AROMATHERAPY

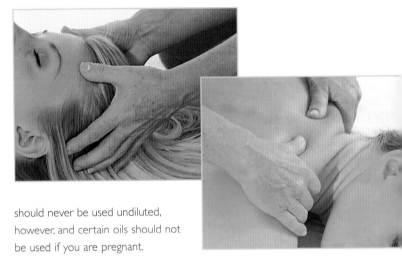

For hundreds of years, the essential oils of various plants have been enjoyed for their scents, which can relax the mind and body. Smell is the most developed of our five senses, and when certain scents are inhaled, they can induce feelings of calm or invigoration, as well as toning the skin. Essential oils, therefore, are divided into three categories: calming oils such as cedarwood, jasmine and neroli, which have a sedating effect; uplifting oils such as bergamot, basil or rosemary, which raise the spirits; and toning and regulating oils, such as lemongrass and myrrh. Oils can be heated over a burner. Vaporizing jasmine or lavender essential oil can create a calming atmosphere in your home or office. Oils can be added to baths, face masks, and foot baths, used for steam inhalations or be massaged into your body. They should never be used undiluted, however, and certain oils should not be used if you are pregnant.

ESSENTIAL OIL	USE
Camomile	Relieves stress and insomnia
Sandalwood	Soothes tension and anxiety
Lavender	Eases depression and insomnia
Cedarwood	Soothes anxiety
Neroli	Helps relieve anxiety and depression
Ylang-ylang	Stirs the senses and is an aphrodisiac

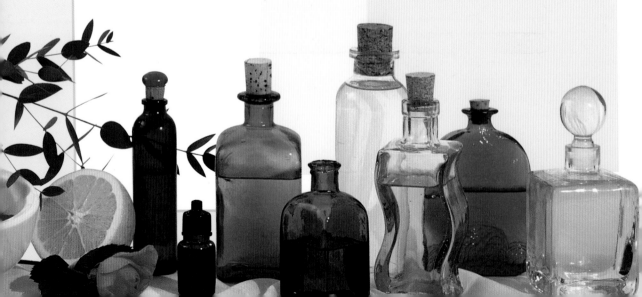

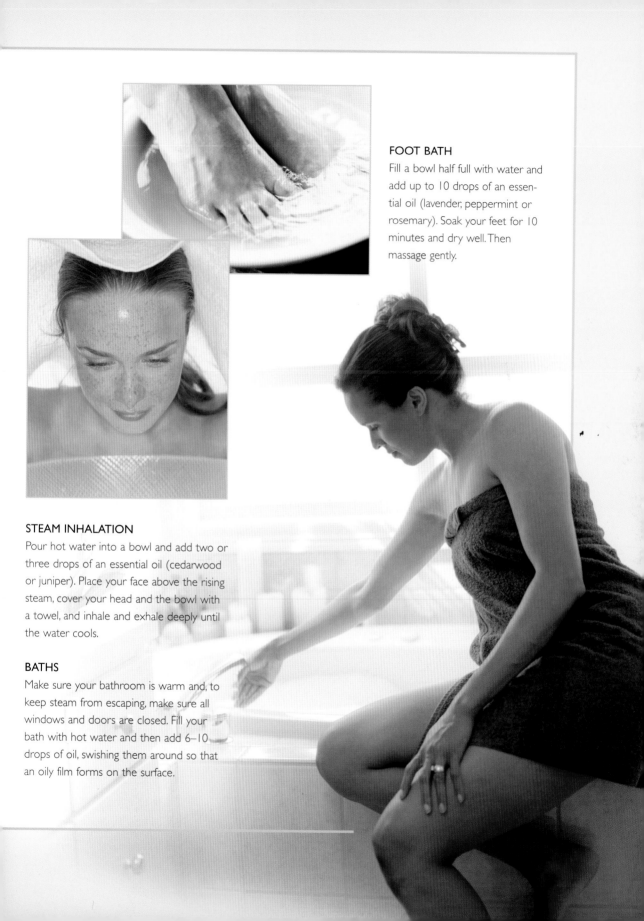

FOOT BATH

Fill a bowl half full with water and add up to 10 drops of an essential oil (lavender, peppermint or rosemary). Soak your feet for 10 minutes and dry well. Then massage gently.

STEAM INHALATION

Pour hot water into a bowl and add two or three drops of an essential oil (cedarwood or juniper). Place your face above the rising steam, cover your head and the bowl with a towel, and inhale and exhale deeply until the water cools.

BATHS

Make sure your bathroom is warm and, to keep steam from escaping, make sure all windows and doors are closed. Fill your bath with hot water and then add 6–10 drops of oil, swishing them around so that an oily film forms on the surface.

▶ STRATEGIES FOR STRESS MANAGEMENT

Homeopathy A number of treatments are available. The recommended prescriptions will depend on the individual's personality and circumstances.

Nutritional therapy Nutritionists believe that stress can lead to weakening of the adrenal glands. Therefore, recommended measures may include treatments such as magnesium supplements, which are said to improve adrenal function and replenish magnesium levels in the body, which may also be depleted by stress.

Massage Massage has been shown to decrease stress levels not only in those receiving massage but also in those giving it. Reflexology may also have a calming effect on people who are stressed.

Acupuncture Acupuncture may be helpful when there are anxiety symptoms and sleep problems. It is also said to improve general well-being.

Biofeedback In biofeedback, information about the functioning of some internal organs is presented visually or by means of a sound. One use for biofeedback is the relief of stress, which may be measured by sensors monitoring skin temperature, production of sweat by the skin or the tension in muscles. For example, sensors may be placed over the muscles of the forehead or around the jaw. As tension increases, a buzzing sound may get louder. The individual tries to relax the muscles in order to quieten and eventually silence the noise altogether. The aim is to be able eventually to reproduce the effects without the use of a machine.

Herbal Remedies

Several herbs may be used to help the body cope with stress. They include Siberian ginseng (see pages 196–197), St. John's wort (see page 197) and vervain (see page 198), which also helps with sleep. Infusions made from lemon balm, rosemary, vervain or camomile (see page 193) are also found to help with relaxation, mood changes and irritability.

ways to combat stress

If, despite the general measures described earlier in this chapter, you still feel stressed, you may also find the following helpful:

- ▶ Seek support from friends and relatives.
- ▶ Think about the sources of your stress and what is causing you to worry. Divide the reasons into those you can do something about and those you can't. Then think what positive steps you can take and give yourself a realistic programme for achieving them.
- ▶ Establish a routine so that you feel in control of your circumstances.
- ▶ Try to face problems directly.
- ▶ Anticipate sources of stress that are likely to arise and think how you will deal with them.
- ▶ Don't be too hard on yourself; give yourself a pat on the back when you think or act in a positive way.
- ▶ Take time for yourself and make sure you have opportunities to relax and enjoy yourself every day.
- ▶ Continue to take regular exercise.
- ▶ Make sure you get enough rest.
- ▶ Restrict your alcohol intake – it is all too easy to depend on alcohol in times of stress.

RECOGNIZING DEPRESSION

Stress and anxiety are often associated with depression. This condition is common around menopause as well as at other times of hormonal change. Depression can sometimes overwhelm even the most optimistic and cheerful of us at any stage in our lives; it is one of the most common mental problems and affects twice as many women as men.

Depression sometimes follows a stressful event, such as a bereavement or the loss of a job – or even a joyful event such as a birth – but often there is no obvious reason.

Symptoms of Depression

The psychological features of depression may include feelings of sadness (often worse in the morning), tearfulness, feelings of guilt, lack of self-esteem, lack of interest, problems enjoying activities, impaired concentration, being indecisive, early morning wakening and a lack of interest in sex. You may also feel anxious. Depression often affects physical well-being too, causing a lack of energy and poor appetite.

If some of the symptoms described apply to you and your depression persists to the point that it is affecting your life, talk to your healthcare professional. Often, people who are depressed find it difficult to imagine feeling well again. This is understandable with an illness that is associated with feeling negative. However, there are many treatment options available and experienced people who are there to help.

Treatment Options

Certain lifestyle changes may help to lift the symptoms of depression. The most effective changes are reducing alcohol intake, as alcohol may aggravate depression, and taking exercise, which is known to improve mood and general well-being. Good diet is another important element (see pages 106–127). Foods containing selenium (found in oysters, mushrooms and Brazil nuts), zinc (found in eggs, seafood and shellfish) and chromium (available as a supplement) have also been shown to have a positive effect on depression.

The support of family and friends is an important part of the recovery process. Depression is often made worse by being hidden. Talk to your family and let them know how you are feeling – or, if you feel you can't share your feelings, try a support group. Many people find it helpful to exchange with others who have similar difficulties.

Counselling may also be helpful in resolving particular underlying issues. Other forms of psychotherapy may also be recommended, in particular cognitive therapy, which aims to change an individual's perceptions of him- or herself and the close environment. It will help to identify and change thoughts that are contributing to the depression.

Drug treatment may be recommended in more severe cases. Many different drugs are available, and they all work by affecting the neurotransmitters in the brain, especially serotonin, noradrenaline and dopamine, the three neurotransmitters that play a central role in many brain functions. Your healthcare professional will take into account various factors, including the nature and severity of your symptoms when selecting a medication. Symptoms may start to improve after about two weeks. As with all drugs, antidepressants can cause side effects – so make sure you discuss any possible side effects with your doctor.

PERSONALITY AND ASSERTIVENESS

Philosophers, scientists and researchers have many different ways of classifying personality, and most of these have a health component. In other words, human beings can be divided into different categories – most scientifically, by the traits they exhibit (such as introvert and extrovert) – and, depending on their 'type', each individual may be more prone to particular health problems. This is also true of stress; some individuals are more likely to become stressed and tend to suffer more because of it. Such people are generally passive and suppress the anger they feel.

BECOMING ASSERTIVE

When difficult situations present themselves, the most effective way to deal with potential anger is not to suppress or control it, but to avoid it by making sure your feelings are known before a danger point is reached. The technique for this is known as assertiveness training, in which participants are taught to speak up to ensure that their needs are addressed. An invaluable technique, it can help improve communication with your partner, other family members and your employer. It will also make you feel better about yourself. Classes are available, but there are a number of things you can do yourself.

Being assertive does not mean riding roughshod over others. It means acknowledging the rights of others and still being able to express your own needs and desires. It can be as simple as using more 'I' sentences such as 'I would like you to wash the dishes', and 'I feel I'm not being listened to', and being more clear about what you want to happen.

It also helps to practice the technique by mentally rehearsing conversations. You might try going over a conversation with your partner in advance, in which you discuss something he or she does that annoys you, or one with your employer, in which you ask for some changes to be made to your job description. In the latter case, it can help to write down a list of the plus factors you bring to your job. Look at the diagram (left) and use the stages to identify the problem and come to a resolution.

WAYS TO GET YOUR VIEW ACROSS

- Make eye contact. Averting your eyes makes you look submissive, so look at the people you're speaking to.
- Speak in a firm voice; do not mumble, shout or raise your voice.
- Stick to the point; avoid long explanations.
- Be polite but don't start a sentence with 'I'm sorry'.
- Listen to the other's point of view but be persistent.

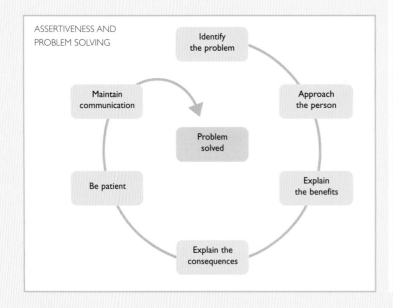

ASSERTIVENESS AND PROBLEM SOLVING

Identify the problem

Approach the person

Explain the benefits

Explain the consequences

Problem solved

Be patient

Maintain communication

KICKING HARMFUL HABITS

The way women experience menopause varies from one individual to another. This is due to many factors, some of which, such as genes, cannot be changed. However, there are things that we can adopt, adapt or avoid, and they can influence both the symptoms you may experience and the way you approach this time of change.

Menopause can be a time when we may be left in no doubt of the harm certain habits do to our bodies and our outlook. It can be very empowering to take control of a habit and experience the positive effects on your body and overall well-being.

CAFFEINE

This is a central nervous system stimulant – meaning it stimulates the brain – and is found in tea, coffee, caffeinated drinks such as cola, and chocolate. Moderate amounts of caffeine (less than about 400 mg per day; see page 37 for information on the caffeine content of various beverages) are thought to be acceptable. However, larger amounts can be associated with undesirable effects, including headaches, anxiety, irritability and having heart palpitations (being aware of the heartbeat, which may be rapid). Frequent urination may also occur as

caffeine is a diuretic. Problems sleeping, in particular getting to sleep, may also occur (see also page 37).

A high intake of caffeine can cause dependence, with symptoms such as headaches, fatigue, anxiety, and even feelings of drowsiness occurring if caffeine is stopped. If you are taking in more than 400 mg of caffeine per day, you may need to cut down.

ALCOHOL

Alcohol has a range of effects, both mental and physical. Small amounts may provide benefits in terms of protecting against coronary artery disease and strokes. However, larger amounts can cause many detrimental effects.

Alcohol is absorbed from the stomach and small intestine into the bloodstream. It is then transported to the liver where it is broken down either to be used as energy or to be stored as fat. Some is also exhaled when we breathe out.

How quickly alcohol is broken down depends on a number of factors, including our weight and whether we have recently eaten.

Effects on the Brain

Alcohol acts on the brain to reduce anxiety and inhibitions. In moderate amounts it helps with relaxation as well as increasing confidence in social situations. However, as a sedative it can also slow down reactions and affect coordination and concentration. Even small amounts can impair an individual's ability to operate machinery and to drive. Larger amounts of alcohol can lead to loss of control, drowsiness and eventually to loss of consciousness. Continued excessive alcohol consumption may be associated with anxiety and depression as well as increasing the risk of developing dementia.

Effects on the Body

Alcohol acts as a diuretic and stimulates the appetite. It causes dilatation (widening) of the blood vessels in the skin, which can be associated with excessive

5 ways to cut caffeine intake

- ► Try to replace some of your caffeinated drinks with decaffeinated ones or other drinks.
- ► Drink instant coffee and weak tea as they contain less caffeine.
- ► Drink smaller and/or weaker caffeinated drinks.
- ► Try drinking more water.
- ► Remember to cut down gradually to avoid unwanted side effects.

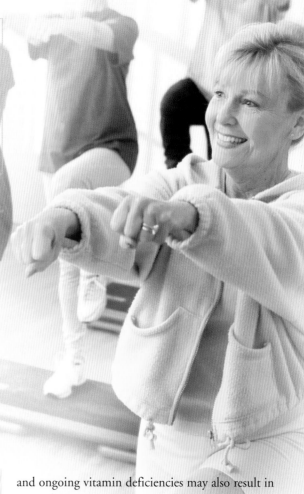

sweating, flushing and loss of heat from the body. Bouts of heavy drinking lead to hangovers with headaches, nausea and a dry mouth. Hangovers are due to the effects of alcohol and other chemicals in alcoholic drinks. Drinking large amounts can lead to loss of memory and loss of consciousness. Many regular drinkers find they put on weight.

Long-term excessive consumption may be associated with many disorders, including stomach ulcers, certain heart and liver diseases, high blood pressure and strokes. It also increases the risk of certain cancers, such as cancer of the mouth, throat and oesophagus, particularly in those who also smoke. Brain function may be affected and related

ways to cut down on alcohol

- ▶ Make sure you have at least two alcohol-free days each week.
- ▶ Avoid drinking during the day at work.
- ▶ When socializing, make sure every other drink is non-alcoholic.
- ▶ Decide in advance how much you want to drink and stick to it.
- ▶ Finish your drink before refilling your glass so you know how much alcohol you have had.
- ▶ Put your glass down between sips to help you drink more slowly.

and ongoing vitamin deficiencies may also result in nerve damage.

Alcohol can also lead to various other problems; it can interfere with an individual's social life as well as affecting work and relationships. Dependence is a common and serious problem; affected individuals find they need to drink, and they keep drinking even though they know it will harm them. Their bodies can tolerate increasing levels of alcohol and they experience symptoms if alcohol is stopped.

It can be difficult to keep track of alcohol consumption. It may be worth trying to keep an alcohol diary for a couple of weeks to give you an idea of how much you're drinking. You should also use a shot glass or drink measure when pouring drinks at home to avoid overgenerous portions. If your level of alcohol consumption is above the recommended limit, it is time to cut down.

The Next Step

The CAGE questionnaire (above) assesses your dependence on alcohol. It gets its name from the initial letters of the key words or phrases in the questions – 'cut down', 'annoyed', 'guilty' and 'eye-opener'. If you answered yes to two or more of the questions seek help as soon as possible.

Your healthcare professional will be able to give you guidance on how to deal with the problem. He or she may refer you to a support organization, such as Alcoholics Anonymous (AA), or suggest that you contact an addiction treatment centre. There are also special clinics that provide help and support. In some cases, medication can be prescribed to help with giving up.

Very heavy drinkers can experience severe and even life-threatening problems if they suddenly stop drinking. In such cases, a period of hospital or clinic care is a possible recommendation. For more information, see page 109.

SMOKING

It is well known that smoking is harmful to health and yet a quarter of all women smoke. It is never too late to benefit from quitting. You will start to feel healthier within a few weeks and, over the long-term, you will have reduced your risk of many serious diseases, including cancers, heart diseases, strokes and lung diseases. It is of particular interest to perimenopausal and menopausal women that smoking also increases the risk of osteoporosis, contributes to hot flushes and sleep disorders and is toxic to the ovaries, bringing on menopause two years earlier than with nonsmokers. It also accentuates skin changes, particularly wrinkles around the lips and dark circles under the eyes.

What Is in Cigarettes?

Cigarette smoke contains nicotine, which causes the addiction, as well as various other chemicals. Many of these, including tar, can cause cancer and other diseases.

Giving Up

Cigarette smoking is not only a habit; the nicotine in cigarette smoke also causes a physical addiction.

Most people need the support of their family and often specialist help if they are to succeed in giving up. Smoking cessation clinics can also provide helpful information and support.

Methods

There are many options available for giving up smoking. Using nicotine replacement therapy helps many people; it has been shown to double the chances of giving up. There are prescription and over-the-counter forms. As with other methods, the smoker must first want to give up.

Like nicotine itself, these therapies can cause a number of effects including nausea and headaches. They may also be associated with sleeping problems. Medical advice should be sought by smokers who have a history of cardiovascular disease.

Forms of Nicotine Replacement Therapy

A frequently used medication called Zyban (bupropion) is available on prescription. It is not certain how the active ingredient in bupropion works to help stop smoking, but it may involve the neurotransmitters noradrenaline and dopamine in

5 tools to help you quit

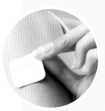

Patches are available in various strengths; they slowly release nicotine into the bloodstream, providing a constant level in the blood to reduce cravings.

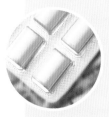

Gum containing nicotine is available in two strengths; it gives the mouth something to do instead of smoking.

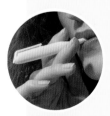

An inhalator involves sucking on a white plastic device that releases a combination of menthol and nicotine; it acts as a substitute for sucking on a cigarette.

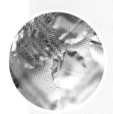

Lozenges and under-the-tongue tablets are also available. Lozenges are available in two strengths.

Nicotine nasal spray is available over-the-counter and can be used up to twice an hour for 16 hours a day. After eight weeks' treatment the dose is gradually reduced.

the brain. (Neurotransmitters are chemicals that transmit impulses from one nerve to another.) A healthcare professional will check a patient's medical history before prescribing bupropion, as it cannot be used in certain conditions, such as the presence of liver disease. Bupropion is associated with possible side effects, which the physician should explain. It can be prescribed for a maximum of 7 to 9 weeks.

Herbal remedies such as chewing gum with herbal extracts may help. Herbal cigarettes are available, but they don't seem to help people to give up smoking, and tar and carbon monoxide are inhaled in the smoke, so they're probably best avoided.

Make it your goal to give up rather than cut down. If you simply reduce the number of cigarettes you smoke, you are still a smoker with the risks that entails. Also, the number of cigarettes smoked is likely to gradually creep up again.

Filters are available that can be fitted over the end of cigarettes to reduce the amount of nicotine and tar inhaled. However, these harmful substances are still being inhaled in significant amounts and again, the person continues to be a smoker.

Hypnotherapy has been helpful to some people. It aims to influence the subconscious and reduce the desire to smoke.

Another useful technique is cognitive therapy. The smoker works with a therapist to understand smoking patterns and the trigger points that act as cues to the habit. You may be asked to keep a smoking diary, listing the cigarettes you had in the day and what you were doing when you had them. The aim is to look for alternatives to smoking a cigarette in response to that cue.

Acupuncture may also help – but as with all quitting aids, the smoker needs to want to give up smoking. It has been estimated that around 30 percent of people give up right away.

After You Give Up

You may experience the symptoms of nicotine withdrawal, which start within 24 hours of the last cigarette. You may feel anxious, low, irritable, have difficulty concentrating and have problems sleeping. These symptoms should last no more than two weeks.

You are likely to produce more phlegm and to cough more because the cilia, the tiny hairs lining the airways that beat to propel mucus and debris out of the lungs, start to work again.

People often put on weight after giving up smoking, as a result of boredom and a need to replace cigarettes with fatty or sugary high-calorie snacks (although the average increase after quitting smoking is under 10 pounds). This can be avoided by chewing sugar-free gum, snacking on fruits and vegetables, drinking plenty of water, following a healthy diet and taking regular exercise.

What Happens If I Have a Relapse?

Most relapses occur within the first three months after quitting. Don't be discouraged: try again – most people attempt to give up smoking several times before they finally quit. Think about the strategies you used the last time you tried – what worked and what didn't – and try to use your most successful ideas again.

There are, however, some 'trigger' scenarios you should try to avoid when you give up smoking. Cut down your alcohol intake, as smoking often goes together with drinking, and you are most likely to relapse in this social setting.

Try to stay clear of other smokers. This can be difficult if you live in a household of smokers, but being around smoke can make you want to smoke again, so ask your family and friends for their help. Perhaps they'll be willing not to smoke or leave cigarettes around you.

Many smokers will gain weight when they quit, but you can do a lot to prevent this – namely by eating a healthy diet and staying active. It's useful to remember that you would need to put on at least 34 kg (75 lb) to cancel out the health benefits of quitting smoking. Don't let a little weight gain become an excuse to deflect you from your primary aim.

Some smokers use bad mood or 'depression' as an excuse to have another cigarette. There are many more efficient ways of brightening your mood other than smoking. De-stress with a hot bath, read a book, get busy with a job you've been putting off – you'll feel better in so many ways!

5 ways to manage your menopause

▶ **Be informed** It seems that finding out about menopause – understanding what happens to the body and why – helps smooth the passage through this stage in life for many women. Know what symptoms you can expect and what you will be able to do about them.

▶ **Be in control** To prevent things from overwhelming you, take care of your body and emotional health, keeping them both in shape. This includes eating healthily, exercising regularly, and taking measures to stay happy.

▶ **Manage stress** Women who are stressed may be more likely to suffer troublesome menopausal symptoms. It is important to learn to manage stress effectively.

▶ **Seek support** You will know many women who have gone through this in the past or are going through it now. Talk to them; share your fears and concerns. It is also worth contacting self-help organizations and women's health groups for information and support.

▶ **Think positively** Try to welcome this new phase in your life and make the most of new-found freedom, whether by making changes in your career or your leisure time.

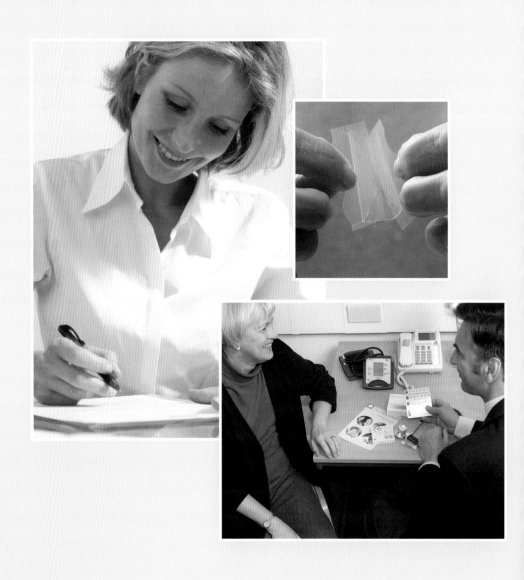

8

HORMONE THERAPY

Choosing whether or not to use hormone therapy is an important health decision, but with ongoing research sending out confusing – and sometimes conflicting – information, it's difficult to know what to do. The most important thing is to be aware of your options before you discuss HT with your healthcare professional. This chapter aims to put you in a better position to ask the right questions, understand the issues and make an informed decision.

UNDERSTANDING HORMONE THERAPY

The most commonly prescribed medications used for treating menopausal symptoms are replacement hormones. They are used to replenish the levels of the female sex hormones – oestrogen and sometimes progesterone – which decrease at menopause.

Although this treatment is commonly known as HRT (hormone replacement therapy), the amount of oestrogen contained in the drugs is well below that produced by the premenopausal ovary, so the term 'replacement' is misleading, and in the United States it is considered a misnomer. Hormone therapy (HT) has been used by millions of women for the relief of menopausal symptoms. Previously it was also used for long-term prevention of osteoporosis, but research has shown that the risks of taking long-term HT may outweigh the benefits.

The Committee for the Safety of Medicines (CSM) in the UK now advises that the lowest effective dose should be used for the shortest duration. Treatment should be reviewed at least once a year, and alternatives should be sought for the treatment of osteoporosis. Every woman considering HT needs to look at what the treatment can offer her and balance these potential benefits against any possible risks. All women should be helped in this with information and advice from their healthcare professionals.

WHAT IT IS
The chief components of HT are oestrogens. Natural oestrogens (estradiol, estrone and estriol)

WISE WOMAN
'Short-duration' HT defined

The Royal College of Obstetricians and Gynaecologists defines 'short-duration' hormone therapy as 'the use of HT for up to five years, usually aimed at the relief of menopausal symptoms in women in their early 50s.'

have a better effect than synthetic ones (ethinyl estradiol and mestranol). In the UK synthetic oestrogens are more commonly used for combined oral contraceptives (COC). In the United States, women younger than 50 are sometimes given the COC to relieve menopausal symptoms, but this is not common practise in the UK.

The oestrogens in HT can cause endometrial hyperplasia (thickening of the lining of the uterus). Although this condition is not cancerous, it can develop into cancer. Women who have had hysterectomies can take oestrogen on its own as they are not at risk for this condition. However, women who still have their uterus must also take a progestogen (a synthetic form of progesterone), or a natural progesterone, which counteracts the effects of oestrogen on the uterine lining.

TYPES OF TREATMENT
There are two main types of HT, oestrogen taken alone, and oestrogen taken in combination with a progestogen or natural progesterone.

Oestrogen Therapy
This is suitable for a woman who has had her uterus removed, as in that case there is no risk of endometrial hyperplasia (thickening of the uterine lining).

Oestrogen and Progestogen/Progesterone Therapy
A progestogen or natural progesterone is given with an oestrogen in one of two ways:

Cyclical HT: Oestrogen is usually taken continuously but the progestogen is taken on a cyclical basis, either for 10–14 days in every month or for a similar period every three months. The progestogen will induce a withdrawal bleed, like a period, in which the thickened lining of the uterus is shed. With new extremely low-dose oestrogen regimens, the natural progesterone may be needed only every six months.

Cyclical HT is preferable for women who are still having periods (a progestogen should be taken monthly), and for those who have had a period in the last year (a progestogen should be taken monthly or three-monthly).

Continuous-combined:
Oestrogen and a progestogen are taken every day. This is appropriate if it is more than a year since the last period. If it is taken before that time, this form of HT may cause irregular bleeding. Abnormal bleeding after menopause always needs to be investigated.

THE HORMONES

Two principal hormones are used in supplementary therapy – oestrogen and progestogen (or natural progesterone). In rare cases, an androgen (see page 178) may be prescribed.

Oestrogen

Two main types are used: natural oestrogens (such as estradiol, estrone and estriol) and synthetic oestrogens (such as ethinyl estradiol and mestranol). Of the two, natural oestrogens, which are derived from plants and animals and include estradiol, are closer in structure and actions to the oestrogens produced by the body. They therefore have less effect on the processes occurring in the body, and so tend to cause fewer side effects.

WISE WOMAN
Bioidentical hormones

•

These are manufactured hormones derived from plant sources that are engineered to have an identical molecular structure to those produced in the human body. They are available in some commercial products and may be custom-compounded. Those sold as dietary supplements are not classified as drugs – and therefore are not licensed for medical use.

Progestogen/Progesterone

Traditionally, natural progesterone was not available in tablet form in a way that would allow it to be sufficiently absorbed from the gut into the bloodstream. Therefore, synthetic forms of progesterone (progestogens) were developed.

There are two main types of progestogens: those that are similar to the female hormone progesterone and those that are related to the male sex hormone testosterone. The two types can produce some similar side effects (see page 178), but those that are testosterone-derived can also cause particular effects, such as acne and hirsutism (excessive hairiness).

Recently, natural micronized progesterone products have been developed that can be taken orally and are well absorbed, but these are not yet generally available on prescription in the UK.

▶ TIBOLONE

Available in Europe but not yet in the U.S. or Canada, this is a selective estrogen receptive modulator or SERM that can relieve menopausal symptoms such as hot flashes and is not usually associated with bleeding (although some bleeding may occur). Tibolone also has been shown to prevent osteoporosis and it may improve sex drive thanks to its testosteronelike effects.

Possible side effects of tibolone include fluid retention, headaches, dizziness, increase in facial hair, depression, aching joints and muscles, visual disturbances, acne, rashes and itching. It may also cause weight changes.

FORMS OF TREATMENT

There are various ways of taking hormone therapy. Here, as well as outlining the pros and cons of the various forms, we will give some general information on their use.

OESTROGEN ALONE

Oestrogen-alone therapy comes in two forms. One is a systemic form, such as pills, skin patches or gels, which allow the oestrogen to circulate throughout the body. The other is a local form, such as creams, rings or pessaries, which release only a small amount of circulating oestrogen; their major effect is on a specific or localized area of the body, such as the vagina.

TABLETS

These are the most commonly prescribed form. The hormone is absorbed from the intestines into the bloodstream and transported to the liver, where it is broken down into other forms of oestrogen. A large proportion of the oestrogens are destroyed in this 'first pass' through the liver, higher doses of oestrogens are needed to achieve adequate levels in the blood.

A number of pill strengths are available. Guidelines recommend that the lowest dose that can control the menopausal symptoms be used. According to the Committee on the Safety of Medicines guidelines, the dosage should be assessed at least annually.

Pros and Cons

Many women find tablets easy to take, and they can be readily stopped if the side effects cannot be tolerated. However, it is also easy to forget to take the pills every day, and if they are missed, irregular bleeding can occur. Also, the first pass of the oestrogens through the liver may make side effects more pronounced (although the side effects associated with tablets tend to resolve within a few months in any case). Furthermore, higher doses of the hormone are needed to achieve the desired effects.

PATCHES

These are thin adhesive strips or round patches that contain the natural hormone oestradiol mixed in with the adhesive.

Patches are applied either weekly or twice-weekly. The oestrogen is slowly absorbed through the skin directly into the bloodstream without being broken down in the liver.

The patch should be applied on cool, dry skin on the upper arm or on the torso below the waist. The area should be free of creams, oils and talcum powder. Patches should never be applied to the breasts or to areas that may be rubbed by bra straps or waistbands. The patch can be left in place during

> ▶ TACHYPHYLAXIS

Sometimes, women using implants (see page 176) develop a condition known as tachyphylaxis. They start to develop menopausal symptoms when their hormone levels are still high enough to control them, and an implant is not yet needed. This can lead to their requiring higher doses or more frequent implants and a gradual rise in their hormone levels. It seems that women affected by this become used to the higher levels of oestrogens and begin to experience symptoms as the levels fall rather than when they are low. To avoid this the hormone levels should be checked before the implants are inserted.

swimming and showering, but it should be covered when sunbathing. Sometimes, patches can leave adhesive on the skin, but this can usually be removed by rubbing it gently with baby oil. The patches can cause skin irritation but this should resolve once the patch has been removed. If this occurs, try a different brand, as the adhesives used vary.

Pros and Cons

Many women find patches easy to use. The oestradiol is slowly absorbed from the patch, avoiding the sudden rises in hormone levels that can occur with pills. Some of the side effects (see page 178) may be less pronounced, as the hormone breakdown in the liver does not occur. Also, lower doses may be needed to achieve the required effects. However, the user needs to remember to change the patch and the patches may irritate the skin.

SKIN GELS

These preparations are used for the relief of menopausal symptoms; but not all of them are licensed for the prevention of osteoporosis. The gels are used daily and rubbed into an area of clean, dry, unbroken skin. The gel should be left to dry for about five minutes before being covered with clothing, and the area of skin should not be washed for at least an hour. Contact of the treated area with another person should also be avoided for an hour. The gel must not be applied on the face, in the breast area, around the vulva or come in contact with the eyes. The dosing of the gel used can be increased after a period of time (depending on the product used), if undesirable symptoms have not been controlled.

Pros and Cons

On the plus side, gels are easy to use. The hormones are absorbed directly into the bloodstream, so bypassing the liver. Therefore, as with patches, a lower dose is needed to achieve the necessary blood levels, and the side effects (see page 178) should be

lighter than with pills. Some women, however, find the gels messy. Like patches, gels can cause skin irritation, although this may be resolved by using a different area of skin with each application.

SYSTEMIC OESTROGEN VAGINAL RING

Because they contain enough oestrogen that is absorbed by the vagina into the bloodstream, a vaginal ring can be used to treat hot flushes and night sweats in addition to vaginal dryness and atrophy. The ring is inserted into the vagina and remains there for three months. Progestogen is

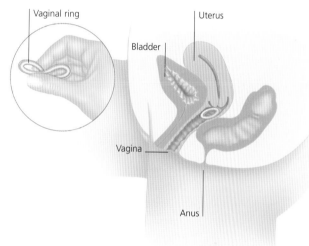

needed cyclically for women who have not had a hysterectomy.

Pros and Cons

Relieves vaginal symptoms, which can be distressing. Easy to insert and remove when necessary.

LOCAL OR LOW-DOSE HORMONE THERAPY

These treatments are inserted into the vagina and are used to treat moderate-to-severe vaginal dryness and atrophy, and in some cases, bladder symptoms. They come as vaginal creams, pessaries and rings. These treatments are not likely to be absorbed into the bloodstream in significant amounts. Short-term use for up to three months is safe – a few weeks of the treatment may be enough to relieve vaginal symptoms, and a further course of treatment may be prescribed if symptoms recur. The low-dose ring and vaginal tablets give minimal blood levels of oestradiol and are considered safe for long-term use. However, it is not known whether significant absorption of oestrogens into the bloodstream could occur with longer-term use. Therefore, cyclical progestogens may be recommended when local treatments are used long-term, as it is possible that the oestrogens could have a significant effect on the uterine lining.

Pros and Cons

These preparations relieve vaginal and urinary symptoms, which can be troublesome and distressing. However, the cream may affect the lining of the uterus if used long-term.

CUSTOMIZED HT PRODUCTS

These formulations can be made by a pharmacist from a healthcare professional's 'custom-made' prescription. They provide women with different types and amounts of oestrogen, as well as different ways of using it. Products include skin creams and gels, vaginal suppositories, sublingual (under-the-tongue) pills, sub-dermal implants and nasal sprays.

IMPLANTS

Implants are pellets that are inserted under the skin of the abdomen or thigh and release oestrogens slowly into the bloodstream over a period of up to eight months, depending on the individual and the dose given. Like patches and gels, they do not get broken down in the liver.

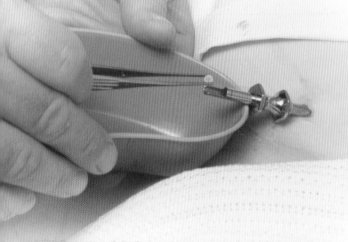

The insertion is carried out under local anaesthetic and takes about 10 minutes. A small incision is made and the pellet is introduced via a cannula through the incision. A small band-aid or a single stitch is used to close the incision. A testosterone implant is sometimes inserted at the same time with the aim of increasing libido.

A woman who still has her uterus must take cyclical progesterone as well, to cause withdrawal bleeds and so protect the lining of her uterus. Once she stops using the implants, she needs to continue her progesterone for some time to protect the lining of the uterus from the effects of the oestrogens that remain in her system.

Pros and Cons

Implants are convenient, as once they are inserted no further action is needed for several months. As the oestrogens are not broken down in the liver, side effects (see page 178) may be less noticeable than with tablets or patches. However, progestogens are needed by women who have their uterus; tachyphylaxis (see box, page 174) may occur, and the effects of an implant take some time to wear off.

NASAL SPRAY

Oestrogen nasal sprays can also be used to treat menopausal symptoms. The treatment starts with a spray of the drug into each nostril at the same time each day. It can be used every day or for 21–28 days, followed by a gap in treatment of 2–7 days. The dose can be adjusted according to the response – up to 4 sprays can be taken daily in divided doses. An additional progestogen is needed if a woman hasn't had a hysterectomy.

Pros and Cons
The spray is easy to use and can be stopped easily. The drug does not pass through the liver so there should be fewer side effects than with pills (see page 178). However, the spray can irritate the lining of the nose; tingling and bleeding may also occur.

COMBINED OESTROGEN-PROGESTOGEN HT
This is used by women who still have their uterus. In addition to oestrogen, progestogen needs to be taken either cyclically or on a continuous basis. Pills and patches that contain both hormones are available.

COMBINED TABLETS
Cyclical Combined HT
In most formulations, oestrogen is taken every day with progestogen added for 10–14 days each month.

In specialist HT clinics, variations to this scheme include 10 weeks of daily oestrogen followed by two weeks of daily combined oestrogen and progestogen and then a week of placebo or drug-free tablets. During this placebo week, premenstrual symptoms and bleeding occur, but only four times a year instead of monthly.

Continuous-Combined HT
Oestrogen and progestogen are combined in a pill that is taken every day. This form of treatment can usually only be taken if a year or more has passed since the last period. Bleeding can occur but it gradually disappears, and after a year of therapy it stops in 90 percent of users.

Intermittent-Combined HT
Provides a daily dose of oestrogen with added progestogen in cycles of three days on, three days off. Bleeding and protection of the endometrium are similar to the effects of a continuous-combined formulation.

COMBINED SKIN PATCHES
These come in various forms: two weeks of oestrogen-only patches and two weeks of oestrogen-and-progestogen patches as continuous-cyclic HT, or oestrogen and progestogen patches as continuous-combined HT. Continuous treatment should not be used until a year has passed since the last period.

> ### PROGESTERONE CREAMS
>
> Progesterone is also available without prescription in skin creams of various strengths (including none at all in some!). However, the most often used non-prescription progesterone cream, Pro-Gest, contains 450 mg progesterone per ounce, the same amount as found in custom-made prescription creams. Some evidence shows that progesterone cream can be effective for mild hot flushes during perimenopause. However, it is not a safe option for protecting the uterus when using oestrogen therapy. On applying the cream to the skin's surface, not enough is absorbed into the bloodstream.

SIDE EFFECTS AND STOPPING

SIDE EFFECTS

HT can be accompanied by side effects. Supplementation with oestrogen may cause nausea, fluid retention and bloating, breast swelling and breast tenderness. Other possible side effects include weight changes, headaches, dizziness, depression, changes in sex drive and finding that contact lenses irritate the eyes. Skin rashes, loss of scalp hair and jaundice (yellow colouration of the whites of the eyes and skin) can occasionally occur.

Possible side effects of progestogens include irregular bleeding, premenstrual-type symptoms such as bloating, tender breasts, weight gain, nausea, headaches, dizziness, sleeping problems and depression. Rashes and loss of scalp hair may also occur. Fortunately, a woman will rarely experience all the possible side effects; though uterine bleeding will occur with HT, this will diminish over time.

Androgen therapy has its own particular side effects (see box, right).

Managing Side Effects

Self-help for many of the unwanted side effects, such as headaches, breast tenderness and bloating, is covered in chapter two. Restricting salt, caffeine and chocolate intake can help several problems such as fluid retention, breast tenderness and mood changes. It's also important to exercise. Many side effects are temporary, and once a woman has adjusted to the hormonal changes, they subside.

Unless the side effects are severe, a trial of at least three months of hormone therapy should be undergone before stopping, lowering the dose or changing the brand. Stopping therapy, however, will show whether side effects are caused by the hormonal treatment or whether there is another cause. One particular thing to remember is that if you are taking HT to ward off hot flushes, these will return if treatment is stopped suddenly and not tapered off gradually.

▶ ANDROGEN THERAPY

Although androgen is primarily a male hormone, women also produce it. Over time its levels can reduce and cause symptoms such as fatigue, mood changes and lowered sex drive.

If an androgen insufficiency is suspected, a healthcare professional may prescribe hormone supplements. However, because androgen taken on its own may cause a woman to suffer adverse effects, it is only prescribed in combination with HT.

Added androgen is given to treat hot flushes when oestrogen therapy is not effective; it is not prescribed to boost a flagging libido although some women find their sex drives are improved by using it.

The long-term risks of using androgen are not known. In too high a dose, it has been known to cause agitation, aggression or depression, as well as excessive facial and body hair, acne, an enlarged clitoris, permanent lowering of the voice, muscle weight gain and changes in cholesterol.

FINDING THE RIGHT PREPARATION

Some preparations are more commonly associated with certain unwanted effects than others, and each woman will respond differently to the preparations. Therefore, if you are having problems with side effects, it is worth asking your healthcare professional to suggest an alternative type or dose. Sometimes changing the progestogen gives a better result, or changing the way the hormones are given – e.g., switching from pills to patches – may reduce unwanted effects. On the opposite page are some strategies you might suggest to your healthcare professional to combat particular problems.

STOPPING YOUR THERAPY

Once you are taking supplementary hormones, you will, at some stage, want to consider when to stop. This is something that you need to discuss with your healthcare professional. Guidelines recommend that HT should be taken for the least time possible to minimize the associated risks. Some data has suggested that the risk of getting breast cancer, for example, increases within 1–2 years of starting HT. Your doctor will take into account your reasons for taking it and the unique set of risk factors you have.

If you are taking HT to relieve menopausal symptoms only, your doctor may recommend stopping your prescription (it should gradually be reduced) to see whether the symptoms recur. If they do, and they affect your quality of life, hormone therapy can be reinstated.

If you suddenly stop taking your medication, this may precipitate a recurrence of symptoms. A better alternative is to slowly taper off over a period of weeks or months. Your healthcare professional may suggest gradually decreasing the dose or extending the time between doses. Matrix dermal patches can be trimmed to provide decreasing doses.

WISE WOMAN
Stopping HT and bone loss

Ending hormonal therapy speeds up bone loss, especially in the first year after stopping. Women at risk for osteoporosis (see pages 68–72) should consult their healthcare professional for other preventive measures or alternative medications.

Combatting side effects

Bloating: Ask for the oestrogen and/or progestogen dose to be lowered. Suggest having another oestrogen prescribed or changing from an oral oestrogen preparation to a skin patch. Ask to switch to progesterone or another progestin.

Breast tenderness: Ask for the oestrogen dose to be lowered or for another oestrogen to be prescribed. Suggest that you switch to progesterone or another progestin.

Headaches: Ask for the dose of oestrogen and/or progestogen to be lowered. Be sure that your medication does not contain medroxyprogesterone acetate (if using continuous-combined and continuous-cyclic pills). Ask to switch to progesterone. Suggest changing to a continuous dosage schedule or a skin patch.

Mood changes: Ask for the progestogen dose to be lowered or whether you can be prescribed progesterone. Suggest changing to a continuous dosage schedule, to a skin patch or to vaginal EPT.

Nausea: Take oestrogen tablets with meals or in the evening with a snack. Ask for the oestrogen and/or progestogen dose to be lowered. Suggest switching to another oral oestrogen or to a skin patch.

Skin irritation under patch: Make sure that the site is very clean. Apply the patch to a different site or ask to be prescribed one with a different adhesive. If the problem continues, you might suggest switching to an oral or vaginal oestrogen.

KEY ISSUES

As well as offering potential benefits, HT has the potential to increase the risk of certain conditions. There are a number of important issues to be aware of when considering whether to take it.

WHAT HT CAN DO

Treatment with supplemental hormones relieves the symptoms of oestrogen withdrawal, including night sweats and hot flushes, as well as more long-term problems associated with the lack of oestrogen.

It also protects against osteoporosis, although for this purpose HT is the preferred treatment only for women who are unable to take other osteoporosis treatments, such as bisphosphonates, or when these other so-called first-line treatments have been unsuccessful. There is evidence that the use of HT is also associated with a reduction in fractures related to osteoporosis. This protection appears rapidly after starting HT and wears off rapidly after stopping it. HT may also reduce the risk of colorectal cancer (cancer affecting the large bowel).

It has often been suggested that supplemental hormonal therapy causes women to put on weight. However, according to some study data, HT probably does not cause a greater weight gain than would normally occur around menopause. There is not enough evidence to say whether its use affects the usual change in body shape that occurs around menopause from pear- to apple-shaped (fat concentrated around the middle rather than on the hips).

CANCER

There is good evidence that HT use increases the risk of breast cancer, cancer of the lining of the uterus (endometrial cancer) and ovarian cancer. The bigger the dose and the longer the treatment is taken, the greater the risk. It's important to know exactly how much greater your risk would be, and to weigh this against the benefits and any problematic side effects.

Breast Cancer

The Women's Health Initiative and other studies have shown that women taking HT have an increased risk of developing breast cancer. This increased risk develops 1–2 years after HT is started. The increase in risk relates to how long HT is taken – the longer it is taken, the greater the risk. Studies have shown that:

- About 32 in every 1,000 women aged 50–65 not using HT are diagnosed with breast cancer over 15 to 20 years.
- With women using HT for five years, the rate increases to 33.5 women per 1,000; for those who use it for 10 years the rate increases to 37 in 1,000. These figures are based on the Million Women Study in the UK. However, the Women's Health Initiative trials of oestrogen-alone therapy in the US suggest that a woman's risk of getting breast cancer decreased, although not statistically significantly, and further research is needed.
- With women using combined HT for five years, the rate increases to 38 women per 1,000; for those who use it for 10 years the rate increases to 51 in 1,000.

When HT is stopped, the increase in cancer risk lessens until 5 years after stopping the treatment, when it returns to the level it would have been if HT had not been taken. As can be seen from these figures, the effect is greater for women who use oestrogen and progesterone combined. The effects on breast cancer risks are shown to be similar with all the different methods used (pills, patches, skin gels and implants), although the data is limited.

Endometrial Cancer

It is known that oestrogen given alone without a progestogen increases the risk of endometrial cancer. There may be a minimal increase with combined HT.

- About 5 women per 1,000 aged 50–64 and not using HT are diagnosed with endometrial cancer every year.

THE MILLION WOMEN STUDY

This British study, a collaboration between Cancer Research UK and the National Health Service (NHS) Breast Screening programme, is looking at the health of some 1.3 million UK women over the age of 50. It is focusing on the effects of HT and other important factors in relation to women's health. Women invited to attend for mammograms at participating NHS Breast Screening Centres were asked to complete a questionnaire, and an impressive 1 in 4 women in the target age group took part. Unlike the Women's Health Initiative trials, this study is observational: all the women are fully aware of what they are taking.

Taking account of research carried out, most doctors think the following advice is reasonable:

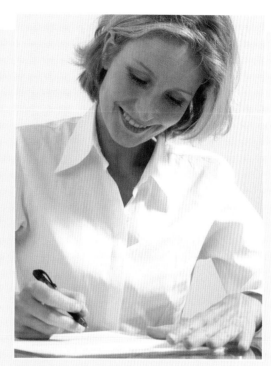

- ▶ A comparison of the potential benefits and the risks of HT is favourable for the short-term treatment of menopausal symptoms. The minimum effective dose should be used for the shortest time possible, and women should have a checkup at least yearly.
- ▶ A comparison of the benefits and risks is unfavourable for the first-line treatment of osteoporosis. HT should only be used for the prevention of osteoporosis when other first-line treatments cannot be tolerated or have not worked.
- ▶ The comparison is generally unfavourable for the use of HT in healthy women who have no symptoms.
- ▶ HT may be used in younger women who have experienced an early menopause (before the age of 50) for treating menopausal symptoms and preventing osteoporosis

(women who have an early menopause are at increased risk for the disease). At the age of 50, the doctor may recommend stopping therapy or taking an alternative medication for osteoporosis prevention.

THE WOMEN'S HEALTH INITIATIVE TRIALS

These trials looked at the use of combined HT in over 16,000 women between the ages of 50–79 who had not had hysterectomies, and of the use of HT in over 10,000 women of similar age who had had hysterectomies. Effects on hip fracture, breast cancer and heart disease were investigated and health in general was assessed.

These trials were double-blind, randomized and controlled; the women were randomly assigned to one of the two groups; one group received HT and the other used a placebo. Neither the patients nor doctors running the trial knew who was receiving a drug and who was taking a placebo.

- With women using oestrogen-alone therapy for five years, the rate of endometrial cancer increases to 9 women per 1,000; for those who use it for 10 years the rate increases to 15 per 1,000.
- With women using combined HT, the rate is estimated as 7 per 1,000 women after 10 years of use.

Ovarian Cancer

Prolonged use of oestrogen-alone therapy may be associated with a slightly increased risk of developing cancer of the ovary. Short-term use may also cause a very small increase in the risk. It has not yet been established whether using combined HT preparations increases the risk of ovarian cancer.

- About 9 women per 1,000 aged 50–69 and not using HT are diagnosed with ovarian cancer every year.
- With women using oestrogen-alone therapy for five years, the rate increases to 10 women per 1,000; for those who use it for 10 years the rate increases to 12 per 1,000.
- The risks of ovarian cancer with combined HT use are not known.

INTELLECTUAL FUNCTIONING

In some studies on healthy postmenopausal women taking HT the scores on cognitive function tests were higher than in the control group, particularly on tests of verbal memory. However, in elderly women who start treatment years after menopause, HT may actually increase the risk of dementia.

BLOOD CLOTS AND HEART DISEASE

There is evidence that the use of both oestrogen-alone and combined HT causes an increase in the risk of venous thromboembolism, particularly during the first year of use. For both oestrogen-alone and combined HT users, this translates as about 18 more blood clots per 10,000 women per year.

Venous thrombosis is the term used when a clot forms in a vein; the deep veins of the legs are most often affected. Fragments of the clot can break away and travel in the circulation to other parts of the body such as the lungs (causing a pulmonary embolism).

WISE WOMAN

Travel

Journeys that involve long periods of immobility (more than five hours) may increase the risk of deep vein thrombosis (a blood clot formed in the leg) in women taking HT. This risk may be reduced by taking exercise during the journey and wearing special stockings.

As the risk of thrombosis can be increased by major surgery, many doctors recommend that HT be stopped 4–6 weeks before some operations, and this should be discussed with your doctor. If HT is continued, special stockings may be worn and drugs given to reduce blood clotting.

The use of HT is also associated with a slightly increased risk of strokes (blood clots in the brain).

- About 3 women per 1,000 aged 50–60, and 11 per 1,000 aged 60–70 and not using HT suffer strokes every year.
- With women using HT for five years, the rate increases to 4 women per 1,000 aged 50–60, and to 15 women per 1,000 aged 60–70.
- Also, there is no evidence of a beneficial effect on heart disease as was previously thought. In fact, HT may increase the risk of coronary artery disease in the first year of treatment. Overall, the increased risk for women using combined HT is 29 percent for such events as angina and heart attacks. This translates as 7 more cases per year in 10,000 women.
- About 3 women per 1,000 aged 50–60, and 8 women per 1,000 aged 60–70 and not using HT are diagnosed with venous thromboembolism every year.
- With women using HT for five years, the rate increases to 7 women per 1,000 aged 50–60, and to 17 women per 1,000 aged 60–70.

SEEKING HELP

GUIDELINES ON HT USE

Taking into account a number of studies, including the Women's Health Initiative and the Million Women Study (see page 181), recommendations have been made on the use of HT. While these studies have produced valuable data, they don't provide all the answers. As the research continues, more will become known about the potential risks and benefits of hormone therapy.

Before making your decision you will need to talk this over with your healthcare professional. The charts on pages 184 and 185 may also help you with your deliberations.

Your healthcare professional will be able to give you an idea of the potential risks of your taking HT once he or she knows your medical history and is aware of any risk factors you may have.

CONTACTING A HEALTHCARE PROFESSIONAL

If you are not consulting your regular doctor, then the first appointment will be an opportunity for any new healthcare professional to find out about you: whether you are a candidate for HT and whether it is likely to benefit you. This visit is also an opportunity for you to fill in the gaps in your knowledge by asking questions. However, it is worth remembering that it may not be possible to answer every question and that research into the effects of HT is ongoing.

Your healthcare professional is likely to ask you about your medical history (if you have any current illnesses or a history of certain diseases, such as coronary artery disease). He or she will also ask about your family's medical history as well as checking your risk factors for certain diseases (in particular osteoporosis, breast cancer, venous thrombosis, pulmonary embolism, coronary artery disease and strokes). You will also be asked to describe your symptoms – including whether you have hot flushes, night sweats, vaginal dryness and soreness or bladder symptoms. He or she may also ask about how you are feeling generally.

Your blood pressure and weight will be checked. Usually a breast examination will be recommended, and possibly a cervical smear if one is due or if symptoms suggest that it should be done. A pelvic examination will also usually be performed.

If you decide to go ahead with HT, your healthcare provider will probably initially give you a prescription for three months of treatment. This will allow time for your body to get used to the treatment and for any side effects to settle. You may be given a prescription for six months at the next consultation, and then yearly prescriptions if all is well.

MONITORING

If you decide to use HT, you will have regular assessments to monitor your response to the treatment and to re-evaluate your need to continue it. Your doctor is likely to check your blood pressure and weight. Blood tests may be done, including a cholesterol check or blood glucose. A bone density assessment may be recommended for those at risk of osteoporosis (see page 67). Screening mammograms are offered every three years to all women between 50 and 65, whether they are taking HT or not. If you have a high risk of developing breast cancer you may be screened more often (see page 226).

THE FINAL WORD

Deciding whether to use HT is complex, and any decisions should be reviewed periodically. You and your healthcare professional will need to think about your reasons for considering it, your general health, family medical history and lifestyle in the context of research data and the Committee on the Safety of Medicines' recommendations. We know that HT can be beneficial in symptom relief and osteoporosis prevention, but this must be balanced against its potential drawbacks.

ARE YOU A CANDIDATE FOR HT?

HT may be appropriate in the following situations:

▶ If you are suffering symptoms of oestrogen withdrawal, such as hot flushes and night sweats, and they are severe enough to interfere with your everyday life.

▶ No alternative methods relieve your symptoms (see chapters 2 and 9).

▶ If you are at an increased risk of osteoporosis and have not responded to, or cannot take, other first-line treatments for osteoporosis prevention (see page 68).

▶ If you have had a premature menopause and are less than 50 years old.

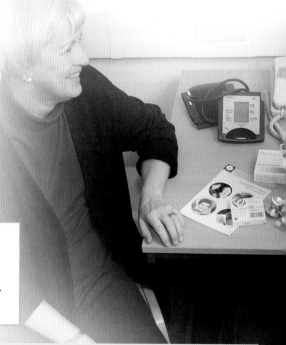

> As with all medications, you need to weigh up the possible benefits, side effects and risks. Your healthcare professional will offer advice and answer any questions.

WHEN HT SHOULD NOT BE TAKEN

There are certain reasons why a woman should not take HT. These are called the contraindications and may include:

▶ Being pregnant.

▶ Breastfeeding.

▶ Having an oestrogen-dependent cancer (cancers that grow in response to the hormone oestrogen, such as endometrial cancer – cancer of the lining of the uterus).

▶ Having breast cancer or having had breast cancer in the past.

▶ Having a venous thrombosis (clot formation in a vein), or having had a thrombosis in the past; also having a pulmonary embolism in which a fragment of clot travels to the lungs.

▶ Having angina or having had a recent heart attack or stroke.

▶ Having certain liver diseases.

▶ Having vaginal bleeding when the cause has not yet been found.

▶ Having endometrial hyperplasia (thickening of the lining of the uterus) that has not been treated.

WHEN HT MAY BE USED BUT WITH EXTRA CAUTION

Some circumstances do not necessarily preclude the use of supplementary hormones but special care should be taken. These include:

- Having fibroids (swellings in the wall of the uterus) as they may grow in response to HT (see also page 59).
- Having endometriosis (in which pieces of the tissue that normally lines the uterus are found in other areas of the pelvis), as the condition may worsen.
- When there is an increased risk of thromboembolism (predisposing factors for this include a personal or family history, severe varicose veins, obesity and prolonged bed rest).
- When there is an increased risk of coronary artery disease or stroke (predisposing factors for this include a personal or family history, diabetes, high blood pressure, smoking and obesity).
- Having migraine or migraine-type headaches, which may worsen.
- Having a family history of breast cancer if it is suggestive of oestrogen-dependent breast cancer.
- Having otosclerosis (a condition that affects the middle ear and causes

worsening hearing impairment), as the condition may worsen.
- Having a history of certain liver diseases, which may worsen.
- Having gallbladder disease, as gallstones may be more likely to form.
- Having diabetes, as blood sugar control may be disrupted.
- Having had endometrial hyperplasia in the past.

HT should only be used with extra care in various other medical conditions, including certain kidney diseases, asthma and epilepsy.

In addition, combined HT should be used with particular caution by women who have impaired liver function or depression.

These are not exhaustive lists. Circumstances vary and healthcare professionals will advise on an individual basis, taking into account existing medical conditions and other risk factors.

WHEN TO STOP TAKING HT

In the following circumstances, HT should be stopped immediately and medical advice sought.
- Pregnancy
- Sudden severe chest pains
- Sudden shortness of breath or a cough with blood in the sputum
- Severe pain in a calf
- Severe stomach pains
- Unusual prolonged severe headache
- Sudden partial or complete loss of vision
- Sudden hearing disturbance
- Sudden speech disturbance
- Fainting attack or collapse
- Unexplained seizure
- Weakness or numbness in an area of the body
- Hepatitis (inflammation of the liver) or jaundice (yellowing of the skin and whites of the eyes)
- Severe depression
- High blood pressure

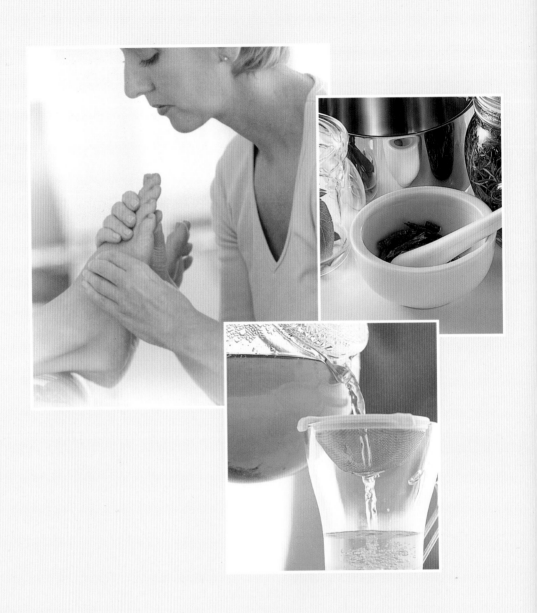

9

ALTERNATIVES TO HORMONE THERAPY

There are many women for whom traditional, chemical hormone therapy is not an option. Complementary approaches to menopause generally centre around dietary changes, as some plants and foods are considered beneficial in maintaining levels of, or even replacing, certain hormones, lifting your spirits, and aiding digestion or memory function, among other things. Holistic practitioners also offer several therapies and techniques that will enhance your overall well-being, health and vitality.

NATURAL REMEDIES

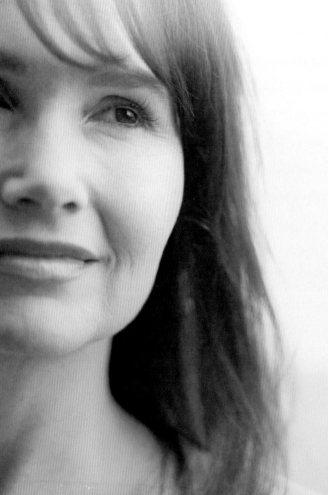

There are many natural foods and herbs that can help women during menopause. In some traditional cultures there is no word for menopause. If symptoms do occur, they are treated by reference to energetic principles just as any other condition would be, using herbs and other therapies that adjust the balance of the body naturally with no invasive side effects. Menopause is simply the onset of another phase of life; it has its own special needs, but otherwise it is just a natural part of life.

It is perhaps a comment on the way we live in our modern world that women experience such disruption at this stage in their lives. The ability to pass through menopause with ease and comfort depends to a large extent on how we have treated our bodies during our lives up until then. Symptoms at menopause may be indications that certain other systems and organs of the body have reached a state of crisis or exhaustion and are in need of support. It is possible that in more traditional cultures this level of wear and tear simply does not occur. Food is more natural and less saturated with additives, processed fats and sugars; water and air are cleaner; and there is less exposure to other environmental pollutants such as radiation, petrochemicals, electromagnetic frequencies and noise.

Perhaps the true extent to which these factors may have placed extra stress upon us can only be guessed at, but common sense tells us that they have a part to play in increasing the levels of certain diseases, diseases that, perhaps like menopausal symptoms, are virtually unknown in so-called underdeveloped societies. As these societies adopt the Western lifestyle, so, too, do they begin to develop diseases more common in the West. If we want to find solutions to these problems, we will need to somewhat revise our lifestyle choices in addition to simply choosing 'natural' remedies. And maybe menopause is a very good time to take stock of some of these factors and make changes – after all, it is called 'The Change'!

It is also probable that in choosing the 'natural' way, we are all too often thinking in the same modern way: that there is some magic pill that will take away all our symptoms and make our lives effortlessly comfortable. The truth is that the natural response to health and to life does demand some effort on our part. Other parts of this book present some very solid suggestions about how to begin this process of taking responsibility for your own health. In this chapter, you are also invited to consider that menopausal symptoms are nature's way of bringing certain imbalances to your attention, and encouraging you to understand yourself in a new way.

WHAT IS 'NATURAL HT'?

The notion of hormone therapy does not really begin to describe how herbal and natural solutions work for menopause. The emphasis on replacing hormones only addresses the fact that levels of oestrogen and progesterone decrease at this time of life. Certainly, there are plenty of foods and plants that can help to maintain levels of these hormones (see pages 112–114), or at least ease the decline, which in some women is sudden and can cause discomfort.

However, herbal medicine, where the practice of polypharmacy, or the combining of several herbs in one formula, addresses the whole picture of individual health, can do far more than simply supply extra hormones. A herbal practitioner can make an assessment of the individual woman in all her complexity and provide support for her whole system, perhaps targeting those organs or systems that have taken the toll of general wear and tear. In doing so, herbal medicine contributes not merely to the reduction of symptoms, but to enhancing her level of health and vitality, which surely is the birthright of any woman at any age.

It is not widely known, for example, that the liver and the adrenals, in particular, have vital roles to play at this time of a woman's life, and if these have become depleted, they will inevitably contribute to problems in menopause. Healthy adrenals will take up some oestrogen production at menopause, thus to some extent cushioning the drop in oestrogen produced in the ovaries. The liver, on the other hand, has been found to be an important factor in treating hot flushes. No one is quite sure why this is, except that it seems to have a role to play in temperature regulation.

Even when adjusting hormones, herbs can do more than simply supply extra. Some herbs can affect the pituitary, the master endocrine gland in

WISE WOMAN
Holistic health

A herbal practitioner will not only look at your current physical symptoms, but review your physical, mental and emotional state, probably going back some years to gain an accurate impression of your current and future needs.

the brain, thus influencing the output of certain hormones. This approach is one of the best treatments in any imbalance of the female hormone system and will usually form the basis of a herbal 'HT' formula.

Then there is the matter of bone loss: this, too, can have a variety of influences. Once again, in addition to treating the hormone levels, herbs and foods can help in supplying additional calcium (see the bone, flesh and cartilage formula on page 192) and can also improve the absorption and utilization of calcium via the digestive system.

A herbal menopause formula can thus address and adjust many different aspects of the body, targeting both 'routine' and specific requirements, and so create greater harmony throughout the whole system.

WHO CAN TAKE IT?

Herbal treatments for menopause are suitable for most women because they can be helpful for a number of related health problems, and if one approach is contraindicated for some reason, there are still benefits to be obtained from others.

This approach is particularly useful if for some reason – either because of contraindications or because of intolerance – your doctor will not prescribe pharmaceutical HT. In other cases, a woman may find she feels worse for taking HT, and her doctor may respond by changing the prescription to another kind. However, sometimes these too may continue to cause a woman to feel unwell. In such circumstances, herbal hormone treatments are well worth trying.

It also sometimes happens that for some medical reason a doctor feels that conventional HT is contraindicated after a woman has been on it for some time. If hormone therapy is withdrawn at short notice, a woman can experience a great deal of discomfort. A herbal solution at a time like this can be a welcome rescue remedy.

CONTRAINDICATIONS

The main contraindication to herbal treatment is that if you have had breast cancer and are taking tamoxifen, you should not take herbs containing phyto-estrogens. The reason is that, since tamoxifen suppresses the production of oestrogen in hormone-driven cancers, it may be rendered less effective in the presence of HT, and thus the level of protection against the recurrence of the cancer may be reduced. In fact, phytoestrogen use is controversial for women who have had oestrogen-dependent cancers (breast and endo-metrial) or are at high risk of them.

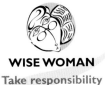

WISE WOMAN
Take responsibility

The more actively you are involved in your own health management the more empowered and successful you will feel. Choose methods that you can become involved in and read around subjects so you are better informed.

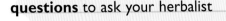

questions to ask your herbalist

- ▶ How long have you been in practice?
- ▶ Where did you study herbalism and what are your qualifications?
- ▶ How are herbal products regulated in this country?
- ▶ How long will it be before I see the benefits of this herbal supplement?
- ▶ Should I tell my doctor that I'm using herbal supplements?
- ▶ Will the herbal formulas you recommend interact with my prescribed medication(s)?

Apart from this, if you are taking other prescription medications you should check whether any of the herbs you wish to take have been cited in any herb/drug interactions. A well-known example of such interactions is the case of St. John's wort, which, studies have shown, can have adverse reactions with a number of drugs, including anti-depressants, hypertensive drugs, anticoagulants and the contraceptive pill. This herb has been used successfully for many years, and in that time very few problems have been reported among its users. However, until it is cleared of all implications, if you are taking any prescribed medications it is important that you check with your healthcare professional or a qualified herbalist before using St. John's wort.

The herbs listed here come with a list of contra-indicated drugs and conditions. They represent a selection of the plants that are considered to be the most useful in treating perimenopausal and menopausal women. They are also discussed as traditional extracts, that is to say, teas, powders or tinctures (water and alcohol extracts). As such, they are safe (except where contraindications are listed), and also widely available. The use of standardized extracts – preparations where the presumed 'active constituents' are guaranteed at a specific level generally larger than that originally intended in nature – is not generally recommended without professional advice.

SEEING A QUALIFIED HERBALIST

The best way to find out which herbs are specifically suited to your individual purposes is to consult a herbalist. He or she has been trained to make a proper assessment of your needs, and these will be more than simply the relief of symptoms, which themselves will, to an expert eye, suggest deeper imbalances and deficiencies.

A professional herbalist will start by taking a case history, to familiarize him- or herself with all aspects of your medical history and lifestyle. This will give an idea of what factors have contributed, or continue to contribute, to your discomfort. As we have noted, wear and tear during your life so far will have an impact on your health as you reach menopause, particularly if you have overindulged in terms of your diet or other habits such as drugs, tobacco or alcohol. It is highly likely that some revisions will be suggested, even if you are basically normal and healthy.

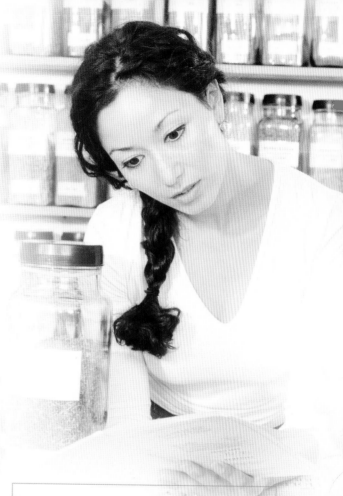

In addition to listening to your case history, a herbalist may well use other diagnostic methods, such as pulse or tongue diagnosis, or iridology. Iridology is a method of assessing your hereditary health tendencies, strengths and weaknesses, and possible levels of intoxication caused by improper diet or under-functioning organs of detoxification and elimination. This last item is especially important, since build-up and congestion in certain areas may well be responsible for some of the symptoms you are experiencing.

A herbalist is also trained to know when you should *not* take certain herbs. As we have seen, there will usually be a way to circumvent contraindications, but expert advice is needed to determine which route can safely be taken.

Herbal remedies will then be chosen to suit your individual profile, and these will usually be combined in a formula, a blend of perhaps four or five herbs that each tackle some aspect of your symptom picture and your constitutional requirements.

Regulating Bodies

In the UK qualified herbal practitioners go through rigorous training and are well versed in the human sciences and biomedical considerations. It is expected that herbalists in the UK will shortly be accorded statutory self-regulatory status, and thus be recognized as primary healthcare specialists.

There are several non-governmental bodies – such as the National Institute of Medical Herbalists – that seek to set standards of training, practice and quality of herbal medicine and offer professional membership and certification.

The Professional Herbalist

Do some research on the herbalists in your area before you decide which one to consult. Check up on their professional qualifications and the range of services they offer. Ask for a personal recommendation from friends and colleagues.

SOME USEFUL HERBAL FORMULAS

The following formulas may be particularly useful at the time of menopause. However, because of the holistic nature of herbal medicine, you should seek the advice of a qualified herbalist if you want to try them. Herbal practitioners go through a rigorous training course, so they will be better able to ensure that a particular formula is right for you.

More information on many of the herbs used here is given in the Menopause Herbal on pages 194–198.

'SUPER-SEXY' FORMULA

This formula can revive a flagging libido and help you to feel more confident in yourself. Take 25 drops of the tincture three times daily.

Ingredients
equal parts of:
Damiana
Siberian ginseng
Gotu kola
Rose
Vervain

BONE, FLESH AND CARTILAGE FORMULA

The herbs in this formula, based on that devised by the late Dr. John Raymond Christopher, are chosen for their high calcium content and other bone-building properties. This is a versatile formula that can be used for injuries and wounds, as well as in the maintenance of healthy bone density. Some of the herbs are also powerful nerve tonics and relaxants (the nervous system uses a lot of calcium). Osteoporosis is becoming more common in our society. Simply consuming foods high in calcium does not appear to reduce or prevent bone loss altogether. Calcium management is a complex issue that also depends on other nutritional factors, as well as on the ability of the individual digestive system to absorb and distribute calcium effectively. In herbs we find a high 'bioavailability' of nutrients, often in combination with other properties that can assist digestion and absorption. The formula below is best prepared as a powder and mixed into a fruit smoothie (see page 116).

Ingredients
2 parts Marshmallow root
2 parts Oak bark
2 parts Mullein
2 parts Oat seed
2 parts Horsetail
1 part Valerian
1 part Skullcap
1 part Wormwood

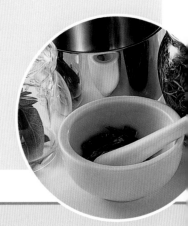

HEART AND
CIRCULATION TONIC

Strengthening the heart can be invaluable to anyone at this time of life, and the stresses and strains of hormonal instability may indeed place extra pressure on the heart. Use 25 drops of the tincture three times daily.

Ingredients

2 parts Hawthorn
1 part Red clover
1 part Motherwort
⅛ part Cayenne
¼ part Ginger

HERBAL HT

This is standard herbal hormone replacement therapy. That is to say, it can be used instead of HT, and is especially useful for assisting withdrawal from HT, should that be necessary or desirable. Use 20–25 drops of the tincture three times daily.

Ingredients

equal parts of:
Dong quai
Chaste tree berry
Black cohosh
Red clover
Siberian ginseng
Motherwort

DEPRESSION AND MOOD CHANGES

Anxiety, depression, irritability and moodiness can affect many women around the time of menopause, but there are herbs you can take regularly that will lift your spirits. Try a tea made with lemon balm, rosemary or vervain for a quick lift. Valerian and passionflower are effective for severe nervousness or panic attacks.

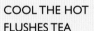

COOL THE HOT
FLUSHES TEA

Hot flushes and night sweats are common and can be very irritating. Both these herbs are excellent for relieving hot flushes, so drink this tea frequently throughout the day, or have some on hand by your bedside.

Ingredients

equal parts of:
Sage
Motherwort

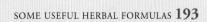

A MENOPAUSE HERBAL

The following pages will give you greater insight into the way herbal remedies may be applied at the time of menopause. The suggestions here (and in the formulas on the previous pages) are usually offered by herbalists as tinctures, which are alcohol extracts taken in a small amount of water. These are easy to administer, quickly absorbed and have the advantage of having a long shelf life, being quite stable at room temperature. Some herbalists, however, prefer to work with infusions – hot or cold, depending on the herb in use – and decoctions, and if you are alcohol-sensitive, either these, or other extracts not made with alcohol,

would be preferable. Alternatively, some, though not all, of these herbs may be available as capsules or tablets. Always follow the dosage instructions on the product label.

When using herbal remedies keep in mind that the 'results' might not be as immediate as with pharmaceuticals, but in some cases they are safer, more effective and longer-lasting.

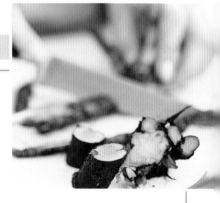

PREPARING HERBS

There are several ways to prepare herbs for use, each designed to make the most of the different parts of the plant that may be used.

Tinctures
These are alcohol extractions and are very concentrated. They are available from herbal practitioners, and the larger health food and herbal shops. The dose depends on the strength of the extract used, but a rough guide for a tincture is one teaspoon up to three times a day.

Herbal Infusions
Use this method for dried leaves, 'tips' of herbs and flowers.

1 Place 1 heaped dessertspoon of the herb or herbs in a pan.

2 Add 1 litre water, bring to a boil and simmer for 10 minutes, then leave to steep overnight.

3 Strain the herbs, squeezing out all the moisture, and drink 2–4 cups a day, hot or cold, storing in the refrigerator.

Decoctions
Use this method for roots, seeds, barks and berries.

1 Place 1 dessertspoon dried herbs in a pan.

2 Add 500 ml water, bring to a boil and simmer for 10–15 minutes.

3 Strain and drink.

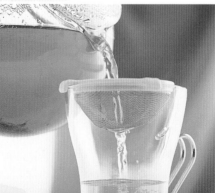

BLACK COHOSH (*Cimicifuga racemosa*)

This herb is known as an all-round helper for women's problems. During menstruation it helps to ease menstrual pain and cramping. It is anti-inflammatory and anti-spasmodic and contains phytoestrogens, thus making it a true 'herbal HT'. It is therefore a good all-round choice. In addition, it helps to relieve arthritic pain and can assist in spasmodic conditions of the bowel, or irritable bowel syndrome (IBS). The root is used.

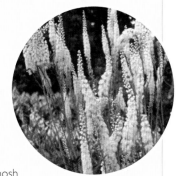

Contraindications: Because of its oestrogen effect, black cohosh should not be used with tamoxifen.

CHASTE TREE BERRY (*Vitex agnus-castus*)

A very well-known women's herb, chaste tree berry is a hormone balancer, working on pituitary gland secretions. It has the ability to promote higher secretions of progesterone. It, too, can be used at any time in a woman's life cycle, and it is often chosen to relieve menstrual symptoms. It has a particular role to play in relieving adolescent acne (in both girls and boys), but at menopause it is a gentle hormone balancer that brings the female system into equilibrium whatever the symptom picture.

Contraindications: Possible harmful interaction with bromocriptine.

DONG QUAI (*Angelica sinensis*)

They say one billion Chinese women can't be wrong! This herb from the Chinese herbal repertoire has been described as the most popular herb on the planet. Like chaste tree berry, it is thought to work on the pituitary gland as a hormone balancer, but it is also known in Chinese medicine for its ability to 'move and nourish the blood'. It is a member of the umbelliferaceae – a large group of plants that also includes fennel and Sweet Cicely, as well as the English variety *Angelica archangelica*, which is chiefly known as a digestive remedy, but can be substituted for dong quai if necessary. Dong quai is good in the treatment of fibroids. The root is used.

Contraindications: Dong quai should not be used alongside anticoagulants.

MOTHERWORT (*Leonurus cardiaca*)

This is a herb with a wide range of applications for women. It is known as an emmenagogue (promotes or brings on menstrual flow). It also protects the heart (note its Latin name, *cardiaca*), which it does partly by virtue of its cholesterol-lowering powers and its calming and relaxing properties. It is indicated wherever tension and anxiety are associated with menopause. The ariel parts of the plant are used. It combines particularly well with hawthorn for assisting with high blood pressure and protecting the heart.

Contraindications: Possible harmful interaction with antipsychotic drugs and non-steroidal anti-inflammatory drugs.

LADY'S MANTLE (*Alchemilla vulgaris*)
A very useful uterine astringent, lady's mantle can slow down and even stop profuse heavy bleeding and flooding. As some women approach menopause, periods begin to come more frequently and are heavier. Sometimes they may get to the stage where there is no gap between one period and the next, and they are bleeding constantly. Lady's mantle might help. This herb, combined, for example, with dong quai and black cohosh, can rectify the situation quite quickly – although you should bear in mind that 'quickly' in terms of herbal medicine may mean a week or two. However, it has helped save some women from having a hysterectomy. Add cayenne if the bleeding is severe, and consider iron-rich herbs also, such as raspberry leaf and yellow dock root.

Contraindications: None known.

RED CLOVER (*Trifolium pratense*)
Clover belongs to the same plant family as the pea, which is known for high content of phytoestrogens. Hence, like black cohosh, it is considered as a true herbal HT. Its other properties include the ability to cleanse and even thin the blood, as it contains coumarins, which have a mild anticoagulant effect. In fact, if you are taking a pharmaceutical anticoagulant, even large doses of aspirin, you should avoid this remedy. It is also known as an anti-cancer agent and appears in many herbal cancer formulas.

Contraindications: Because of its oestrogen-promoting activity, it is contraindicated in some forms of breast cancer, and where tamoxifen is being taken. Also, because one of its pharmacological effects is to thin the blood, it should not be used alongside anticoagulants.

SIBERIAN GINSENG (*Eleutherococcus senticosus*)
The adrenal glands become very important at menopause, and no herbal HT formula would be complete without some attention to them. Siberian ginseng (not related to Korean, Chinese or American ginseng) is described as an 'adaptogen', which means that it helps the body to adjust to stress and to periods of change, imparting increased energy. Perhaps because of this, it is also known as an antidepressant and can be used to help restore a lost libido.

Contraindications: Care should be taken if you have high blood pressure, and it should not be used with anticoagulants. Do not use if you are on a digitalis, such as digoxin, and take care if you use sedatives as it can cause excess sedation.

ST. JOHN'S WORT (*Hypericum perforatum*)

These days we know St. John's wort as an antidepressant. This is because of certain articles that appeared in the medical press, which set it up immediately in competition with Prozac and the like. However, herbalists throughout the ages have known this plant to be a gentle yet powerful healer of any trauma – physical or mental. At menopause, it can ease any feelings of low spirits and loss of self-esteem, and help to calm and relax the nerves.

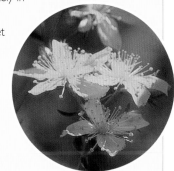

Contraindications: Do not use if you are taking heart drugs, other antidepressants (especially SSRIs) or a birth control pill: ask your doctor, a pharmacist or preferably a herbalist if you wish to take this remedy.

GOTU KOLA (*Hydrocotyl asiatica*)

A restorative, tonic herb, this remedy is in the same class as Siberian ginseng. At menopause it is particularly valued for its ability to help counteract the loss of mental function and memory that some women experience at this time of life.

Contraindications: May cause excess sedation if mixed with sedative drugs. Not to be used in pregnancy or by people who suffer from epilepsy.

LICORICE (*Glycyrrhiza glabra*)

Oestrogen- and progesterone-balancing, adrenal-enhancing and a great digestive remedy, this herb is often overlooked in hormone treatments, yet it is one of the most useful all-rounders. A topical cream made from the root has proved extremely effective in counteracting dryness of the vagina, not only by acting as a lubricant, but also, over a period of time, assisting a return to near-normal levels of secretion.

Contraindications: Not for internal use in cases of heart weakness or high blood pressure, though it can still be used vaginally. Possible adverse reactions with several types of pharmaceutical medications, especially heart drugs, are suspected: check with your health care practitioner before using.

SAGE (*Salvia officinalis*)

Symptomatic relief for hot flushes is the main contribution of sage at menopause. It can be added into a formula if hot flushes are a major problem, but it is generally preferable to take sage as a separate remedy so that you can dose yourself as and when you need to. If a hormone corrective treatment is being given as well, you should find your need for sage decreases over the period of a couple of months or so. Tip: add 20 drops to a glass of water and keep on your bedside table at night. If you are awakened by hot flushes, take a few sips immediately.

Contraindications: Possible add-on effects if used with sedatives.

ROSE (*Rosa damascena*)

The petals of damask rose have long been considered a favourite women's herb, and because it is also an extremely pleasant-tasting extract, it is enjoyable to take as a separate remedy. That way the whole experience of taking rose becomes a special treat! Rose is for regulating the menstrual cycle, treating uterine congestion and fibroids, and also for fertility; at menopause it is also useful as an aphrodisiac and antidepressant.

Contraindications: None known.

DAMIANA (*Turnera diffusa*)

This herb has a traditional reputation as an aphrodisiac. It is commonly considered a male remedy, but at menopause it is thought to be equally useful for stimulating libido in women. It is considered a tonic for the nervous system and is a safe stimulant with no known side effects.

Contraindications: None known.

VERVAIN (*Verbena hastata*)

This nerve strengthener and tonic has a wide range of applications and is known for its ability to impart strength and stamina. This it does partly through its action on the digestion, which again is tonic and bitter – stimulating the production of digestive secretions. It is also a significant mood-enhancer and antidepressant, and it was used by the wise women of olden times to assist dreams and visions.

Contraindications: None known.

OTHER SUPPORTIVE THERAPIES

As you will no doubt have gathered by now, the natural approach to menopause consists overwhelmingly of supporting and conditioning the whole system so that all its parts can continue to work in harmony as nature intended. There are, of course, many different approaches to this goal, most of which will also offer specific treatments for the hormonal system at this crucial time of your life. You will need to consult an appropriate professional practitioner in order to take proper advantage of these methods.

It can be confusing to find the right approach for yourself when there is so much to choose from. However, the brief descriptions that follow will perhaps be useful.

ACUPUNCTURE

An ancient healing art developed in Asia over 5,000 years ago, acupuncture uses a system of 14 energy pathways, called meridians, that run through the body in order to identify blockages in vital force (chi). Then, by the insertion of very fine needles at certain known acupuncture points, acupuncture restores the flow of chi throughout the system to achieve optimum health. Traditional acupuncturists use pulse diagnosis to determine where the energy is blocked. This is a holistic approach: symptoms are important more for the information they reveal about where the blockages in vital energy have occurred than as indicators of a specific 'disease'.

Benefits

Many people experience feelings of well-being and heightened energy levels as a result of being 'balanced'. Organs function in harmony, as they are 'unblocked' and are now supplied with vital energy in the right measure.

Disadvantages

Some people are understandably squeamish about needles. In fact, acupuncture needles are so fine they can hardy be felt; however, some discomfort may be experienced as the 'point' itself is penetrated. This is thought to be due to the release of stuck energy, rather than to a purely physical reaction.

HOMEOPATHY

The administration of extremely small amounts of substances (herbal, mineral or animal), which may even be toxic in large amounts, in order to stimulate the body's healing responses. The doses are known as 'potencies', and may be so small as to be

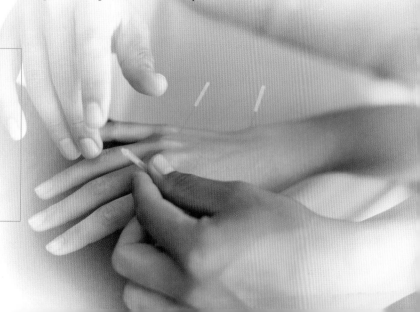

Acupuncture

According to the World Health Organization, there is good evidence that acupuncture is beneficial for joint pain caused by menopausal symptoms, lower back pain, rheumatoid arthritis and other persistent pain.

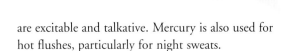

pharmacologically undetectable. However, the more dilute the preparation, the higher the potency and the stronger the effect. The founder of homeopathy, Samuel Hahnemann, worked on the premise that 'like cures like', and selected remedies that, given in large doses, would cause the same symptoms as those he sought to cure. Remedies are chosen by reference to 'constitution', that is, an assessment of the whole person – traits, common symptoms, personality and emotional factors. It is sometimes said that each individual has her own unique constitutional remedy.

Benefits

Remedies are easy to take, usually being a small tablet dissolved on the tongue, with no strong taste. Homeopathy treats the whole person.

Disadvantages

You will be asked to avoid certain foods and drinks that may be an 'antidote' to homeopathic remedies. These commonly include peppermint (including the flavouring in toothpaste) and coffee.

Some Useful Homeopathic Remedies

Generally, a homeopath needs to prescribe for the person, not the problem. If you wish to use homeopathic remedies, research them first to see whether you fit the general profile for the remedy. For example, sepia is used for low libido and low energy. 'Sepia' people exhibit a tendency to push others away and are prone to fatigue. Lachesis is sometimes used for hot flushes. 'Lachesis' people

are excitable and talkative. Mercury is also used for hot flushes, particularly for night sweats.

REFLEXOLOGY

This gentle technique, which dates back to the ancient Egyptians, is based upon stimulating 'reflex points' on the feet, which correspond to the organs of the body according to a 'reflex chart'. It is used to restore and maintain the body's natural equilibrium. It is said to be effective for back pain, migraine, sleep disorders, hormonal imbalances and stress-related conditions. Some reflexologists also talk of breaking down and releasing 'crystals' of uric acid or other impurities in the soles of the feet in order to 'decongest' and thus benefit the organs.

Benefits

Reflexology is usually an extremely pleasant and relaxing therapy in the hands of a competent professional. The massage is conducted so as to give attention to all organs of the body, while paying particular attention to those that need it, thus producing a balancing and stimulating effect on the whole system. Reflexology can also function as a diagnostic tool, by identifying spots on the feet that are painful and referring to the reflexology chart to pinpoint the organ concerned.

Disadvantages

There may be occasional pain when blocked organ reflexes are touched. This will indicate the need to unblock the energy, and any discomfort is usually short-lived.

NEUROLINGUISTIC PROGRAMMING

The basic premise of neurolinguistic programming (NLP) is that the words we use (and our non-verbal communication) reflect our subconscious perception of our 'problems'. If these words and perceptions are inaccurate, the underlying problem will persist as long as we continue to use them. For example, if you repeatedly find yourself saying 'I'm so tired', the likelihood is that you will act tired and stay tired, no

SHIATSU FOOT MASSAGE

Shiatsu – a type of acupressure massage – is a great way to wind down. Like acupressure, shiatsu works on the flow of chi through the body, using the 14 meridians or pathways. The following steps for a stress-busting self-massage will relax your feet and keep them flexible. When you have completed steps 1–5 on one foot, swap feet and repeat on the other foot.

1 Sit on a chair and place one foot on the opposite thigh. Rub a little massage oil or body lotion onto your foot. With your thumbs on the sole of your foot, apply pressure and work from the bottom of your arch up to the top, near your big toe. Repeat 5 times.

2 Press your knuckles into the bottom of your foot, moving up from your heel to your toes. Repeat 5 times.

3 Massage each toe by holding it firmly and moving it from side to side, then stretch each toe away from your foot. Apply pressure to the areas between your toes.

4 Hold your toes in one hand and bend them towards you, holding them for 5–10 seconds. Then bend them away from you and hold for 5–10 seconds. Repeat 3 times.

5 Roll your thumbs and press between the bones of the ball of your foot.

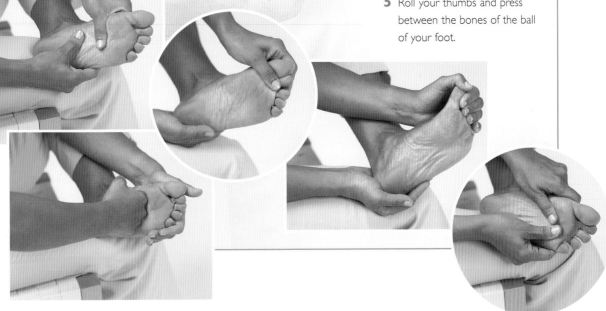

matter how much restful sleep you actually achieve.

With NLP, the therapist will analyse the words you use in describing your symptoms, as well as examine your facial expressions and body movements. After determining possible problems in your perception, the therapist will help you to understand the root cause and, with reference to how others have successfully dealt with similar situations, guide you in remodelling your thoughts and mental associations, replacing your old notions with positive thoughts and patterns that promote wellness.

Benefits

By showing you how others have successfully responded to the particular situation you are facing, NLP highlights the differences in approaches to 'problems' and outcomes, and encourages you to make positive changes to your behaviour voluntarily.

WISE WOMAN
Bach flower remedies

Prepared from the flowers of wild plants, bushes and trees, bach flower remedies help to resolve emotional and psychological disturbances and, combined with supportive herbs, can be excellent in balancing the emotions and increasing vitality.

ways to boost your energy

▶ Deep breathing – oxygen is a great source of energy that we don't use to its full potential.

▶ Drink water – dehydration is a common energy drainer, aim to drink eight glasses a day.

▶ Take a shower, alternating the water temperature between warm and cool to get your circulation going.

▶ Try a shiatsu massage (see box, page 201).

▶ Go for a brisk walk instead of slumping in front of the television.

▶ Take a siesta – a 20-minute mid-afternoon rest can revitalize mind and body.

Disadvantages

There should be no drawbacks to NLP, but as it is a 'talking therapy' it is important that you find the right therapist for you.

DIETARY CONSIDERATIONS

Diet is a crucial factor in achieving and maintaining good health at any age, but as we grow older we may become more sensitive to foods of a low nutritional value (see pages 106–127). Usually this sensitivity will register as some minor discomfort, perhaps in the digestive system itself, or perhaps in our general state of health.

A good test to see whether a particular food or meal is being well tolerated is to observe how you feel 30 to 40 minutes after eating it. If you feel fine, full of energy and clear-headed, then your body is happy with that food. If, on the other hand, you feel a distinct sluggishness, an uncomfortable fullness in the digestive tract or a sense of being fuzzy-headed and tired, this would strongly suggest that this food, at this time, does not suit you.

There is no one right diet for everyone – even at menopause. What supports your system, and what is tolerated by it, will be different from what the next woman needs. However, there are some foods that can be particularly useful at this time. Obviously, foods that have an oestrogen value, such as soya and members of the pea and pulse families, are strong favourites, so you might want to think about adding more lentils, peas, split peas, chickpeas and beans to your diet. There are many varieties of beans, all with their particular, individual flavour, and some with other health-enhancing properties as well. Aduki beans, for example, are great for the kidneys and adrenals, as are mung beans. Kidney beans, as well as being shaped like a kidney, are also said to be supportive of that organ.

There is also a range of foods that have come to be known as 'superfoods' (see pages 115–116). These are plant foods with highly beneficial nutritional profiles, which can be eaten either to supply particular nutrients or be used in combination with other foods to boost your intake of essential nutrients.

EXERCISE

Studies show that 1–3 hours of exercise a week may reduce hot flushes, so now is a good time to look at the amount of exercise you take. Exercise is vital for the support and strength of the cardiovascular system in particular. Other benefits include stress management, muscle strength and coordination and weight loss. Start with something gentle and consult your healthcare professional (see also chapter 6).

Yoga

Although yoga is known mainly as a system of exercises, it also has some quite specific therapeutic indications, and therefore can be a powerful way to support the body through the most radical of changes (see box, right and pages 144–145). Again, yoga should be viewed as a holistic system that tones and revitalizes the entire system; however, some postures may be practised to work on particular parts of the body. Consult a qualified teacher for guidance and advice about possible contraindications.

Dance

An advantage of dance as a form of exercise is that it is also very creative and good fun. Some dance styles are especially liberating to the menopausal woman. These include Arabian dance (Raqs Sharqi, bellydance), which celebrates and empowers the female at all ages, and other forms of dance that emphasize spontaneity and free expression.

Yoga for Menopause

Yoga stretches can benefit both the body and the mind, bringing energy and balance – particularly useful to women at this time because of their changing hormonal levels and fluctuating body chemistry. A gentle, slow-paced yoga practice is recommended. Lower-back bending poses such as the Locust tone the kidneys, nourish the adrenals and alleviate fatigue, while stretches such as the Tree can strengthen bone mass by increasing weight-bearing on the legs, hips and spine.

Working with a partner can be very rewarding, not only in correcting each other's postures, but in synchronizing with the other's breathing and feeling a genuine and peaceful togetherness with your partner.

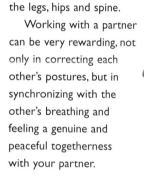

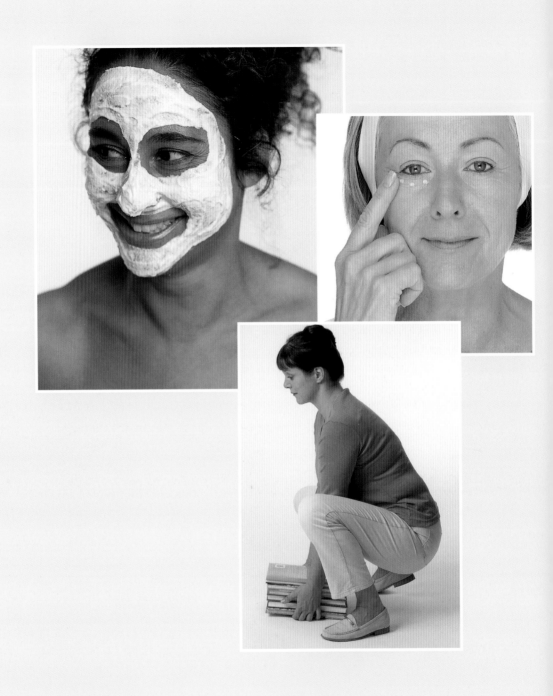

10

LOOKING AFTER YOUR BODY

For most women, menopause takes place at a time when their bodies are naturally aging. The combined effect of a loss of hormones with the normal aging process can lead to unwelcome changes in appearance. It's important for your self-esteem to feel and look good during this time. This chapter covers the many self-help measures and treatments available, along with useful self-checks you should carry out on a regular basis to safeguard your health.

TAKING CARE OF YOUR SKIN

Gradual skin changes (see pages 52–54) are among the recognized side effects of menopause. However, the loss of your skin's elasticity and flexibility and the emergence of wrinkles and lines can, to some extent, be minimized by proper skin care. Depressing as these changes may be, it's worth remembering that they don't happen overnight, so the sooner you increase your skin care the better.

Moisturize

Your skin needs to be hydrated from the outside, which is why moisturizing is especially important for dry, mature skin. Moisturizers contain water, which is absorbed by the skin cells, and a form of lubricant that then seals the moisture into the skin, giving it a softened surface. The best time to apply moisturizer is after a bath or shower while your skin is slightly damp, as this will give the skin cells a better chance to absorb the moisture. Pay particular attention to your elbows, knees and shins, as these areas don't produce as much natural lubricant as other areas of the body and this, combined with a depletion of collagen, makes them more prone to dryness. Moisturizers worn during the day will also help protect your skin against environmental damage – make sure you use one with an SPF of at least 15 to protect against sun damage, as well. At night, cell renewal is at its most active. It's a good idea to apply moisturizer at bedtime so it can nourish your skin while you are asleep.

Cleanse and Tone

Regardless of whether you wear make-up, cleansing and toning your face and neck should be done every morning and evening. Cleansing creams and lotions dissolve make-up and remove surface dirt, while toners remove any excess grease and restore the pH balance of the skin. Choose a toner that doesn't contain alcohol, as it can be very drying. Make sure you cleanse and tone behind the ears, under the hairline and down the neck to the collarbone.

Avoid Sun Damage

There's no doubt about it; too much exposure to the sun's ultraviolet (UV) rays can inflict a great deal of harm on your skin. UV rays destroy the skin's collagen fibres and also cause a build-up of abnormal elastin that causes the skin to stretch and wrinkles to form. In fact, most of the symptoms of premature skin aging can be blamed on the sun. Of course, it's impractical to suggest that you keep out of the sun altogether – you need sunlight for the production of vitamin D, which is essential for healthy bones – but protecting your skin from UV rays will certainly help prevent an increase in the signs of aging.

Fake It

Fake tans are an ideal way to give yourself a healthy glow without damaging your skin. There are a number of products you can buy over the counter to use at home, or you may prefer to go to a beauty salon where a number of different fake tanning treatments are available. These range from fake-tan

5 ways to protect your skin from sun

▶ Wear make-up that contains both UVA and UVB sunscreens.

▶ Always use a moisturizer that contains sunscreen with an SPF factor of at least 15.

▶ Apply sunscreen at least 15 minutes before going out in the sun and replenish it at least every two hours.

▶ During the summer months avoid being in the sun from 11 a.m. to 3 p.m. when the sun's rays are at their strongest.

▶ Wear a sun hat and sunglasses to protect your face, neck and eyes when it's sunny.

creams that are massaged onto your skin, to standing in a cabinet that sprays the fake tan all over your body. Fake tans can be topped up with repeated applications. If you are concerned about using fake tan on your face, you may prefer to try one of the after-sun creams that contain a 'tan prolonger'. These are moisturizers that have a small amount of fake tan in them so that they give a natural-looking, healthy colour.

Exfoliate

Removing dead skin cells (exfoliation) is one of the most effective ways of improving the quality of your skin. You can use a natural-fibre body brush or pad, or you may prefer to try one of the many exfoliating products that are on the market. If you use a brush or pad, always use it on dry skin – if it's wet, mature skin can be stretched by brushing vigorously – brush towards the heart with long, firm strokes, starting at your ankles and working upwards. Don't forget your hands when you body-brush; exfoliating them will remove dead skin and make them look younger. It's also necessary to exfoliate before applying fake tan – particularly on ankles and knees. Exfoliating washes are used with water and contain particles that take off dead skin cells. Whichever method you choose, for it to be effective, you will need to exfoliate at least twice a week.

Eat Right

Eating the right food and drinking plenty of water – at least eight glasses a day – can go a long way towards keeping your skin healthy. Include plenty of fresh fruits and vegetables in your diet, as they will give you a natural intake of vitamins A, B and C – all of which are essential for healthy skin. It's also recommended to include two or three portions of oily fish, such as salmon, sardines or mackerel, each week or take a cod-liver oil supplement. Oily fish contains omega-3 fatty acids that are good for your skin and joints. Vitamin E, found in avocados and wheat germ, or taken as a supplement, will help to rehydrate the skin. If you think you may not be getting enough of these vitamins from the food you

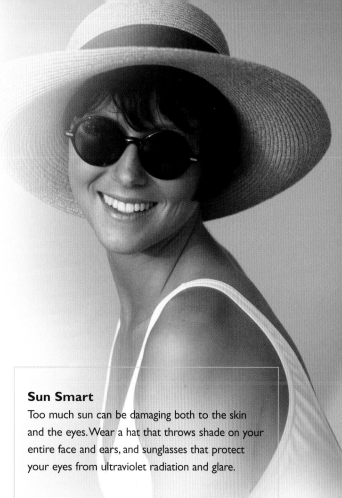

Sun Smart

Too much sun can be damaging both to the skin and the eyes. Wear a hat that throws shade on your entire face and ears, and sunglasses that protect your eyes from ultraviolet radiation and glare.

eat, you can top up your vitamin and mineral intake with a multivitamin and mineral supplement – look for one that has been specially formulated for menopausal women. (See pages 106–127 for more information on diet.)

COSMETIC TREATMENTS

More and more women are turning to specialized procedures to help delay the signs of aging. There is a whole range of treatments specifically aimed at the mature woman. If you are considering such a treatment, find out as much as you can about the doctor or surgeon who will perform the procedure and check out his or her qualifications and areas of expertise. When you visit the doctor, make sure you have a thorough consultation and that you understand exactly what the procedure involves.

NON-SURGICAL TREATMENTS

Botox (botulinum toxin) injections

Small amounts of botulinum toxin are injected into the area around deep lines, such as frown lines, to temporarily paralyse the muscles. After the injection your skin has a smooth line-free surface that lasts about three to four months.

Collagen Injections

A replacement collagen product (there are many different types on the market) is injected into the skin to fill out and smooth away lines and wrinkles, frown furrows and acne scars. The results are instant and last for up to three months. A small amount of redness may occur immediately after treatment, but this soon wears off.

Chemical Peels

Available in varying strengths, from mild to deep, an acid solution is applied to the skin to remove fine lines, wrinkles and skin discolouration in the top layers, and to encourage the regeneration of new tissue and improve skin texture. Initially, you may be left with flaking, reddened skin but this soon wears off, leaving a softer, relatively line-free surface. The effects of a chemical peel can last for up to a year.

Microdermabrasion

This is a mild, mechanical peel that improves the skin's texture by using a stream of crystals and suction to exfoliate the skin. The treatment is used to remove age spots, sun damage and minor imperfections and leaves the skin with a healthy

GIVE YOURSELF A NATURAL FACIAL

Face masks contain properties that draw out impurities and shrink the pores, so they are a really easy way to give your complexion a boost. If you can, have a good soak in a warm bath before you apply the mask as this will help to open up the pores. Alternatively, cover your face with a hot face cloth for a minute or two before applying the mask. Once it has been on for the required amount of time, rinse it off using a face cloth to make sure all traces have been removed, then smooth on your usual moisturizer.

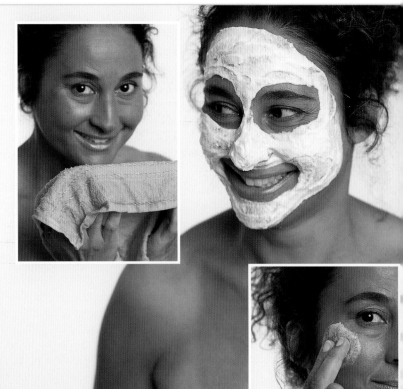

glow. A number of initial treatments will be needed, followed by a longer-term maintenance programme.

Dermabrasion

A moderate to deep mechanical peel, this removes the surface layer of the skin with high-speed sanding. It is used on deep acne scars, lines and wrinkles and isn't suitable for everyone. The treatment is carried out under anaesthesia and requires up to two weeks for recovery.

Laser Skin Resurfacing

Lasers can be used to treat mild to severe wrinkles by resurfacing the skin so that it becomes smooth again. The recovery time is around two weeks. The non-ablative laser, which heats up the dermis without injury to the upper layers of skin, is a new technique that is thought to increase collagen and elastin production and formation.

Intense Pulsed Light Therapy

Also known as IPL Photorejuvenation, this treatment uses high intensity pulses of light to penetrate the skin. Different filters are used to treat particular skin conditions, such as thread veins, fine lines and wrinkles. Four to six initial treatments are required; they produce gradual, natural improvement with good long-term results.

Chickpea flour mask

- 2 tbsp chickpea flour
- a pinch ground turmeric
- 1 small pot live natural yogurt
- 2–3 drops lemon or lime juice (oily skin)
- 2–3 drops sweet almond oil (dry skin)

Mix the flour, turmeric and natural yogurt into a paste. Add in either the lemon or lime juice or sweet almond oil. Smooth over face and neck. Relax for 20 minutes. Splash off with warm water. Repeat 2–3 times a week for at least three months and you'll see visible improvements.

Anti-aging avocado mask

- 1 ripe avocado
- 1 tbsp unpasteurized honey
- 2 capsules evening primrose oil
- 1 tbsp rosewater

Mash up the avocado and mix in the honey. Blend in the oil from the capsules. Pat onto your face and neck. Leave on for 20 minutes. Rinse off with cool water or wipe with a cotton ball soaked in rosewater. Use once a week.

Refreshing sandalwood mask

- 2 tbsp chickpea flour
- 1 tbsp live natural yogurt
- 6 drops sandalwood essential oil

Mix the flour with enough yogurt to make a paste, then add the oil. Massage over your face, avoiding eyes and mouth. Relax for 10 minutes. Splash off with water.

Moisturizing honey mask

- 2 tbsp unpasteurized honey
- 2 tsp freshly squeezed lemon or lime juice

Mix the honey and juice. Pat the mixture onto your face and neck using upward, circular movements. Relax for 15 minutes. Rinse off with warm water. Most effective when applied after steaming your face.

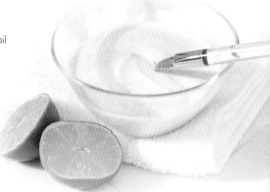

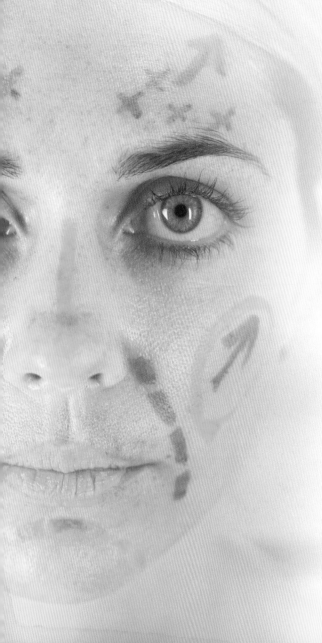

SURGICAL PROCEDURES
Complete Face-lift
If you look in a mirror and put your hands on either side of your face and then pull your skin back, you will get some idea of what can be achieved with a face-lift. This is major surgery, done under general anaesthesia, and involves a stay in a hospital or outpatient facility. Pain, swelling and bruising can be a problem for several weeks after the operation, but the end result usually leaves your face looking 10 to 15 years younger.

Brow-Lift
This opens up your eyes without surgery on your eyelids. Keyhole surgery is used to remove the folds of skin above the eyelid that occur when the eyebrows start to droop. The skin is gently pulled back to reposition the arch of the eyebrow. The operation is carried out under general anaesthesia, and you will normally be treated as an outpatient. All signs of the surgery should have disappeared within three weeks, leaving you with younger and less tired-looking eyes.

Upper Eyelid
Carried out to remove excess fat and skin from your eyelids, this operation is done on an outpatient basis under local anaesthesia. Swelling and bruising can be a problem for a couple of weeks and the scars will need protection from the sun for several months. The result is eyes that look younger and wider.

Lower Eyelid
This operation gets rid of the bags under the eyes. It is done on an outpatient basis under local anaesthesia. Bruising and puffiness occur for at least two weeks afterwards, but the result is eyes that look many years younger.

Lip Augmentation
This is surgical enhancement of the lips. Fat and skin are taken from another part of the body and are used to fill out the lips. It takes from two to six weeks for all signs of surgery to disappear, and even then there will be a small scar, but it can be hidden with lipstick. The result is fuller lips that will last longer than collagen injections.

MID-LIFE MAKE-UP

The right make-up can hide a multitude of skin problems and give you a healthy, glowing look. One of the best products for mature skin is concealer, which can be used to cover dark circles under the eyes and age spots, as well as to lighten the deep lines that run between the nose and mouth. Choose a creamy, yellow-toned concealer that you can pat into the skin.

Foundation should match your natural skin colour as closely as possible – yellow tones are better for mature skins than pinky shades and will give warmth to your skin. Look for foundations that contain built-in moisturizers and light-diffusing particles. Apply only enough to give an even finish; too much foundation cakes on the skin and emphasizes lines and wrinkles. If you use powder to keep your foundation in place, choose one with a superfine texture that won't clog pores and wrinkle lines.

As mature skin tends to lose colour with age, blusher can really give your face a boost. Choose peachy or apricot shades that blend with your natural skin tone.

Lips

Like the rest of your skin, your lips need to be moisturized and protected. Work the moisturizer into your lips and the skin around them to help fill out fine lines. Lip balms are a good way to keep moisture sealed in and they will help to protect your lips during the day. Look for a lip balm that contains a sunscreen. Apply lip balm at night before going to bed so that your lips continue to be moisturized while you sleep.

Lipstick is another good protector. Choose one with a moisturizer in it – matt lipsticks are often too drying for mature lips. A lipstick base under your lipstick will help stop the colour from 'bleeding' into the fine lines around your mouth.

Eyes

Keep eye make-up light and natural-looking – too much will become clogged in the folds of your eyelids and may 'bleed' into the laugh lines at the sides of your eyes. To be flattering to mature skin, eye shadow should be subtle rather than bright. Powder eye shadow is best – cream eye shadow often melts and slips into the creases so it ends up accentuating any lines.

Mascara can work wonders, making your eyes appear bigger and wider than they really are, but avoid black as it may be too harsh against your skin. If you have droopy eyelids use waterproof mascara that won't smudge into the skin.

Eyebrows

Your eyebrows, like your hair, may be getting thinner and losing their colour. Shape your eyebrows, keeping as close to their natural line as possible. Don't be tempted to try and make them dark again; this will only make them dominate your face. If your hair is still dark, aim to make your brows a few shades lighter. If you are grey or light blond try using a grey or light-brown eyebrow pencil, or for a more permanent solution, you may prefer to have them dyed a few shades darker.

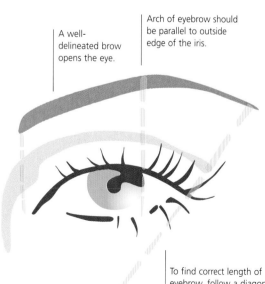

A well-delineated brow opens the eye.

Arch of eyebrow should be parallel to outside edge of the iris.

To find correct length of eyebrow, follow a diagonal line from same-side nostril.

HAIR, TEETH AND NAILS

Like skin, hair, teeth and nails require special attention during menopause.

HAIR CARE

One of the most obvious signs of aging is greying hair – as you get older new hair growth has little or no pigmentation. Although grey hair is just as healthy as pigmented hair, it can be coarse as well as fine, and it has a tendency to be dry and look dull. Oestrogen is needed to nurture new hair cells, so as the levels drop, your hair loses its natural nutrition, becomes thinner and loses volume. Hair loss (see pages 57–58) often results from fluctuating hormones, but once your hormones level off, your hair should become thicker again.

Washing

A build-up of dust and grime will make your hair look lifeless, so it's important to shampoo it regularly – at least every two or three days. Because mature hair is more fragile, the edges of the hair shafts can become rough, giving the hair a 'fluffy' appearance. Washing your hair helps to flatten the hair shafts, which in turn helps to create a smoother,

glossier appearance. Look for shampoos for mature hair that contain polymers, as these help to smooth the hair shaft and add volume.

Conditioning

A good conditioner will give your hair additional body and help to protect it if you use styling aids, such as curling tongs. Use your fingers or a wide-toothed comb to spread the conditioner through the hair. If your hair tends to be greasy, try applying conditioner to the ends rather than over the whole head. Leave-in conditioners will help to give your hair added body, but don't use too much as they can make your hair appear dull and flat. Use a hot oil or intensive-moisturizing conditioner every few weeks for an added boost.

Colour

Although healthy grey or white hair can look really good, especially if it's styled well, not everyone wants to go grey gracefully, and you may prefer to camou-flage this particular sign of aging. If you're Caucasian, avoid using dyes in rich, dark colours as they will not complement your skin tones and, instead of deducting years from your appearance, may actually make you look older. It's best to go a couple of shades lighter than your natural colour, and perhaps add a few lowlights to give an appearance of warmth that will also flatter your skin. Your hairdresser will be able to advise you on the best choice of colours. If you prefer to treat your hair at home, you can choose from a number of different colouring products.

- **Temporary colours** give a colour change that washes out after a few shampoos. They are a good idea if you want to see if a new shade suits you.
- **Semi-permanent colours** will blend the grey into your hair colour so it completely disappears. Over time the darker colour will disappear so it will need to be reapplied every few weeks.
- **Permanent colours** have a chemical base that penetrates the hair shaft so they can't be washed

---

tips for healthy hair

- ▶ Wear a hat to protect your hair from the sun.
- ▶ Cover your hair with a cap when swimming in chlorinated pools.
- ▶ Use a leave-in conditioner to protect your hair, especially if you swim in the sea.
- ▶ Avoid using anything that 'tugs' at the hair or causes it to break, such as narrow-toothed combs and tight hair bands or elastics.
- ▶ Have your hair trimmed regularly.
- ▶ Always use your hairdryer on a cool setting.

out. Look for products that are specifically for grey hair, as they will be less damaging and will give better coverage. Depending on how quickly your hair grows, colour should be applied to your roots every six to eight weeks.

Unwanted Hair

Another side effect of menopause is the appearance of unwanted hair on the face. This can be soft and downy or you may get random coarse hairs sprouting around the mouth and chin. The easiest way of dealing with the soft downy hair that grows on the cheeks, chin and as a 'moustache' on the upper lip is bleaching. This will make the hair much less noticeable – you can further disguise it by using a foundation that gives a matt finish. Avoid using loose powder on your skin as it will cling to the hairs, making them even more obvious.

If a 'moustache' is a problem, you can try removing the hair with specially formulated facial strips. Don't use ordinary waxing strips as they are too harsh for mature skin and could cause damage. Always finish off with a mild antiseptic, such as tea tree oil, to prevent skin reactions.

Alternatively, electrolysis or laser hair removal can be used to get rid of unsightly facial hair. These treatments will eventually remove unwanted hair permanently, but they should always be carried out by a qualified professional, as there are risks involved if the treatment isn't performed correctly.

Individual coarse hairs can be plucked out with tweezers. You will have to repeat the procedure as the hairs grow back, but gradually they may become weaker and less noticeable.

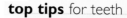

Threading is less damaging to delicate skin, and just as effective as plucking or waxing on areas such as the chin, upper lip and eyebrows. A skilled practitioner can remove a number of hairs in a single twist of the thread.

DENTAL HYGIENE

If you want to keep your teeth into old age, you will need to pay a great deal of attention to your dental hygiene now. Your teeth should be cleaned, using toothpaste that contains fluoride, at least twice a day – in the morning and again last thing at night – but, better still, after every meal. If you suffer from sensitive teeth – when the enamel of the teeth becomes thinner, making them more porous and more sensitive to hot and cold – use a toothpaste specially formulated for sensitive teeth. If you have less saliva than you used to, you can buy a toothpaste formulated for dry mouth that gives the salivary enzymes you need and reduces the risk of bacterial infection.

Avoid using a toothbrush with hard bristles as these will irritate and damage the gums. It's better to go for a soft- or medium-bristled brush, with a compact head size, which should be changed every six to eight weeks. This applies equally to electric or sonic toothbrush heads.

Cleaning between your teeth is as important as brushing their surfaces. Flossing between the teeth each time you brush them will remove any particles that have become trapped. Many people find flossing difficult, so you may prefer to use a tiny interdental brush specially designed for the job. Finish off your cleaning routine with a mouthwash that will help remove any remaining bacteria.

Be sure to visit your dentist every six months for a checkup and a professional cleaning by a dental hygienist. The hygienist will remove plaque and any build-up of tartar, and clean and polish your teeth.

Discoloured or Misaligned Teeth

As you get older your teeth produce more yellow-brown dentine, and the white enamel that covers the outside becomes thinner, leaving the teeth looking discoloured. Although visits to the hygienist will help, you may want to consider having your teeth whitened professionally, or you may prefer to try a home whitening kit.

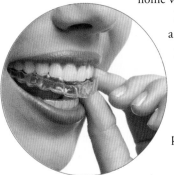

If misaligned teeth are a concern, talk to your dentist about straightening your teeth using almost invisible clear braces called 'aligners' (see photograph).

MAINTAINING NAILS

The loss of oestrogen can make your nails brittle and flaky, so avoid trimming them with scissors, clippers or metal files – use an emery board instead – and massage hand and nail cream into your cuticles daily. Protect your hands when you are doing housework, gardening or other heavy jobs. Hardening of the arteries, which can occur as you get older, causes poor circulation, which can, in turn, lead to nail thickening, so it's important to trim your nails at least once a week. If your nails are very thick keep them short and try to thin them as you cut them. Regular treatment by a chiropodist will help to keep your feet in good condition. (See also page 201.)

False Nails and Extensions

False fingernails can give your hands instant glamour. However, the glue used to attach them could do long-term damage to your own nails if used too often. Nail extensions are an alternative, but should be put on by an expert and shouldn't be worn for too long as they prevent the nails from 'breathing', which they need to do to stay healthy.

NAIL CARE

1 Soft cuticles are less likely to suffer from cuts and infections. Once a week, add some wheat germ oil to warm water and soak your nails.

2 While in the bath, use a pumice stone to remove hard skin on your hands or feet, then rinse and pat dry.

3 Apply a moisturizer or hand or foot cream, really working it into the skin and cuticles so that you give yourself a massage as well.

4 Shape fingernails with an emery board and cut toenails straight across with clippers. Apply a base coat to nourish and protect nails.

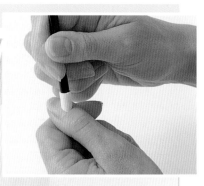

5 Check that your nails are free of infections. *Paronychia*, for example, produces ridged and discoloured nails, or you may have some swelling and tenderness.

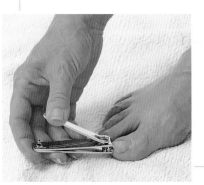

EYES AND EARS

Fluctuating hormone levels can cause alterations in vision and eye shape, which can make wearing contact lenses more difficult. It is also quite common during and after menopause to experience "dry eyes"—your eyes feel dry, gritty, and sore, but not painful. Dry eyes are caused by changes within the constitution of the tears that your eyes naturally produce, both in terms of volume and effectiveness. Tear substitutes, such as eye drops, can alleviate the symptoms, but they won't cure the cause. Always wash your hands before applying eye drops. You may also find that taking an ocular nutritional supplement helps to relieve the symptoms. This lack of lubrication can cause problems if you wear contact lenses, so if you are experiencing problems seek advice from an ophthalmologist.

Make sure, too, that you have regular checkups as glaucoma, cataracts, and macular degeneration—all serious eye problems—become more prevalent as we get older.

Good lighting, both at home and in your workplace, becomes increasingly important as we age, as the pupils react more slowly and inadequately to changes. This also means that bright lights, such as oncoming cars' headlights while night driving, become more dazzling.

Laser surgery

Everyone's eyesight deteriorates as they get older, few people, male or female, reach middle age without needing glasses. Laser surgery can be used to replace the need for distance glasses, but if you are shortsighted this can affect your reading ability. Also, the success rate, even with eyes with normal tears, is still only 90 to 95 percent, which means 5 percent of people could need contact lenses to correct a laser-induced permanent problem. If you want to consider laser surgery you should discuss this in detail with an ophthalmologic surgeon, who will be able to explain the likely outcome of any procedure.

ways to help dry eyes

- ▶ Protect your eyes from sun and wind by wearing sunglasses.
- ▶ Avoid irritants such as smoke, dust and cosmetics.
- ▶ Wear goggles when swimming in a pool to protect your eyes from chlorine.
- ▶ Use artificial tears or a lubricant regularly.
- ▶ Seek medical help if dry eyes persist for more than a week, despite treatment.

AVOIDING HEARING LOSS

Some hearing loss is a natural part of aging. With age, the eardrum stiffens and its ability to vibrate becomes reduced. There also can be degenerative changes in the middle ear bones and a loss of hair cells in the inner ear. Some types of hearing loss even run in families.

The most important thing you can do to maintain your hearing is to protect your ears against noise. That means turning down your music system at home and in the car. When outside, use earplugs when necessary if there is excessive noise from jackhammers or electric saws, for example. Try also not to expose your ears to long bursts of noise.

It's preferable not to remove earwax with swabs as wax protects your delicate eardrum from dust and water. If wax becomes bothersome, however, consult your doctor who will clean your ears or give you a prescription for drops.

Certain medications, antibiotics and aspirin, for example, can produce temporary hearing loss and ringing in the ears. Smoking and coffee both restrict blood flow to the ears, affecting hearing, as will fatty and high-cholesterol foods. Keeping active, however, will help stimulate blood circulation.

BACK CARE AND POSTURE

The changes to your muscles, ligaments and bones caused by the decrease in oestrogen and the effects of 'wear and tear' are likely to make back injuries more common once you become menopausal. Your spine is supported and moved by an intricate network of muscles. Muscles always operate in pairs, so for every muscle that contracts there is an equal and opposite one that relaxes. The muscles of your abdomen work in this way with the muscles of your back to maintain your spine's natural curves. Make sure when you exercise that you work all your back and stomach muscles equally so that there is no danger of an imbalance – a common cause of pain.

Ligaments are broad bands of tough tissue that bind your vertebrae together, allowing your spine to move as one piece. Two long ligaments run down the length of your spine at the front and back of your vertebae. Ligaments may be tough, but they have a poor blood supply and do not heal easily if strained or torn.

The most common cause of back pain is muscle strain. This is particularly likely to occur if you stand or sit still for long periods of time and don't exercise regularly, as the muscles that support your spine will weaken from lack of use. And, when you try to do something a little more strenuous than

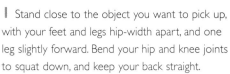

LIFTING AND CARRYING CORRECTLY

1 Stand close to the object you want to pick up, with your feet and legs hip-width apart, and one leg slightly forward. Bend your hip and knee joints to squat down, and keep your back straight.

2 Before lifting, make sure your pelvis is tilted upwards and your abdominal muscles are tight. Bring the object in towards your body and allow your heels to lift slightly off the floor. Pick up the items as centrally as possible, so that their weight is distributed evenly.

3 Stand up slowly, keeping your back upright. Make your leg muscles do the work of raising you. When you carry anything, keep your back straight and the items close to you. Take care not to twist your body.

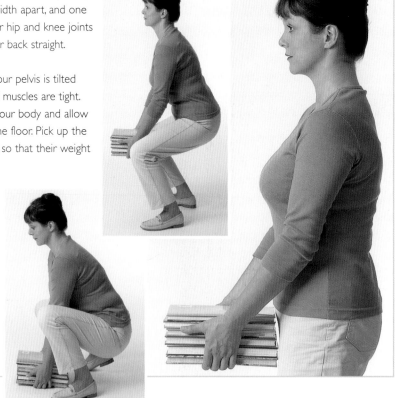

usual, such as lifting a heavy object, your muscles will be unprepared and may strain as a result.

Learning to lift and carry heavy items is essential for maintaining a healthy back. If you lift from the floor with your arms extended and your back bent, your leverage will be poor and the weight borne by your back will be perhaps ten times the weight you are trying to lift. If your muscles are not strong enough, your ligaments will take too much strain and may tear. See opposite for the correct technique.

See opposite for the correct technique.

▶ GET EXPERT HELP

Physiotherapy is the oldest-established conventional manipulative therapy. Practitioners use a variety of treatments, including massage and joint manipul-ation, heat and ultrasound to ease pain and stiffness.

Chiropractic involves hands-on manipulation of the spine, joints, muscles and surrounding tissues with particular attention to the realignment of the vertebrae in your spine. A chiropractor will use sharp, rapid thrusts along with more gentle manipulation.

Osteopathy also uses hands-on manipulation to stretch and loosen muscles and ligaments. Through gentle movements it aims to restore muscles and ligaments to their normal range of movement and alleviate pain.

Shiatsu is an Eastern-based therapy in which a practitioner uses a combination of passive manipulation, stretches and pressure from the hands, thumbs, elbows, knees and feet on pressure points located around the patient's body to stimulate Ki energy and eliminate blockages that are causing pain.

PERFECTING YOUR POSTURE

Posture tends to deteriorate with age because of bad habits, such as slouching and sitting hunched up, which have been developed over many years. Your posture affects your balance and the way your limbs move – if it's good, you will be able to walk and move smoothly with controlled movements; if it's bad, your gait will be uneven and your movements jerky. Bad posture can make you look older than someone who has a relaxed, upright posture. By paying attention to the way you stand, walk and sit, you will not only look and feel younger, but you will also be helping to keep your spine and back muscles in good shape.

Standing Straight

Once you've mastered this way of standing, you will find that your muscles are more relaxed and that your balance is centred. If you've been standing badly for years, then you may need help in achieving good posture. Consider learning Pilates, the Alexander Technique or t'ai chi, all of which will help you unlearn bad habits and teach you how to control your movements so that your body is well balanced and moves freely.

Your shoulders should be relaxed, not hunched.

Your spine should be vertical with no hollow in your lower back.

Try to keep your pelvis slightly 'tucked' under.

Keep your legs straight with your knees soft, not locked.

Your feet should be parallel with your weight evenly distributed between them.

Sitting Well

Always use a chair that supports your lower back; a straight-backed chair is preferable to an easy chair. You could also use a reclining chair that keeps your legs propped up. Try not to sit with your legs crossed and don't sit in one position for too long. When you are on a long train or plane journey, get up every 30 minutes or so to stretch and take the pressure off your back. Whenever you get the chance, lie flat on your back with your knees bent.

The best position is to sit with your weight evenly distributed, your knees slightly apart so that your weight is well supported, and your feet together, underneath your knees. It helps to choose a chair that gives you proper support – especially when looking for a desk chair (see below).

(see below)

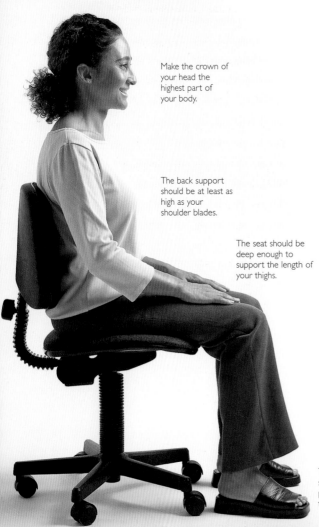

Make the crown of your head the highest part of your body.

The back support should be at least as high as your shoulder blades.

The seat should be deep enough to support the length of your thighs.

The height of the seat should allow you to place your feet flat on the floor comfortably.

Preventing Veiny Legs

After the age of 40, spider veins and varicose veins become much more common, particularly in women. Women are six times more likely to suffer from them, and scientists now think that the female hormones may play a role in their formation. Both pregnancy and menstruation increase pressure on the veins through increased blood flow.

There are certain things you can do to forestall varicose veins:

- Shed some weight, as extra pounds put extra pressure on legs.
- Drink plenty of water to soften stools and eat more fibre to prevent constipation.
- Keep on the move while working: take regular ambulatory breaks to keep blood from pooling.

However, if you already have varicose veins, there are things you can do to keep them from getting worse:

- Elevate your legs as much as possible and sleep with your feet raised to prevent blood from pooling in your legs at night.
- Wear support hose; they can help when there are a few small veins. Their compression helps to keep the veins down.
- Participate in regular rhythmic exercise to keep your blood moving.
- Make sure that your vitamin E intake is sufficient. A deficiency has been associated with the exacerbation of varicose veins.
- If you're on HT, check with your doctor that your dose is correct. Occasionally, women on low-dose oestrogen therapy will suffer from swollen and aching legs and a worsening of existing varicose veins.

SLEEP WELL

One of the best and easiest ways to look good is to get a good night's sleep. Sufficient sleep makes you feel better, perform better and remain emotionally balanced. Moreover, while you are asleep your body releases its greatest concentration of growth hormone, the substance that helps your body repair damaged tissue.

However, with menopause there can be changes to your normal sleep pattern. You may find you need more or less sleep and that it can take longer for you to fall asleep. You may also suffer from sleep disorders. See pages 37–38 for advice on dealing with insomnia and other sleep problems.

Assuming that you are lucky enough to fall asleep easily and stay asleep, the correct position is important, as it can help to prevent muscle aches and stiffness. The best position for sleeping is on your back or side. If you suffer from lower-back pain you may find that placing a pillow between your knees will make you more comfortable, or you may need to change your mattress. If you have only recently started to experience aches and pains in your back it may be because your mattress is too hard or too soft.

As you get older your spine loses mobility and resilience and your mattress needs to compensate for this. Consider buying an orthopaedic mattress specially designed to give the additional support you need. It is recommended that you get a new mattress at least every ten years.

When you wake in the morning, try giving yourself a good stretch before you get out of bed. This helps to lengthen your muscles and relax them. However, be careful not to overdo it, the stretch should feel comfortable and not painful in any way – overstretching can cause muscles to tear.

If you wake up in the morning feeling tired and sluggish, it may be that you've had a disturbed night due to snoring. By age 60, almost 40 percent of women snore. Snoring is more common in the overweight and those with short, thick necks. It can be helpful to stop smoking, lose weight, cut down on alcohol, make sure your nasal passages are clear, and sleep on your stomach or back.

If your insomnia begins to interfere with your daytime functioning, discuss it with your doctor and consider an evaluation by a sleep specialist.

Sleeping Soundly
Don't expose yourself to allergens while sleeping. Natural fibres such as linen and cotton are ideal choices for bed linen. They don't attract dust and they allow your skin to breathe properly. Avoid foam and feather pillows and mattresses made of synthetic fibres.

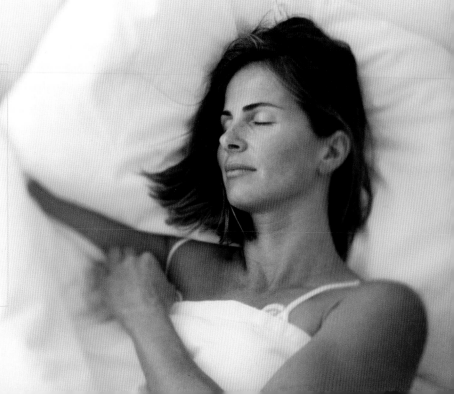

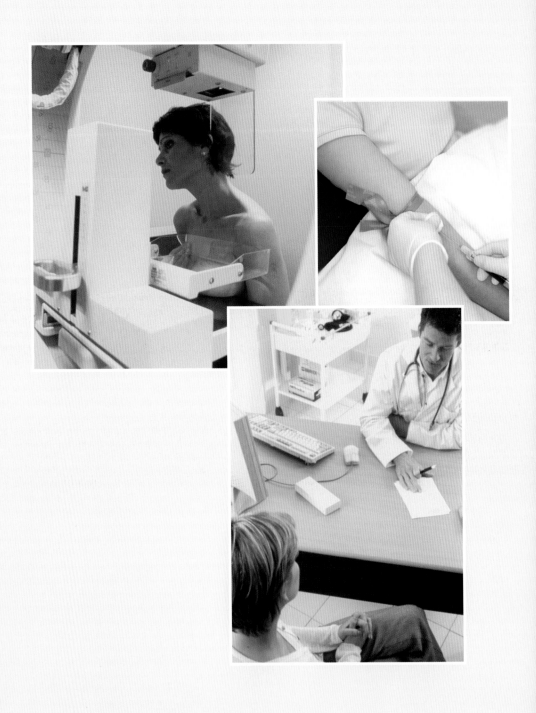

11

SAFEGUARDING
YOUR HEALTH

There are some changes that may occur simply because of the aging process and others that are directly linked to menopause. The important thing is that you feel confident about any necessary tests or procedures you may have to undergo. This chapter looks at the diseases that are most likely to occur around this time and the treatment options that may be offered to you.

BEING BODY AWARE

As we become older, we are more likely to get various diseases. Whether we are affected or not depends to some extent on our genetic make-up; some of us will be at greater risk of getting heart disease or certain types of cancer than others. However, in many cases we can influence our risk by modifying our lifestyle. We can also improve our prospects by looking out for warning signs of disease and by taking screening tests where appropriate; in most cases, the sooner a disease is diagnosed, the better the likely outcome.

In this chapter, we will discuss some common diseases specifically related to the breasts and the reproductive system, as well as some diseases that are more likely to occur after menopause. These include coronary artery disease (which causes angina and heart attacks). We will also cover some of the tests you may encounter either as a part of normal screening or if you have symptoms that need to be investigated further.

Making Informed Decisions

From perimenopause onwards, women often find they are consulting doctors more frequently than they ever did before. Some of the consultations will be about menopause itself, but others may have to do with disorders and diseases that are more common in later age. It pays, therefore, to make sure you are in the best position to make informed decisions about your health, and the best way to do this is to have a good relationship with your healthcare practitioner. There are a number of ways you can make medical appointments more meaningful and get the most from them.

It's a good idea to make a list of problems that are concerning you, so that when you see your health-care professional, you'll be able to cover everything. This is especially important if you are worried about particular symptoms. If you keep a record of what they are and when they seem to occur, you will enable your doctor to give you much better advice. Don't be shy about sensitive topics, such as urinary and faecal incontinence – your doctor is there to help you and the more he or she knows about your situation, the more accurate the diagnosis and treatment will be. If you don't feel comfortable talking about particular subjects with your health-care professional, you should try to find someone else more compatible. And, if there is anything you don't understand about the recommended treatment or screening procedure, make sure you keep asking questions until all the ground is covered.

It's a good idea to be proactive and keep yourself abreast of the latest developments in menopause and treatments of some of its side effects. New products are constantly being introduced. Moreover, if you are not satisfied with the advice you receive, you should feel free to actively seek a second opinion. No woman should settle for less than the best in her healthcare.

BREAST AWARENESS

It is recommended that all women should become familiar with the appearance and texture of their breasts so that they'll notice if any changes occur. Learning how your breasts feel at different times will help you to know what's normal for you. Before menopause, normal breasts feel different at different times of the month. The milk-producing tissue in the breast becomes active in the days before a period starts, making some women's breasts feel tender and lumpy, especially near their armpit area. After menopause, activity in the milk-producing tissue stops and normal breasts feel softer and less lumpy.

In the past, monthly self-examination of the breasts was recommended so that problems could be picked up at an early stage. Current thinking is that this formal checking can cause anxiety and guilt if it is missed, so many health professionals advocate a more relaxed approach. However, it is still strongly recommended that women become familiar with their breasts and monitor for changes. If you're not familiar with self-examination, then it is a good idea to examine your breasts every day to start with so that you become really familiar with how they look and feel. Then continue to monitor them regularly. Checking your breasts with a soapy hand in the shower is a good way to examine yourself, but also see the illustrated procedure on page 224.

breast changes to look out for

- ▶ A lump or area of thickening in the breast.
- ▶ Change in the size or shape of the breasts.
- ▶ Dimpling of the skin.
- ▶ Nipple becomes turned in.
- ▶ Discharge from the nipple.
- ▶ Swelling or a lump in the armpit.
- ▶ Skin changes in the nipple or the surrounding areola.

It is important to seek medical advice if you notice any changes in your breasts. However, it is worth remembering that seven out of eight breast lumps are found to be benign.

▶ DIABETES AND MENOPAUSE

Although all women experience some bodily changes at the time of menopause, diabetic women are faced with more specific changes and risks. The fluctuating levels of oestrogen and progesterone at this time have an effect on blood sugar levels. Decreasing oestrogen makes the body more resistant to insulin so that blood sugar levels rise; decreasing progesterone levels, however, result in increased insulin sensitivity, so blood sugar levels drop. These changes may call for diabetes medication to be adjusted. However, many women require up to 20 percent less medication to control diabetes following menopause due to the body's more efficient use of insulin, as well as an increased insulin sensitivity.

There are also some specific health risks associated with diabetes and menopause. The chance of contracting coronary artery disease (CAD) is two to three times higher for post-menopausal diabetic women than for non-diabetics. Diabetic women also incur more vaginitis and vaginal yeast infections. Decreased oestrogen and high blood sugar levels combine to create an environment where yeast and bacteria thrive. A heart-healthy diet (see pages 120–121) and the right exercise programme (see pages 130–151) can help reduce the risk of CAD, while maintaining blood glucose levels, and following the advice on page 47 can help reduce vaginal infections.

1 Look in the mirror and check for any changes in the appearance or position of the nipple. Also look for rashes or patches of dry skin on the nipple or the surrounding area (the areola). Look again while raising your hands above your head.

2 Put your hands on your hips and press them into your hips. Look out for lumps, which may be visible if near the skin, and check for puckering or pulling of the skin.

3 With the pads of your fingers (not the tips) press gently on the breast tissue. Imagine that your breast is divided into four areas and examine each quarter carefully. Then press again but more firmly. Also, examine the tissue that extends from your breast to your armpit. Then check the armpits for swollen glands. Think of the armpit as a pyramid; check the four walls and the apex at the top. The more you do this the quicker you'll get.

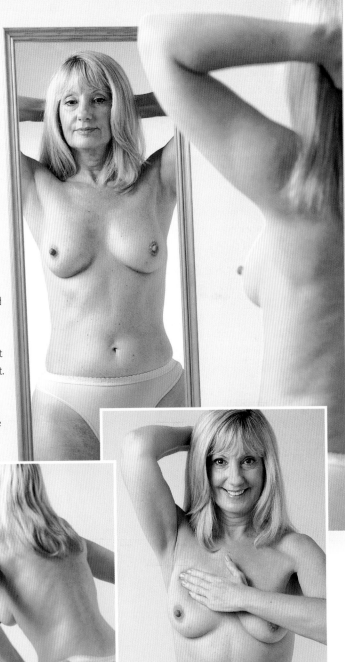

CHECKING YOUR SKIN

The incidence of skin cancer is increasing, particularly in our sun-loving culture, but most forms are easy to cure if caught early enough. You should check your skin every month for new skin lesions and moles and for changes in existing ones. The earlier a skin cancer is detected, the better the prognosis. Look carefully for any changes in the way your skin looks or feels.

When examining your skin, work from top to toe and remember to include the scalp, face, neck, armpits, between the fingers and toes, the nails, soles of your feet and between your buttocks. Use a mirror to examine your back and buttocks.

Many harmless growths, such as skin tags, become much more prevalent with age (see page 54) so it's important that you consult a doctor so that he or she can reassure you as to what is normal and what is not.

5 skin changes to look out for

- ▶ A new skin growth.
- ▶ A skin growth that gets bigger, thickens or changes shape.
- ▶ A skin growth that appears pearly, brown, black or multicoloured.
- ▶ A mole or brown spot that:
  - changes colour
  - changes texture
  - has an irregular shape
  - oozes or bleeds
  - itches
- ▶ A spot or sore that:
  - itches or is painful
  - forms a crust or scab
  - ulcerates or bleeds
  - does not heal within three weeks

3 main types of skin cancer

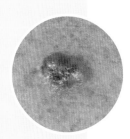

Basal cell carcinoma (also called rodent ulcer) is the most common type of skin cancer, and is most often associated with excessive exposure to the sun. These tumours are usually slow-growing and can be cured in most cases. If left untreated, they eventually erode into nearby structures, but spreading to other areas of the body is very rare.

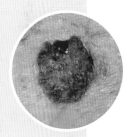

Squamous cell carcinoma is also common. These cancers tend to grow more rapidly than basal cell carcinomas and can spread to other sites in the body. Again, in most cases they relate to sun exposure.

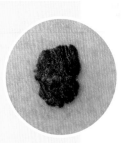

Melanoma is the most serious form of skin cancer as it can spread early to other body sites. However, it can be cured if it is diagnosed early. As with other types of skin cancer, the incidence is rising, probably as a result of excessive sun exposure. About half of malignant skin melanomas arise from pre-existing moles.

SPECIALIST TESTING

The following investigations are offered to the general population to check for signs of certain diseases in their early stages. Some screening tests are offered routinely to all women; others are offered to women at increased risk. Although other tests may not be offered as part of a formal programme, your doctor should carry out screening checks, such as checking weight and blood pressure, or testing urine for sugar, which may indicate diabetes mellitus.

MAMMOGRAPHY

Using special low-dose x-rays, mammography produces images of the breast tissue. The aim is to detect breast cancer in its early stages, thereby increasing the likelihood of successful treatment.

Experts disagree on how early to have a mammogram and how often it should be carried out. In the UK, the NHS Breast Screening Programme offers screening mammograms to all women from the age of 50, and repeat mammograms are offered every three years. Women are recalled until the age of 70 and may choose to continue to have screening mammograms thereafter. Women who have a family history

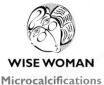

WISE WOMAN
Microcalcifications

These are tiny deposits of calcium in the breast that can't be felt but can be seen on a mammogram. A cluster of microcalcifications can be an early warning sign of cancer.

or an increased risk of breast cancer should consult their GP, who will refer them to a Breast Clinic for risk assessment. Women with a righ risk may be offered annual mammograms.

When hormone levels are high, as they are in perimenopausal women, breasts appear denser on mammograms and they can be more difficult to read, resulting in more false positives. In such cases, the timing of the mammogram should be scheduled just following menstruation, or, if you are on contraceptives, during the week of any withdrawal bleed.

Women with implants or fibrocystic or lumpy breasts also have denser breasts, and for them, mammography may not be able to accurately detect abnormalities.

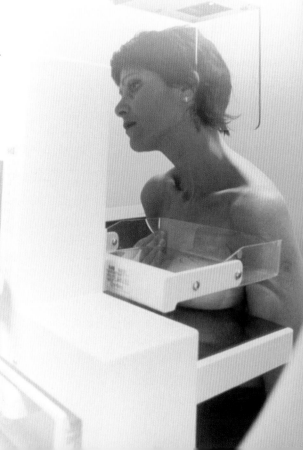

Mammograms

Although mammograms have some limitations and cannot detect all types of cancer, regular mammograms are the most effective way to detect cancer early. A radiologist reading the resulting films will look for several types of changes – calcifications or microcalcifications, a 'mass' or a cyst.

What Happens During a Mammogram

First one breast and then the other is placed on the x-ray machine and then compressed with a plastic plate. Two views are usually taken of each breast. Mammography may cause some discomfort, but the test lasts only a few minutes.

In most cases, the x-rays will be normal. If an abnormal area is shown, you will be asked to attend further breast assessment. This does not necessarily mean that cancer is suspected – mammograms can detect other breast abnormalities. In a few cases, mammograms need to be repeated for technical reasons, including lack of clarity of the images.

Special mammography views that give clearer images of an abnormality, or magnified or enlarged views of the breast, can also be done. Spot compression views look at one small area of the breast and are used to assess microcalcifications.

ULTRASOUND

High-energy sound waves are bounced off internal breast tissues to determine if there are lumps, and if so, whether they are solid or cystic (containing fluid). This can help to provide information on whether an abnormality is benign or cancerous. Gel is applied to the breast and a small ultrasound probe is run over the breast tissue. This test is painless and takes only a few minutes. Because the waves are unaffected by breast density, ultrasound may be helpful for women who have denser breasts (see above). Ultrasound cannot, however, consistently detect microcalcifications.

IMAGE-GUIDED BIOPSY

If a lump has been detected and an ultrasound or MRI can't determine if it's benign, a sample of tissue may be removed. Using ultrasound or x-ray, the doctor will locate the lump and make a small incision to remove a small sample of tissue from the affected area (core biopsy) or draw out cells and fluid through a small, fine needle called a fine needle aspiration, or FNA. Both are performed under local anaesthetic. If a cyst is present, the lump may disappear once the fluid is withdrawn. If a solid lump is present, a sample of cells may be taken. In both cases, the samples are sent to the laboratory for examination. The sampled area may be tender and bruised for several days afterwards. In some cases, the whole lump is removed under either general or local anaesthetic. This is usually arranged on an outpatient basis, but it may occasionally require an overnight stay in hospital.

In the majority of cases further investigations will prove negative or will show benign breast disease. However, if breast cancer is detected, further treatment will be necessary (see pages 242–245).

CERVICAL SMEARS

Also known in the United States as Pap smears (after Dr. George Papanicolaou, who first developed them), these are done to examine samples of cells taken from the cervix. Specialists check both for abnormalities which, if left untreated, may develop into cervical cancer in the future, and for infections.

What Happens During a Cervical Smear

The doctor or nurse will insert a speculum into the vagina to keep the vaginal walls open, allowing the cervix to be seen clearly. Cells are collected from the cervix using a small spatula or brush and are spread on a glass slide or put in a jar with a special liquid, which is sent to the laboratory for examination.

Smears may pick up a variety of abnormalities. Often, these will be due to an inflammation or infection that may require treatment. Some medications can cause changes in the appearance of cervical cells (you should mention to the doctor any drugs you are taking). However, sometimes the changes are caused by cervical intraepithelial neoplasia, also called CIN (see page 228). This condition is not cancer but may develop into cancer in the future if left untreated. Therefore, such changes may need to be investigated further. The smear report may refer to these abnormalities as dysplasia. Cervical smears can also sometimes detect early cervical cancer but this is much less common. Rarely, endometrial cancer cells may also be seen in postmenopausal women.

COLPOSCOPY

This test allows the doctor or nurse specialist to look at the cervix in more detail with a special microscope. As with a cervical smear, the walls of the vagina are kept apart with a speculum. The cervix is coated with a special fluid that highlights the abnormal area, enabling the examiner to take samples of the abnormal cells. The test usually takes up to 20 minutes. If the abnormal areas cannot be seen clearly, a cone biopsy may be required.

3 types of CIN

Cervical intraepithelial neoplasia (CIN) is graded from 1–3, depending on how deeply it extends into the surface layers of the cervix. If cancer is present, the abnormal cells extend deeper into the cervix.

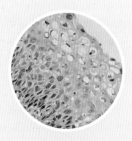

CIN 1: As mild changes often return to normal on their own, a repeat smear may be performed 6–12 months later.

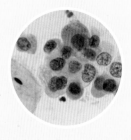

CIN 2 and CIN 3: A colposcopy will be arranged.

CONE BIOPSY

This test is carried out under local or general anaesthetic and involves removing a cone-shaped sample of the cervix that contains all the layers of tissue needed for microscopic examination.

Treatment Options

CIN 1 does not usually require treatment. CIN 2 and CIN 3 may be treated in various ways, all of which involve either removing or destroying the abnormal cells. In large loop excision, a common method, a thin wire is used to remove the abnormal area after the cervix is anaesthetized locally. Alternatively, the abnormal area may be removed by cone biopsy.

Methods of destroying the abnormal cells include laser treatment, in which a laser beam is directed at the affected area, and heat treatment, which involves the use of a hot probe. Both of these procedures can be carried out under local anaesthetic.

Rarely, a hysterectomy may be recommended for women who do not wish to become pregnant and have a more severe abnormality.

A smear test will usually be repeated after six months, or in some cases a colposcopy will be arranged. Smear tests will then be repeated at least every year for 5–10 years. Hysterectomy is followed by vault smears; these are similar to cervical smears but the cells are taken from the top of the vagina.

GENERAL TESTS

The body usually tells us when something is wrong by presenting symptoms. Doctors use the information we tell them about our symptoms, as well as what they find when they examine us, to guide them in making a diagnosis. Tests will often be needed to back up these findings. Here, we describe some of the investigations commonly used.

Testing Those at Increased Risk

Particular screening tests are sometimes offered to those who may be at increased risk of certain diseases. Examples include blood lipid tests for people who are obese or have a family history of raised blood lipids, and colonoscopy for those with a family history of bowel cancer. In a colonoscopy, a viewing instrument is passed up the bowel to examine its lining. Samples of tissue may be taken for examination under the microscope.

If you think a disease may run in your family, see your doctor. He or she may recommend screening tests and also suggest lifestyle changes that should lower your risk of getting the disease.

BLOOD TESTS

FULL BLOOD COUNT

A blood count measures the levels of red blood cells (which carry oxygen to the tissues), white blood cells (which fight infection) and platelets (which help the blood to clot). As well as testing for specific disorders, the blood count is used as a measure of general well-being.

THE SEX HORMONES

Luteinizing hormone (LH) and follicle stimulating hormone (FSH) play a key role in the control of the menstrual cycle. They are produced by the pituitary gland (see pages 14–15) and stimulate the production of oestrogens and progesterone by the ovaries. Around menopause the ovaries fail to respond to these hormones and oestrogen levels fall. The production of LH and FSH increases in an attempt to stimulate the ovaries. Therefore, doctors sometimes check blood levels of LH, FSH and estradiol (a type of oestrogen) to help them diagnose menopause. After menopause, FSH and LH levels will be high, whereas estradiol levels will be low. In perimenopause and the early stages of menopause these levels may be normal.

CHOLESTEROL

Increased cholesterol levels, associated with an increased risk of coronary artery disease, have been linked to a fatty diet. However, a lipid blood test can

WISE WOMAN
Gene testing

Some of the genes responsible for increasing the risk of particular diseases have been identified, including some of those associated with breast, colon and ovarian cancer. For example, the BRCA-1 and BRCA-2 genes are known to be associated with an increased risk of breast cancer. Therefore, gene testing may be possible for some individuals with a family history of a particular disease.

measure not only cholesterol levels, but also the levels of triglyceride (another type of fat in the blood) and certain types of lipoproteins (the particles that transport cholesterol and triglycerides in the blood). The lipoproteins can be separated because they have different densities. Two that are particularly important are the low-density lipoprotein (LDL) particles and the high-density lipoprotein (HDL) particles. High LDL concentrations are associated with an increased risk of coronary artery disease, whereas higher concentrations of HDL particles have a protective effect. Very high levels of triglycerides are associated with an increased risk of acute pancreatitis (a very painful and potentially life-threatening condition in which the pancreas becomes inflamed) and retinal vein thrombosis (blockage of a blood vessel in the eye that can cause impaired vision). Other risk factors for coronary artery disease are taken into account when the results are evaluated by the doctor.

Ideally, cholesterol should be less than 5mmol/l, but should be evaluated in conjunction with the values of LDL and HDL.

BLOOD GLUCOSE LEVELS

These are often checked as a screening test for diabetes mellitus.

INVESTIGATING THE REPRODUCTIVE TRACT

ENDOMETRIAL BIOPSY

Endometrial biopsies may be taken to investigate abnormal vaginal bleeding and to look for evidence of endometrial cancer. A sample of tissue is taken from the lining of the uterus (the endometrium) for microscopic examination. It may be taken during a hysteroscopy (see below), D&C (see right) or with a suction device, usually in conjunction with transvaginal ultrasound (ultrasound scanning in which the probe is placed in the vagina). Transvaginal ultrasound enables the examiner to measure the thickness of the endometrium, which may help in the diagnosis of endometrial cancer.

A simple outpatient procedure, an endometrial biopsy takes only a few minutes. A speculum is used to keep the vaginal walls apart and a thin, flexible tube is passed into the uterus. Suction is used to draw an endometrial sample into the tube.

DIAGNOSTIC LAPAROSCOPY

This procedure allows the doctor to examine the pelvic organs. A small hollow needle is passed through the abdominal wall and carbon dioxide is passed through it. This distends the abdomen and allows a trocar (a rigid hollow tube) to be passed in without damaging the pelvic organs. The laparoscope (a viewing instrument) is then passed down the trocar into the pelvis. Many operations can be performed laparoscopically.

HYSTEROSCOPY

Using a viewing instrument (the hysteroscope), the doctor can take samples of the lining of the uterus (called endometrial biopsies) and look inside the uterus. The uterus is filled with a liquid passed through the hysteroscope. This allows the interior to be seen clearly. The procedure can be carried out under general or local anaesthetic and takes about 15 minutes.

DILATATION AND CURETTAGE (D&C)

This is another method for taking samples from the lining of the uterus. It is carried out under general anaesthesia or local anaesthesia with intravenous sedation. The cervix is widened by passing rods of increasing width through and then the lining of the uterus is scraped. This procedure has largely been replaced by hysteroscopy, which allows the inside of the uterus to be examined.

INVESTIGATING BONE DENSITY
BONE DENSITOMETRY

Known as DXA (dual-energy x-ray absorptiometry), bone densitometry uses very low doses of radiation (less than 10 percent the radiation dose of a chest x-ray) to measure bone density, which accounts for 70 percent of bone strength, in order to diagnose osteoporosis (see pages 68–71).

The lower spine and the hips are usually assessed. However, small devices can be used for screening

Bone Densitometry

Like cholesterol level and blood pressure, bone density is a risk factor that can be changed. You can't do much about factors such as genetics, sex or age, but your doctor can use the results of a DXA test to prevent or treat osteoporosis.

and to assess other parts of the body, such as the wrists or heels.

Bone densitometry diagnoses bone loss which may be mild (osteopenia) or more severe (osteoporosis). Combined with other risk factors the density measurement is used to assess the risk of developing fractures in the future. It is also used to monitor the response to treatment in people with osteoporosis.

What Happens During Bone Densitometry

You will lie on a padded examination table, below which is an x-ray generator that sends x-ray beams through your body. Above, there is a detector arm that passes over the body taking measurements. The test takes 10–30 minutes. The smaller machines sometimes used for screening are basically box-like structures into which the foot or forearm is placed.

You will be given two scores. The T-score indicates the bone density compared to a young woman with peak bone mass. Above –1 is normal;

WISE WOMAN
T-scores

Most older women will have a T-score below the standard. However, bone changes very slowly so the test should only be repeated after a year.

between –1 and –2.5 indicates that significant bone thinning has occurred but not enough to be classed as osteoporosis; below –2.5 gives the diagnosis of osteoporosis. This score is also used to assess the fracture risk.

The Z-score indicates the bone density compared to other women of a similar age and size. If it is very high or low, further tests may be recommended.

INVESTIGATING THE CARDIOVASCULAR SYSTEM
ECG (ELECTROCARDIOGRAPHY)

The ECG test records the electrical activity in the heart. The contractions of the heart are triggered by electrical impulses that start in the right atrium (one of the heart's two upper chambers) and spread across the heart muscle. Electrodes placed on the chest wall, wrists and ankles detect these electrical impulses, which are then represented visually as an echocardiogram. The test may show an abnormal heart rhythm or evidence of a previous heart attack.

STRESS ECG (TREADMILL TEST)

This test is often used to look for evidence of coronary artery disease. The electrical activity of the heart is recorded when the heart is put under stress, often by the individual walking on a treadmill with an adjustable slope.

ANGIOGRAPHY

This test is used to detect narrowings or blockages in the arteries that supply the heart muscle with blood (the coronary arteries). A thin, flexible catheter (a tube) is passed into the femoral artery at the groin and then up the aorta (the biggest artery in the body) to a coronary artery. Dye is injected through the catheter and its passage through the coronary arteries is observed on a screen and recorded on a series of x-rays.

reasons to have DXA

- ▶ If you have had menopause and are taller than 5' 7" or weigh less than 57 kg (125 lb).
- ▶ If you have sustained a hip fracture or a vertebral fracture.
- ▶ If you had a fracture following a minor injury.
- ▶ If there is a family history of osteoporosis or hip fractures.
- ▶ If you smoke or have smoked in the past.
- ▶ If you take or have taken drugs known to cause bone loss, such as oral corticosteroids.
- ▶ If you have type I diabetes mellitus, kidney disease, liver disease or thyroid disorders, such as hypothyroidism.

REPRODUCTIVE ORGAN DISEASES

CERVICAL POLYPS

These benign, non-cancerous growths are most common on the cervix around the age of 40, but they may develop earlier or later. The reasons why they develop are not known.

Cervical polyps may cause abnormal bleeding, either after intercourse, between periods or after menopause. However, in many cases they cause no symptoms at all. They can be seen during examination with a speculum and in most cases can be easily removed without the need for a general anaesthetic. They sometimes recur.

UTERINE POLYPS

These non-cancerous growths are common in the uterus and are rarely a cause for concern. What causes uterine polyps is not known. Women who have not had children are at increased risk.

Symptoms may include bleeding between periods or after menopause. In a few cases, uterine polyps become cancerous.

They may be shown by ultrasound scanning (see page 227) or during a hysteroscopy (see page 230). They can also be removed during a hysteroscopy and then be sent to the laboratory and checked for cancer cells. Like cervical polyps, they can recur.

OVARIAN CYSTS

In most cases, these fluid-filled swellings in the ovaries are not cancerous. However, in some women benign cysts can develop into a malignant tumour. There are various types of cysts. The reasons why they develop are not understood.

Ovarian cysts can cause a number of symptoms but they often produce no symptoms at all. Possible complaints include pain during intercourse, discomfort in the abdomen and, in premenopausal women, irregular periods.

Occasionally, cysts grow very large and put pressure on other structures, such as the bladder, in which case an affected individual may need to pass urine more often than usual. Sometimes a cyst can

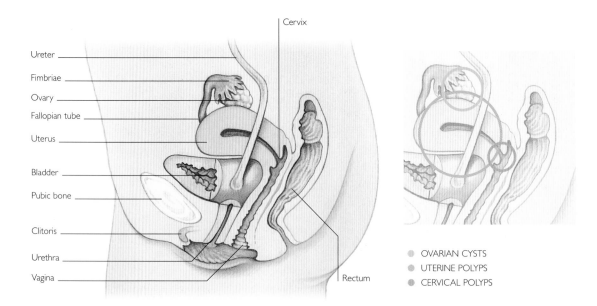

Cervix

Ureter

Fimbriae

Ovary

Fallopian tube

Uterus

Bladder

Pubic bone

Clitoris

Urethra

Vagina

Rectum

- OVARIAN CYSTS
- UTERINE POLYPS
- CERVICAL POLYPS

become twisted or burst. These complications cause severe abdominal pain and require urgent treatment.

How Are Ovarian Cysts Diagnosed and Treated?

Large cysts may be detected during a pelvic examination. The diagnosis will be confirmed by ultrasound scanning (see page 227) and sometimes during a laparoscopy (see page 230).

Cyst growth can be checked regularly by ultrasound scanning. In some cases, cysts disappear without treatment. However, in others, cysts are drained of fluid or removed.

Ovarian cysts can recur and further treatment may become necessary in the future.

POSTMENOPAUSAL BLEEDING

Vaginal bleeding that occurs at least six months after periods have stopped may have a variety of causes. Atropic vaginitis, in which the walls of the vagina become dry and inflamed due to low oestrogen levels after menopause, is one possible cause, as is inflammation of the cervix. However, in some cases cancer of the endometrium (the lining of the uterus) or the cervix may be present. Therefore, such bleeding requires investigation.

How Is Postmenopausal Bleeding Investigated and Treated?

A pelvic examination will take place, the cervix viewed and a cervical smear taken (see pages 227–228).

If further examination is necessary, a transvaginal ultrasound (see page 230) may be recommended. Alternatively an endometrial biopsy (see pages 229–230) is taken and the sample is sent to the laboratory for examination. The biopsy may be taken during a hysteroscopy (see page 230), when

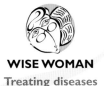

WISE WOMAN
Treating diseases

Whether drugs, surgery or other treatment options are recommended, it is important to consider the potential benefits against any possible side effects or complications. All drugs can produce unwanted symptoms and may interact with other medications; operations are associated with risks. Your doctor should discuss possible side effects and risks with you so that you are able to make an informed decision about what should happen.

the lining of the uterus is also examined. The underlying cause will be treated. For atrophic vaginitis, this may include applying oestrogen cream to the affected area.

UROGENITAL DISORDERS
PROLAPSE

The lowering of the uterus or walls of the vagina from their usual position due to weakness of the supporting structures is a very common condition that tends to affect older women. The degree of prolapse varies from the uterus lying low within the vagina to the more severe cases when the uterus protrudes out of the vagina. The type of prolapse can also vary depending on the area of vaginal wall that is weakened. If the front wall is weak, the bladder may bulge inwards into the vagina to form a cystocele; if the weakness lies below the level of the bladder, the urethra, which carries urine from the bladder to the outside, will bulge inwards (a urethrocele). When a rectocele is present, the rectum bulges into the weakened back wall of the vagina. In many women, both the uterus and the vagina have prolapsed.

What Are the Causes of Prolapse?

Women who have had one or more vaginal deliveries are more at risk of developing a prolapse. The low oestrogen levels present after menopause may contribute to the weakening of muscles and ligaments. It is also possible that some women have an inherited genetic tendency.

Certain conditions increase the pressure placed on the supporting ligaments and so increase the risk of a prolapse. These include obesity, a chronic cough or a job that requires heavy lifting. Occasionally, a prolapse is caused by a growth in the abdomen putting pressure on the ligaments.

What Are the Symptoms of Prolapse?

There may be no symptoms. However, some women complain of a feeling of fullness in the vagina and sometimes a dragging feeling in the lower abdomen. If the front vaginal wall is weakened there may be a problem with urination, such as leakage of urine or a need to pass urine frequently, usually related to coughing, sneezing, laughing or running. If the back vaginal wall is affected, symptoms may include constipation.

How Is Prolapse Diagnosed and Treated?

Prolapses are diagnosed from a vaginal examination. Rarely, an ultrasound scan (see page 227) of the pelvis may be arranged to look for a possible cause.

Weight loss is advised – where appropriate – and physiotherapy may have a role to play in some cases. A physiotherapist will certainly be able to provide pelvic floor and Kegel exercises to strengthen the muscles (see page 50). Many women are happy to take no action.

Some women choose to have a pessary, a plastic device that is placed into the vagina to support the sagging tissues. Others have surgery – either a hysterectomy or a procedure that aims to strengthen the weakened tissues and restore the uterus and vagina to their original position. However, surgery does not always completely resolve the problem, or the pelvic relaxation may recur years later.

PROLAPSED UTERUS

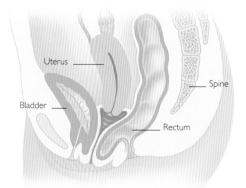

Uterus

Bladder

Spine

Rectum

> THYROID DISEASE

A significant number of women suffer from a thyroid imbalance after menopause, particularly hypothyroidism, an underactive thyroid gland. Some of the symptoms of thyroid disease are very similar to those of perimenopause – hot flushes and night sweats, fatigue and difficulty sleeping, mood swings, loss of interest in sex and lack of concentration – so it needs to be ruled out and treated correctly. Your healthcare professional can test the levels of thyroid-stimulating hormone in the blood to detect either of the two main conditions.

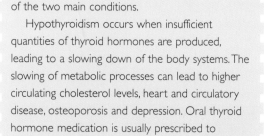

THYROID GLAND

Trachea

Hypothyroidism occurs when insufficient quantities of thyroid hormones are produced, leading to a slowing down of the body systems. The slowing of metabolic processes can lead to higher circulating cholesterol levels, heart and circulatory disease, osteoporosis and depression. Oral thyroid hormone medication is usually prescribed to replenish the supply.

Hyperthyroidism, which is the less prevalent of the two, occurs when too many thyroid hormones are produced by the thyroid gland. This excess of thyroid hormones speeds up metabolic processes, which can cause heart palpitations as well as bulging eyes (exophthalmos) and goitre (a swollen lump on the neck). Medication and surgical techniques are available to block the excessive production and release of thyroid hormones.

REPRODUCTIVE ORGAN CANCERS

CANCER OF THE VAGINA

Malignant vaginal tumours are rare, accounting for 2 percent of cancers affecting the reproductive tract. Vaginal cancer particularly affects women between the ages of 50–70 but can affect other age groups.

Cancer can also spread to the vagina from other nearby structures, such as the cervix, uterus, bladder or bowel. This is called secondary cancer and is more common than primary cancer, which begins in the vagina.

Possible symptoms include abnormal bleeding (after menopause or following intercourse) and discharge. A lump or ulcer may also be noticed.

Some women have urinary symptoms, such as a frequent need to pass urine, urinating at night or blood in the urine. There may also be pain during intercourse or pain in the rectum. However, these common symptoms are almost always caused by benign conditions.

How Is Vaginal Cancer Diagnosed and Treated?

A vaginal examination is carried out as well as a cervical smear (see page 227). The vagina will be inspected closely with a colposcope (see page 228) and a biopsy will be taken to be examined for cancer cells. If cancer is present, the type of cancer cell will be identified and the cancer 'staged' (an assessment that takes account of the tumour size and whether it has spread). Tests designed to look for possible cancer spread include a chest x-ray, a CT scan and an MRI (see page 236). This information will be used to determine the most appropriate treatment option.

Treatment is usually carried out with radio-therapy. This may be delivered by a machine outside the body daily for several weeks. The treatment is painless and lasts for a few minutes. Alternatively, an applicator containing a radioactive substance may be inserted into the vagina. In some cases, tiny

---

female cancers danger signs

In all types of cancer the earlier the diagnosis is made, the better the outlook. Look out for the following:

- ▶ Abnormal vaginal bleeding (after menopause, after intercourse or between periods)
- ▶ Discharge
- ▶ Lumps or ulcers affecting the vulva or vagina
- ▶ Discoloured patch on the vulva
- ▶ Vulval itching or soreness
- ▶ Bleeding or discharge from the vulva
- ▶ Abdominal pain or swelling
- ▶ Pain during intercourse

Remember, there may be another reason for your symptoms, but you should see your doctor as soon as possible in case a cancer is present.

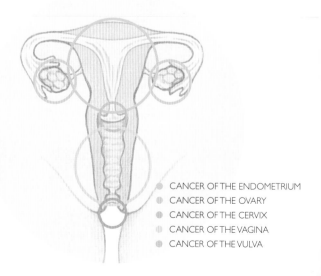

CANCER OF THE ENDOMETRIUM
CANCER OF THE OVARY
CANCER OF THE CERVIX
CANCER OF THE VAGINA
CANCER OF THE VULVA

CT (computerized tomography) scanning, also called CAT scanning, produces cross-sectional and in some cases three-dimensional views of the body.

The machine, which is shaped like a doughnut, rotates around the patient, who lies on a movable table. X-rays emitted from one side pass through the body to detectors on the other side. These detectors register the amount of x-rays absorbed by the tissues. This information is analyzed by a computer to produce the images viewed on the screen. The images produced allow detailed examination of many areas of the body and aid the diagnosis and investigation of many disorders, including strokes, head injuries and tumours. CT scanning may be used to look for evidence of cancer spread.

MRI (magnetic resonance imaging) also produces cross-sectional or three-dimensional images using a magnetic field and radiowaves. The patient lies inside a scanner machine consisting of a large magnet, a radiowave producer and a radiowave detector. A second magnet is placed around the part of the body being investigated. The first magnet generates a magnetic field that causes the atoms of the body to form lines. Bursts of radiowaves directed at the site briefly disrupt these parallel lines. As the atoms line up again, they give out tiny impulses that are detected by the scanner and are used by a computer to generate the image. Like CT scanning, MRI forms detailed pictures of areas of the body. It is particularly useful for imaging the brain and spinal cord and takes up to an hour to perform.

Both tests are commonly done after an injection of an intravenous contrast medium.

radioactive needles are also inserted into the surrounding area under general anaesthetic. The needles are removed at the end of the treatment. Sometimes surgery or chemotherapy is recommended.

CANCER OF THE VULVA

Vulval cancer, a malignant tumour in the area around the entrance to the vagina, accounts for about 5 percent of cancers affecting the reproductive tract. It is most common after the age of 60 and may be preceded by a condition called vulval intraepithelial neoplasia (VIN). This condition, which is linked to some types of the human papilloma virus (a wart virus), is graded I to III according to its severity. This condition, which is not cancer but needs to be treated as VIN III, can eventually develop into vulval cancer if left untreated. Cigarette smoking can increase the risk of VIN and vulval cancer.

Two skin conditions that can affect the vulva, *lichen sclerosus* and *lichen planus*, can occasionally develop into vulval cancer after a long time. These skin conditions sometimes run in families.

Possible symptoms of vulval cancer include itching, bleeding, soreness, pain or discharge. A lump, swelling or ulcer may be present. A thickened or discoloured area (red, white or darkened) may be noticed. There may be soreness on urinating. A mole that changes shape or colour should also be checked, as melanomas (see page 225) can occasionally occur in the vulval area.

How Is Vulval Cancer Diagnosed and Treated?

A vaginal examination is performed and possibly a cervical smear taken (see page 227). A biopsy will be taken from the affected area to make the diagnosis. The vulva may be inspected closely by colposcopy (see page 228). If cancer is confirmed, an assessment will also be made to see whether cancer cells have spread to surrounding tissues or to other parts of the body. This may involve an internal examination under general anaesthesia (to avoid any discomfort) as well as a chest x-ray, CT scan or an MRI (see opposite). Treatment will then be recommended, taking account of these results and the size of the tumour (together known as the tumour stage). Treatment usually includes surgery to remove the abnormal tissue and some surrounding healthy tissue. In some cases, the lymph nodes in the groin are also removed. Some women are treated with radio-therapy and chemotherapy.

CANCER OF THE CERVIX

Up to one-third of all female reproductive tract cancers develop in the cervix. Each year, about 3,000 women are diagnosed with cancer of the cervix, a malignant tumour affecting the neck of the uterus. It is most common in women over 45.

Cervical cancer is preceded by the condition cervical intraepithelial neoplasia (CIN, see page 228), in which there are abnormal cells in the surface layers of the cervix. CIN, which is detected on cervical smears, is not cancer but may eventually develop into cancer if it is not treated. CIN and cervical cancer have similar causes and risk factors. Both conditions can be related to the human papilloma virus, which is sexually transmitted. The herpes simplex virus may also play a role.

Sometimes, there are no symptoms and the disease is detected by an abnormal smear. Otherwise, there may be bleeding after intercourse, between

WISE WOMAN
Tumour markers

These are proteins produced by cells in some tumours. If your blood shows evidence of tumour markers, regular checks may be arranged to monitor the response to chemotherapy.

periods (for premenopausal women) or after menopause. Discharge may also be noticed. Sometimes there is pain during intercourse. Left untreated, the disease may cause other symptoms due to spread of the cancer to other tissues. These symptoms may include blood in the urine, rectal bleeding and pain.

How Is Cervical Cancer Diagnosed and Treated?

Cervical cancer is usually diagnosed by a cervical smear and confirmed by colposcopic biopsy. The tumour may be visible as a lump or an ulcer during a speculum examination, although early tumours are usually not visible. If cancer is confirmed, an assessment will be made to see whether spread to other tissues has occurred. This may involve an examination under anaesthesia (an internal examination that is performed under general anaesthesia to avoid any discomfort) and a CT scan or an MRI (see opposite).

Early disease may be treated by cone biopsy (see page 228) or sometimes a hysterectomy (see pages 240–241). More advanced disease may also require removal of nearby tissues and lymph nodes. Surgery may be followed by, or in some cases replaced by, radiotherapy. In more advanced cases, radiotherapy will be used, possibly in combination with chemotherapy.

CANCER OF THE ENDOMETRIUM

This malignant tumour affecting the lining of the uterus is the most common type of cancer affecting the female reproductive tract. It mainly affects women between the ages of 50 and 64.

These cancers are all related to the hormone oestrogen. If you have not had a hysterectomy and are taking HT, you must take progesterone with the oestrogen to protect the endometrium from an increased risk of cancer developing. While taking combined HT for up to 5 years is not thought to

risk factors
CERVICAL CANCER

▷ Many sexual contacts, particularly at an early age.
▷ Cigarette smoking.
▷ Impaired immunity.
▷ History of genital or cervical warts.

risk factors
CANCER OF THE ENDOMETRIUM

▶ Obesity
▶ Polycystic ovary syndrome
▶ Not having children
▶ Late menopause

increase the risk of getting this type of cancer, taking it for more than 5 years may slightly increase the risk, although this finding is controversial.

The most common symptom is bleeding after menopause. Premenopausal women may notice irregular or heavy periods, or bleeding between periods or after intercourse. Some women have pain in the lower abdomen or during intercourse.

How Is Endometrial Cancer Diagnosed and Treated?

A biopsy is taken from the endometrium during an office endometrial biopsy, hysteroscopy or a D&C (see page 230). A pelvic examination may also be carried out under general anaesthetic. If the diagnosis is confirmed, further tests, such as a chest x-ray, CT scan or MRI may be arranged to look for evidence of tumour spread.

The treatment recommended depends on whether the cancer has spread. It usually includes removal of the uterus, fallopian tubes and ovaries. The upper vagina may also be removed as well as nearby pelvic lymph nodes. Surgery may be followed by radiotherapy. The hormone progesterone may also be used and, in some cases, chemotherapy.

CANCER OF THE OVARY

Malignant tumours affecting the ovary account for around 35 percent of all reproductive tract tumours. They most commonly affect women over 60.

Non-cancerous cysts may rarely develop into ovarian cancer. Risk factors for the disease include an early onset of periods, a late menopause, never

having had children and, possibly, the long-term use of hormones. Breastfeeding and having several children are thought to have a protective effect. Sometimes, ovarian cancer runs in families, due to inherited genetic defects.

There are usually no symptoms initially. Later, the abdomen may become swollen or a lump may be felt in the abdomen. Occasionally, pain in the lower abdomen, frequent urination or abnormal bleeding, such as irregular periods, may be present.

How Is Ovarian Cancer Diagnosed and Treated?

The diagnosis is usually made by pelvic examination or ultrasound scanning (see box, below), which is also used to look for evidence of tumour spread. Other tests may include liver function tests, a chest x-ray, a CT scan or an MRI.

Surgery is needed to remove the uterus, tubes, ovaries and all of the cancer if it has spread in the abdomen or to the regional lymph nodes. This is usually followed by chemotherapy or radiotherapy.

In about 80 percent of cases the blood levels of a tumour marker CA 125 are found to be elevated.

▶ ULTRASOUND SCANNING

This test uses high-frequency sound waves to create pictures of tissues. The sound waves pass into the body from a transducer passed over the skin in the area to be investigated. The echoes produced are detected by the same transducer and converted to electrical impulses that are analyzed by a computer. Ultrasound is particularly good for examining soft tissues; it can also be used to image hollow organs and moving structures, such as the heart (echocardiography is the specialized form of ultrasound used). Ultrasound scanning can distinguish between solid and cystic lumps (those containing fluid) and helps to judge whether a solid lump is benign or malignant.

CANCER TREATMENTS

Gynaecological cancers and breast cancer can be treated in a number of ways and often with a combination of methods. Treatment method, or methods, selected depend on a number of factors, including the type of cancer, its size and whether it has spread. A woman's general health and other medical conditions are also taken into account.

Tumours can originate from different types of cells within the same organ or tissue. The treatment recommended and the prognosis are in part determined by this.

'Staging' (see also page 244) is the term used to take account of the tumour size and whether it has spread. A number of tests may be performed to look for evidence of cancer spread, including a chest x-ray, ultrasound scanning of the liver (see page 227 and box left), CT scanning and MRI (see page 236).

CANCER TREATMENTS AVAILABLE

Cancer treatments may aim to cure cancer, slow the growth of a tumour or relieve the symptoms it causes. The treatments available include:

Surgery

Often used to treat solid cancers, surgery is particularly useful when cancer is diagnosed early. A margin of tissue surrounding the tumour is also likely to be removed. This surgery aims to increase the probability of removing all the cancer cells and decrease the chances of spread or recurrence of the tumour. Nearby lymph nodes may also be removed and examined under the microscope to look for cancer cells. Sometimes, surgery is performed to relieve symptoms.

One or more other treatments may be given as well as surgery. Sometimes they are given first to shrink a tumour before surgery. Often, they are given after surgery with the aim of destroying any remaining cancer cells. The treatments most commonly used are radiotherapy and chemotherapy, both of which aim to destroy cancer cells by damaging their genes.

Radiotherapy

High-intensity radiation is directed at the tumour. Radiotherapy may be given as multiple treatments either delivered by a machine outside the body or by radiation sources placed in or near the cancer. Vaginal cancer is often treated in this way.

Chemotherapy

In chemotherapy, anticancer drugs are used to destroy cancer cells, and more than one drug is often prescribed. However, as well as destroying cancer cells, chemotherapy drugs can affect other cells that rapidly divide. This explains some of the side effects, such as hair loss, that can occur with certain drugs. Some of these drugs may also affect the production of blood cells by the bone marrow, causing anaemia and increasing susceptibility to infections. Other possible side effects include nausea, but very effective anti-nausea drugs are now available.

Hormone therapy

Treatment with hormones can be used for certain cancers, such as breast cancer (see pages 242–245).

PALLIATIVE CARE

An important aspect of treating individuals with cancer is relieving their symptoms, whether they are caused by the cancer itself or by the treatment. Palliative care may include analgesics for pain or anti-nausea drugs for sickness caused by chemotherapy.

Cancer care also needs to consider the emotional needs of the individual – being diagnosed with cancer is a difficult, often devastating, experience. The support and understanding of partners, relatives and friends, as well as the medical and nursing teams, is key to coming to terms with the diagnosis and coping with the treatment. Support groups and counselling can also be a source of comfort.

The outlook for individuals with cancer depends on a number of factors, including the cell type and how early the cancer is diagnosed. In order to realize an early diagnosis, it is important that women attend screening appointments and report worrying symptoms to a doctor at an early stage.

HAVING A HYSTERECTOMY

WHAT IS A HYSTERECTOMY?

A hysterectomy involves removal of the uterus and can be carried out in three main ways:

- through an incision in the vagina (vaginal hysterectomy),
- through an incision in the abdomen (abdominal hysterectomy),
- by the use of laparoscopic techniques and removal of the uterus through the vagina.

Hysterectomy is a very common procedure; around 1 in 5 of all women will have a hysterectomy at some time for one of a variety of reasons.

WHY ARE THEY DONE?

Possible reasons include heavy periods (in premenopausal women), severe pelvic infections, large or symptomatic fibroids, prolapse of the uterus (as part of a prolapse repair operation) or cancer affecting the cervix, uterus, fallopian tubes or ovaries.

HOW ARE THEY DONE?

Vaginal hysterectomy An incision is made near the top of the vagina and the uterus is removed through the vagina. Less painful than the abdominal hysterectomy, there is no visible external scar. A hospital stay of 1–3 days is advised, and the recovery time is about four weeks.

Abdominal hysterectomy An incision, typically horizontal but sometimes vertical, is made just above the pubic hair, and the uterus is removed. The cut usually heals well with a neat scar. A hospital stay of 3–5 days is advised, and the recovery time is between 4–8 weeks.

Laparoscopic hysterectomy A viewing instrument is passed through a small incision in the abdomen, and surgical instruments are then passed through other small incisions. The uterus is removed through the vagina. The hospital stay is usually one day, and the recovery time is about two weeks.

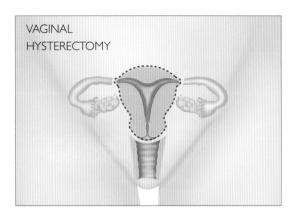

VAGINAL HYSTERECTOMY

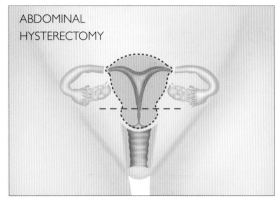

ABDOMINAL HYSTERECTOMY

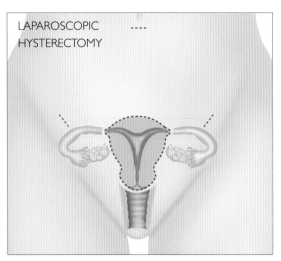

LAPAROSCOPIC HYSTERECTOMY

WHAT TYPES ARE THERE?

In a total hysterectomy, the uterus and cervix are removed. This is the type most often performed. Sometimes, the cervix is left in place (a sub-total hysterectomy). Women who have these procedures may experience menopause earlier than they would have done. In some cases, the ovaries and fallopian tubes are removed as well (called a bilateral salpingo-oophorectomy, or BSO). Women then become menopausal after the operation.

Sometimes it's necessary for more tissues to be removed to treat cancer. In addition to the uterus, cervix, fallopian tubes and ovaries, the upper vagina, some lymph glands and some pelvic tissue may also be removed.

WHAT HAPPENS AFTER A HYSTERECTOMY?

Six weeks' convalescence is usually the minimum recommended recovery time following a hysterectomy. Heavy lifting should be avoided for up to 12 weeks after the operation. Individuals vary, but most women return to work after about 6 weeks. However, it is very important to listen to your body and only do what you feel able to do. It may take several months for you to feel completely back to normal.

You are likely to notice a vaginal discharge for a few weeks after the operation. If the discharge becomes smelly, bright red or heavy, you should seek medical advice.

If the hysterectomy was performed for reasons other than cancer and the cervix was removed, no further cervical smears will be needed. However, if the cervix has been left in place, regular cervical screening should be continued.

EXERCISING

You can start gentle exercise once the stitches have been taken out. Leaflets will be available at the hospital or your doctor's surgery to advise on appropriate exercises. Walking is a good way to improve mobility. Start with about 10 minutes a day and gradually increase the time as you feel able.

SEX

Gentle intercourse may be possible about six weeks after the operation. Some couples prefer to wait until after the hospital checkup to ensure that the vaginal scar has completely healed. Most women find that their enjoyment of sex is unaffected by the operation.

EMOTIONS

How women feel after a hysterectomy varies greatly between individuals. Many feel content that the operation is over and that symptoms may be relieved. However, some women feel depressed and experience a real sense of loss. Such feelings may be less likely among women who have a clear understanding of what the operation will involve and have come to their decision about it ahead of time. It is also helpful to seek support by talking to a partner, a friend or a healthcare practitioner. You should also fully discuss what will happen with your gynaecologist and ensure that any questions you have are answered.

BREAST DISEASES

BREAST CYSTS

Fluid-filled lumps, or cysts, within the tissue of the breasts are rarely a cause for concern, but medical advice should be sought to exclude the presence of breast cancer.

Breast cysts particularly affect women between the ages of 30 and 50.

It is not known why breast cysts develop, but they are related to the female sex hormones. The cysts are often felt as lumps close to the surface of the breast or deeper in the breast tissue. Breast cysts tend to be painless, although pain may occur in some cases. Often, more than one cyst is present. Very rarely, there may be cancerous cells in the wall of a breast cyst.

How Are Breast Cysts Diagnosed and Treated?

Mammography (see page 226) or ultrasound scanning (see page 227) of the breast may be used to confirm the diagnosis. The fluid within the cyst may be withdrawn using a fine needle and syringe. It may then be sent to the laboratory and tested to make sure no cancer cells are present. Breast cysts can usually be treated successfully by draining them, but they can recur.

Another common type of benign breast lump is a fibroadenoma. These tend to occur in young women under the age of 30.

BREAST CANCER

A malignant tumour in the tissue of the breast is the most common type of cancer to affect women.

Around 1 in 10 women who get breast cancer have inherited a gene that increases their risk. Two of those identified, BRCA-1 and BRCA-2, account for about two-thirds of cases of inherited breast cancer. The following may indicate the presence of a faulty gene:

- Relatives developed breast cancer under the age of 50.
- Several relatives have had breast cancer.
- Relatives have had the disease in both breasts or have a history of certain other cancers, including cancer of the ovaries or colon.

Special clinics are run for women who think they may be at increased risk of breast cancer. Your doctor can advise on this.

TYPES OF BREAST CANCER

DUCTAL CARCINOMA IN SITU

In this condition, also known as noninvasive or intraductal carcinoma, the cancer cells develop in the lining of the ducts. They are completely contained within the ducts and there has been no spread to the surrounding breast tissue. Without treatment, there may eventually be some spread of the abnormal cells to the breast tissue.

ANATOMY OF THE BREAST

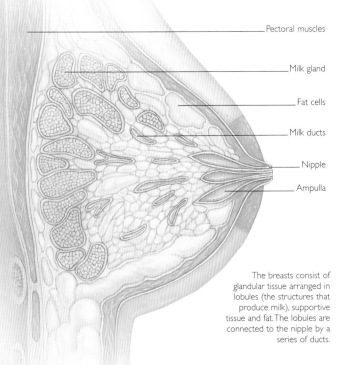

Pectoral muscles

Milk gland

Fat cells

Milk ducts

Nipple

Ampulla

The breasts consist of glandular tissue arranged in lobules (the structures that produce milk), supportive tissue and fat. The lobules are connected to the nipple by a series of ducts.

How Is Ductal Breast Cancer Diagnosed and Treated?

This usually shows on mammograms as areas of tiny spots of calcium. However, it should be noted that this 'microcalcification' is often seen on mammograms and is not caused by cancer cells in most cases.

A sample of cells is taken and examined under the microscope. This will give an indication as to how likely the cancer cells are to spread and, together with information on the extent of the abnormal area, will be used to determine what treatment would be best. In many cases, excision of the affected area and a normal margin of tissue around it will be recommended. Yearly checkups will be arranged to ensure that there is no recurrence or, should the condition recur, that it is picked up and treated at an early stage. If the abnormal area is large and microscopic examination indicates it is more likely to spread, mastectomy may be advised. No additional treatment is usually necessary, but regular mammograms of the other breast will be arranged. However, if the abnormal area is large, lymph glands may be removed from the armpit and checked for cancer cells.

Sometimes, cells in the affected area are found to be the type that grow in response to the female hormone oestrogen. In these cases, tamoxifen or one of the newer medications that block the action of oestrogen, may be prescribed.

LOBULAR CARCINOMA IN SITU

With lobular carcinoma, the abnormal cells are confined to the lining of the lobules. This is not cancer but there is a small risk that it may eventually develop into cancer. No treatment is needed in most cases, but regular checkup examinations and mammograms will be arranged as a precaution.

PAGET'S DISEASE OF THE BREAST

In this condition, there is usually a patch of abnormal skin resembling eczema on the nipple or the surrounding area of darkened skin (the areola). It is often associated with a cancer in the breast tissue, which may be invasive or intraductal.

How Is Paget's Disease Diagnosed and Treated?

Cells are taken from the abnormal area and from a lump, if present, for microscopic examination. If a large area is affected or the abnormal area is some distance from the nipple, a mastectomy will be recommended. If the area is small or close to the nipple, it may be possible to conserve some of the

> A patch that is scaly and red
> Crusting, bleeding or soreness of the patch
> Formation of an ulcer
> Turning in of the nipple
> Nipple discharge
> A lump in the breast tissue

breast tissue, removing the nipple area, underlying tissue and a surrounding margin of normal tissue. Radiotherapy, hormonal treatment and chemotherapy may be recommended in some cases.

INVASIVE BREAST CANCER

With invasive breast cancer, the abnormal cells are in the tissue of the breast, and they can spread to lymph nodes and eventually to other parts of the body.

Treatment

A number of factors are taken into account when selecting the most appropriate form of treatment. The tumour is staged (see below) by assessing its size and whether it has spread. It is also graded, to assess how quickly it is likely to spread. This is determined by examining the cancer cells under the microscope. High-grade tumours are more likely to grow or spread than low-grade tumours.

The surgical treatment recommended depends on the site of the tumour and whether it has spread.

CANCER STAGING

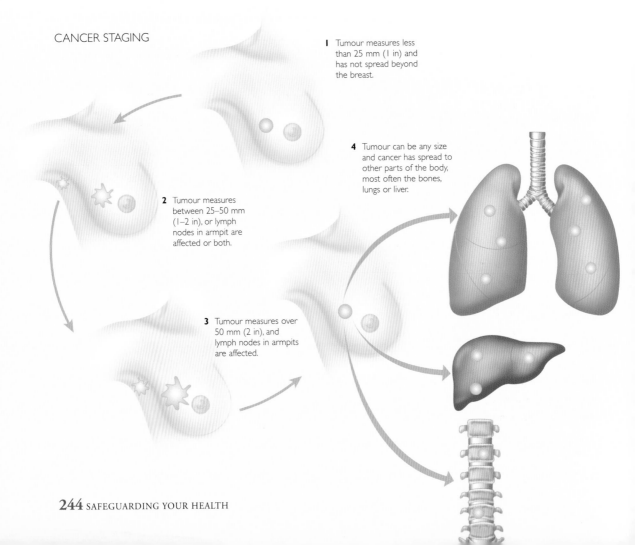

1 Tumour measures less than 25 mm (1 in) and has not spread beyond the breast.

2 Tumour measures between 25–50 mm (1–2 in), or lymph nodes in armpit are affected or both.

3 Tumour measures over 50 mm (2 in), and lymph nodes in armpits are affected.

4 Tumour can be any size and cancer has spread to other parts of the body, most often the bones, lungs or liver.

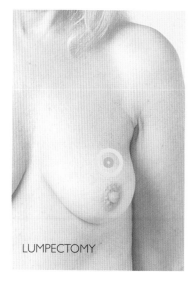

LUMPECTOMY

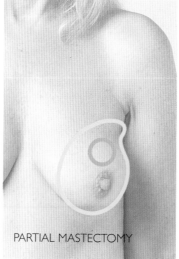

PARTIAL MASTECTOMY

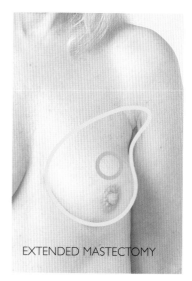

EXTENDED MASTECTOMY

Tests may be arranged to look for evidence of cancer spread. These may include a chest x-ray, ultrasound scanning of the liver (see page 227) and an MRI (see page 236). A bone scan may also be performed; a mildly radioactive liquid is injected into a vein in the arm, and then the body is scanned a few hours later.

Early breast cancer may be treated by removal of the lump (lumpectomy) together with a margin of tissue around the lump. This will probably be followed by radiotherapy. If cancer cells are found to be present at the edge of the removed tissue, more tissue will need to be removed and a mastectomy (removal of all the breast tissue) may be recommended. In some cases, a mastectomy may be arranged right away. A few lymph glands will be removed from the armpit at the same time and tested for cancer cells. If this test is positive, the remaining glands will be treated with radiotherapy or removed. Sometimes, all the glands in the armpit are removed (called axillary clearance).

Some women decide to have a breast recon-struction, which can be carried out either at the

WISE WOMAN

Breast reconstruction

Your surgeon will explain which reconstructive options are best for you after studying your general health, age, body type, lifestyle and goals, but ask questions and make sure you are fully informed about your options.

same time as the mastectomy or at a later date.

Other treatments, such as chemotherapy, hormonal therapy and radiotherapy (see page 239), may be recommended either following surgery or, sometimes, with the aim of shrinking a large tumour before surgery.

THE IMPORTANCE OF SUPPORT

From the time the diagnosis of breast cancer is made and throughout the treatment, the support and understanding of relatives, friends and the medical team is vital. Breast care nurses, who specialize in the care of women with breast cancer, are available at many hospitals to answer any questions and give support. Counselling may also be very valuable, as may self-help and support groups. Ask your healthcare team for information on counselling options and support groups active in your region.

CARDIOVASCULAR DISEASES

According to studies in the US and Canada, while a man's risk for heart disease increases significantly after the age of 45, a woman's risk increases after menopause, whatever her age. Heart disease rates in postmenopausal women are two to three times higher than those in premenopausal women of the same age, leading researchers to suggest that the body's oestrogen level provides some protection.

Heart disease is often detected later in women than in men due to a difference in symptoms. Apart from the classic symptoms of chest pain or pain in the left arm, women also complain of nausea, heartburn, indigestion, fatigue and shortness of breath – all of which are not immediately recognized as symptomatic of heart disease. And when the fact that women are less likely than men to receive treatment for heart disease is added to this equation, it's perhaps not surprising that after the age of 55, more than half of all deaths in women are caused by heart disease.

HYPERTENSION

Blood pressure levels normally vary with activity and various other factors, including stress. However, if blood pressure is persistently elevated (hypertension) and left untreated it can lead to a variety of compli-

risk factors
HYPERTENSION

- A family history
- Stress
- Drinking too much alcohol
- A high-salt diet
- Being overweight
- Certain kidney and hormonal disorders
- Some drugs, including corticosteroids

cations, including heart attacks and strokes, as well as damage to other organs such as the eyes and the kidneys.

Blood pressure is recorded as two figures: the upper, or systolic, figure reflects the pressure of the blood when the heart contracts to pump blood around the body; the second, or diastolic, figure represents the pressure between heart contractions. What is considered an acceptable blood pressure varies, but in general blood pressure that is persistently 140/90 or over is considered to be high.

Hypertension tends to run in families and to occur as people get older.

What Are the Symptoms of Hypertension?
In most cases of hypertension there are no symptoms. However, if the blood pressure is very high, headaches, dizziness, visual disturbances and nosebleeds may result.

How Is It Diagnosed and Treated?
If a patient's blood pressure is found to be high, it is usually taken on a number of occasions to see whether the problem persists. Depending on the level of the blood pressure, the doctor may carry out a more general examination and arrange tests to look

4 ways to lower your blood pressure

- Bring your weight within the healthy range.
- Ensure your diet is low in salt and high in vegetables and fruits.
- Drink alcohol in moderation (one drink per day for women).
- Take regular exercise, such as brisk walking.

for evidence of underlying causes and for signs of damage caused by the high pressure.

If blood pressure is elevated, lifestyle measures alone may be recommended in the first instance and blood pressure will be frequently checked to see whether it is coming under control. If the blood pressure remains elevated, medications will be prescribed. These may include certain diuretics and a choice of antihypertensive drugs. The diuretic bendroflumethiazide is commonly used; it causes the kidneys to release more salts and water from the body and so decreases the volume of blood in the system. Antihypertensives work in a number of ways, including reducing the force with which the heart contracts and causing the blood vessels around the body to widen. These drugs include beta-blockers, angiotensin-converting enzyme (ACE) inhibitors and calcium-channel blockers. Some patients may be advised to take a 75 mg aspirin

every day, particularly those at high risk of coronary artery disease and strokes.

CORONARY ARTERY DISEASE (CAD)
The muscle of the heart walls is supplied with oxygen-rich blood by the coronary arteries, a network of blood vessels that branch from the aorta, the main artery of the body. In coronary artery disease, the arteries become narrowed as a result of atherosclerosis, a condition in which fatty deposits form on the lining of the arteries.

In most cases, the blood delivered to the heart muscle is sufficient at rest, but when the activity of the heart increases, perhaps as a result of stress or exercise, the blood supply can be insufficient to supply adequate oxygen. This shortage can result in chest pain (called angina). If one of the arteries is blocked, an area of heart muscle is perman-ently damaged (a heart attack).

Coronary artery disease can run in families and tends to occur as people get older. Women are at a lower risk of coronary artery disease than men until the age of 60 when the risk becomes the same for men and women. The sex hormone oestrogen is thought to protect women from the disease until menopause (when oestrogen levels fall), after which time this protective effect will gradually wear off.

RESTRICTING BLOOD SUPPLY TO THE HEART

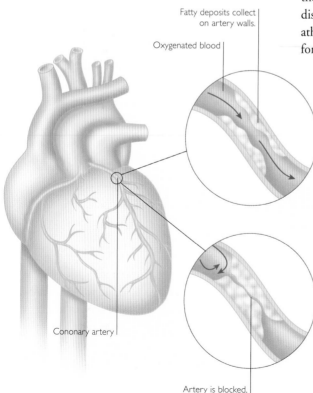

Fatty deposits collect on artery walls.

Oxygenated blood

Cononary artery

Artery is blocked, restricting bloodflow.

What Are the Symptoms of CAD?

Mild coronary artery disease may cause no symptoms. However, angina (pain in the chest that can spread to the neck and arms) may later develop, usually on exertion or in response to stress, but also in cold or windy weather. Shortness of breath may also occur. If the disease becomes more severe, chest pain may occur at rest.

In addition to heart attacks, coronary artery disease may also cause disruptions of the heart rhythm (arrhythmia) and heart failure, a condition in which the heart is unable to pump blood around the body effectively.

How Is CAD Diagnosed and Treated?

An ECG (see page 231) is usually arranged, although the results are likely to be normal when no

ways to reduce the risk

- Stop smoking.
- Eat a diet low in saturated fat.
- Cut down on alcohol.
- Lose weight, if necessary.
- Take regular exercise (under medical advice).

symptoms are present. This is usually followed by a stress ECG, which records the electrical activity in the heart during exercise on a treadmill or exercise bike. This will usually show characteristic changes if coronary artery disease is present.

The functioning of the heart may be assessed by a special ultrasound scan called an echocardiogram. The coronary arteries may be examined in detail by coronary angiography (see page 231). In addition to these heart tests, blood tests may be arranged to look for associated disorders, such as diabetes.

Lifestyle measures will be strongly recommended to people with coronary artery disease. In fact, everyone might consider following the same suggestions to reduce their risk of coronary artery disease (see box, left).

Daily low-dose aspirin (75 mg) may be recommended, as it has been shown to reduce the

▶ METABOLIC SYNDROME

Also called Syndrome X, this is a group of metabolic disorders that affects approximately 40 percent of people over the age of 40 (the American Heart Association estimates that about 47 million adults in the United States have metabolic syndrome). It can increase an individual's risk for heart disease, stroke and diabetes. Diabetics, women with high blood pressure who have high insulin levels as a result of resistance to the action of insulin in their tissues, and are usually overweight but have normal blood glucose levels, are the most at risk. The exact cause of the disorder is unknown but many researchers believe that it is a combination of genetics, a poor diet and insufficient activity.

Menopause is a particularly significant time, as the incidence of the syndrome increases by about 60 percent at this time. This may be due directly to the hormone changes that occur or simply the result of normal aging. Many middle-aged women have increased blood sugar and insulin levels, fluctuations in blood cholesterol levels and increased centralized abdominal fat. One of the criteria for diagnosis of this syndrome in women is central obesity as measured by a waist circumference of more than 88 cm (35 in).

You can lower your risk for metabolic syndrome by ensuring the following:
- You achieve and maintain an acceptable body weight;
- Your diet is low-calorie, low-cholesterol and contains lots of fruit and fibre;
- You perform aerobic exercise for at least 20–30 minutes four times per week.

risk of heart attacks. However, aspirin is not suitable for everyone. Lipid-lowering drugs may also be recommended.

Medications may be prescribed to treat angina when it occurs and to prevent it from occurring. These work in various ways, including reducing the heart-rate and the force with which the heart muscle contracts, as well as relaxing the muscle in the walls of the coronary arteries to allow more blood to pass through. Some drugs also widen arteries around the body, making it easier for the heart to pump blood. (Anti-anginal drugs include nitrates, beta blockers and calcium channel blockers.)

In some cases, angioplasty is recommended. A catheter with a balloon at its end is passed though an artery in the groin up to the affected coronary artery. Here, the balloon is inflated several times to widen the narrowed area. In this illustration (above) the inflated balloon is coloured orange while the whip-like catheter is in red. In some instances a permanent 'stent' – a small, wire mesh tube – is inserted into the artery in order to keep it open. In other instances coronary artery bypass grafting is offered; a vein is taken from the leg and used to bypass the narrowing.

The occurrence of a heart attack is confirmed by a series of ECGs and blood tests. Treatment may involve drugs that aim to break down the clot blocking the artery, followed by medications that prevent angina and improve the prognosis.

INDEX

ACKNOWLEDGEMENTS

Additional consultant: Dr. Lesley Hickin

Production Director: Karol Davies
Computer Management: Paul Stradling
Picture Researcher: Sandra Schneider
Proofreader: Geoffrey West
Indexer: Madeline Weston

Illustration: David Nicholls, Amanda Williams
Photography: Jules Selmes, David Yems

Carroll and Brown would like to thank:
Marie Stopes International; The Water Monopoly;
and Mohini Chatlani, author of *Yoga Flows*

PICTURE CREDITS

P 2 (bottom right) John Henley/Corbis
P 6 (centre) Hybrid Medical Animation/SPL
P 12 (top left) Bild der Frau/Camera Press
P 12 (top right) Biodisc/Visuals Unlimited/Medical-On-Line
P 12 (bottom) Michael Keller/Corbis
P 18 (top) Visuals Unlmited/Medical-On-Line
P 18 (bottom) Biodisc/Visuals Unlimited/Medical-On-Line
P 19 Bild der Frau/Camera Press
P 23 Michael Keller/Corbis
P 25 M. Aymard, ISM/SPL
P 32 Getty Images
P 41 BSIP, Laurent/Laeticia/SPL
P 60 (top left) Getty Images
P 60 (top right) BSIP Roux/SPL
P 62 Getty Images
P 64 SPL
P 66 BSIP Roux/SPL
P 69 (inset) Hybrid Medical Animation/SPL
P 69 Susumu Nishinaga/SPL
P 71 Zephyr/SPL
P 77 Alfred Pasieka/SPL
P 81 Darren Modricker/Corbis
P 99 Getty Images
P 102 BSIP Vem/SPL
P 103 AJ Photo/SPL
P 116 Roger Dixon

P 128 (top left) David Coates/The Detroit News
P 143 Powerstock
P 146 David Coates/The Detroit News
P 152 (top left) John Henley/Corbis
P 152 (top right, bottom) Getty Images
P 154 Laureen March/Corbis
P 155 Pasieka/SPL
P 157 Neil Beckerman/Corbis
P 158 Getty Images
P 161 (top, centre) Getty Images
P 166 John Henley/Corbis
P 168 (top) BSIP, Chassenet/SPL
P 168 (second from top, bottom) Cordelia Molloy/SPL
P 168 (third from top) Damien Lovegrove/SPL
P 170 (top right) AJ Photo/SPL
P 170 (bottom) Saturn Stills/SPL
P 174 AJ Photo/SPL
P 176 Jerry Mason/SPL
P 184 Saturn Stills/SPL
P 195 (top) Eric Crichton/Corbis
P 196 Buddy Mays/Corbis
P 199 Lisa M McGeady/Corbis
P 207 Getty Images
P 210 (left) ER Productions/Corbis
P 210 (right) The Harley Medical Group
P 213 Bucks Free Press
P 214 (top) Align Technology UK Ltd
P 219 Getty Images
P 220 (top left) Mauro Fermariello/SPL
P 220 (top right) Samuel Ashfield/SPL
P 220 (bottom) BSIP, Laurent/SPL
P 222 BSIP, Laurent/SPL
P 225 (top, centre) Dr P Marazzi/SPL
P 225 (bottom) James Stevenson/SPL
P 226 Mauro Fermariello/SPL
P 228 (top) SPL
P 228 (bottom) Parviz M. Pour/SPL
P 229 Samuel Ashfield/SPL
P 230 SPL
P 248 BSIP, Villareal/SPL
P 249 CNRI/SPL